HERE'S AMERICA'S FAVORITE DIET GUIDE

CALORIES AND CARBOHYDRATES

THE BOOK THAT MAKES IT FUN TO LOSE THOSE EXTRA POUNDS

Whether you aim to lose five pounds or fifty, the only safe, healthy way is to eat an adequate, well-balanced diet, choosing your calories from many different kinds of foods in order to ensure that you're getting sufficient vitamins, minerals, and other nutrients. CALORIES AND CARBOHYDRATES contains the most accurate and dependable caloric and carbohydrate counts for practically everything you will eat and drink—thousands and thousands of brand names and basic foods, including alcoholic beverages and take-out foods such as your favorites from McDONALD'S or BURGER KING.

So diet—and enjoy it!

Frieda J. Smith

Barbara Kraus

CALORIES
and
CARBOHYDRATES

THIRD REVISED EDITION

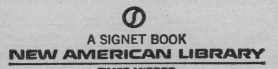

A SIGNET BOOK
NEW AMERICAN LIBRARY
TIMES MIRROR

For Rebecca K. Pecot

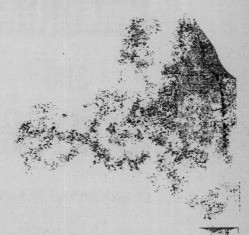

Library of Congress Catalog Card Number: 70-119037

SIGNET TRADEMARK REG. U.S. PAT. OFF. AND FOREIGN COUNTRIES
REGISTERED TRADEMARK—MARCA REGISTRADA
HECHO EN CHICAGO, U.S.A.

SIGNET, SIGNET CLASSICS, MENTOR, PLUME AND MERIDIAN BOOKS
are published by The New American Library, Inc.,
1301 Avenue of the Americas, New York, New York 10019

First Signet Printing, August, 1973
Second Revised Edition, July, 1975
Third Revised Edition, First Signet Printing, March, 1979

16 17 18 19 20 21 22 23 24

PRINTED IN THE UNITED STATES OF AMERICA

Contents

Introduction

This dictionary of foods lists several thousand brand-name products and basic foods with their caloric and carbohydrate content. The calorie yield of your diet versus the amount of energy you expend is the key to whether you maintain your ideal weight, gain too many pounds or lose weight.

Because of the relationship of weight to health, many individuals are "counting calories" at every meal. Interest has also been directed to the carbohydrate content of the diet in relation to weight control. Comprehensive information on these values in basic foods and brand-name products is not readily available in any one source. Nor is the information regularly reported in portions that are usually eaten or bought at the grocery store. To compound the problem, hundreds of new food items appear in our stores every year.

Arrangement of This Book

Foods are listed alphabetically by brand name or by the name of the food. The singular form is used for the entries, that is, blackberry instead of blackberries. Most items are listed individually though a few are grouped (see p. xiii) for example, all candies are listed together so that if you are looking for *Mars* bar, you look first under Candy, then under *M* in alphabetical order. But, if you are looking for a breakfast food such as Oatmeal, you will find it under *O* in the main alphabet. Many cross references are included to assist in finding items called by different names.

Under the main headings, it was often not possible nor even desirable to follow an alphabetical arrangement. For basic foods such as apricots, for example, the first entries are for the fresh product weighed with seeds as it is purchased in the store, then the fruit in small portions as they may be eaten or measured. These entries are followed by the processed products, canned (although it may actually be a bottle or jar), dehydrated, dried and frozen. This basic plan, with adaptations where necessary, was followed for fruits, vegetables and meats.

In almost all entries where data were available the U.S. Department of Agriculture figures are shown first. The Department values represent averages from several manufacturers and are shown for comparison with the values from individual companies or for use where particular brands are not available.

All brand-name products have been italicized and company names appear in parentheses.

Portions Used

The portion column is a most important one to read and note. Common household measures are used insofar as possible. For some items, the amounts given are those commonly purchased in the store, such as 1 pound of meat. These quantities can be divided into the number of servings used in the home and the nutritive values available to each person served can then be readily determined. Of course, any ingredients added to preparing such products must also be taken into account.

The smaller portions given are for foods as served or measured in moderate amounts, such as ½ cup of juice reconstituted, or 4 ounces of meat. Be sure to adjust the calories and carbohydrates to the actual portions you use. For example, if you serve 1 cup of juice instead of ½ cup, multiply the calories and carbohydrates shown for the smaller amount by 2.

Don't fool yourself about the size of portions you use. If you are serious about controlling the calories and carbohydrates in your diet, weigh your foods until you can accurately gauge the weight visually. Remember, the calories and carbohydrates go up with any increase in the weight of foods. Remember, too, that 4 ounces by weight may be very different from 4 fluid ounces or ½ cup. Ounces in the table are always ounces by weight unless specified as fluid ounces, or fractions of a cup or other volumetric measure. Foods that are fluffy in texture, such as flaked coconut and bean sprouts, vary greatly in weight per cup depending on how tightly they are packed into the cup. Such foods as canned green beans also vary when weighed with or without liquid, for example, canned green beans with liquid weigh 4.2 ounces for ½ cup, but drained beans weigh 2.5 ounces for the same ½ cup. Check the weights of your serving portions regularly. Bear in mind that you can cut calories and carbohydrates by cutting the serving size.

It was impossible to convert all the portions to a uniform basis. Some sources were only able to report data in terms of weights with no information on cup or other volumetric measures. I have shown small portions in quantities that might reasonably be expected to be served or measured in the home or institution. Package sizes are useful to show the composition of products as they are purchased and may be divided into the number of serving portions prepared from the entire product, taking into account any added ingredients.

You will find in the portion column the phrases "weighed with bone," or "weighed with skin and seeds" or other inedible parts. These descriptions apply to the products as you purchase them in the markets but the caloric values and the carbohydrate content as shown are for the amount of edible food after you discard the bone, skin, seed or other inedible part. The weight given in the "measure or quantity" column is to the nearest gram or fraction of an ounce.

Data on the composition of foods are constantly changing for many reasons. Better sampling and analytical methods, improvements in marketing procedures and changes in formulas of mixed products, all may alter values for carbohydrates and other nutrients as well as caloric values. Weights of packaged foods are frequently changed. It is essential to read label information to be informed about these matters and to make intelligent use of food tables.

I will be constantly revising and updating this book along with my individual calorie and carbohydrate annual guides (*The Barbara Kraus 1979 Calorie and Carbohydrate Guides to Brand Names and Basic Foods*) to help keep you as up-to-date as possible.

Calories

What is a calorie? It is not a nutrient nor is it a good guide to the nutritive value of a food. It is more like a yardstick to measure the energy that a food will yield in the body. You need energy for your body functions as well as for exercise.

If your diet contains more calories than your body uses for these purposes, the extra "energy" will be stored as fat.

If your plan is to cut down on calories, the easiest way to do so is to consult the calorie column of this counter and keep an accurate count of your total intake of food and beverages for a period of seven days. If you have not gained or lost weight during that week divide that number by seven and you'll have your maintenance diet expressed in calories. To lose weight, you must reduce your daily or weekly intake of calories below this maintenance level. (To gain, increase the intake.)

One pound of fat is equal to 3,500 calories. Add this number of calories to those you need to balance your energy requirements and you will gain one pound; subtract it, and you will lose a pound.

75 Carbohydrates per Day

The carbohydrate column shows the amount of this nutrient in grams for the quantities of foods indicated in the portion column. Some dietitians are giving special attention to this nutrient at present in connection with weight control. Carbohydrates include sugars, starches, acids and other nutrients. The values in this book are total carbohydrates, by difference, the basis on which calories from carbohydrates are calculated in the U.S. diet. *Conversion of excess to Saturated Fat*

Other Nutrients *56, 61*

Do not forget that other nutrients are extremely important in diet planning—protein, fat, minerals and vitamins. Calories yielded by alcohol must also be taken into consideration. From a nutrition viewpoint, perhaps the best advice that can be given to the dieter is to eat a varied diet with all classes of foods represented. Meat, fish, chicken, fats and oils, milk, vegetables, fruits and grain products are all important sources of essential nutrients and some foods from each of these classes of foods should be included in the diet every day. With the great abundance and variety of foods on the grocer's shelves, there is no reason why the dieter should not enjoy a tasty, nutritious and attractive diet. Just eat in moderation and there is no need to eliminate any one food altogether, except in special conditions under a doctor's directions. Choose wisely and eat well.

Sources of Data

Values in this dictionary are based on publications issued by the U.S. Department of Agriculture and on data submitted by manufacturers and processors. The U.S. Department of Agriculture issues basic tables on food composition for use in the United States. The commercial products from U.S.D.A. publications represent average values obtained on products of more than one company. The figures designated "home recipe" are based on recipes on file with the Department of Agriculture. Data on commercial products listed by brand name in this publication are based on values supplied by manufacturers and processors for their own individual products. Very few supermarket brand names, such as Pathmark or private labels were included in this book inasmuch as they are not usually analyzed under these trade names. Every care has been taken to interpret the data and the descriptions supplied by the companies as fully and accurately as possible. Many values have been recalculated to different portions from those submitted in order to bring about greater uniformity among similar items.

Calories in these different sources are not always on a strictly uniform basis. In the Department of Agriculture, calories are calculated using specific factors, which make allowances for losses in digestion and metabolism. The technical explanation of these factors is given in Handbook 74 of the United States Department of Agriculture. Most manufacturers use average factors of 4, 9 and 4 for calories yielded by each gram of protein, fat and carbohydrate respectively; a factor of 7 is used as an average value to calculate the calories from one gram of alcohol. These differences in procedure will give somewhat different results for products of similar composition. Some manufacturers have adopted the values from U.S. Department of Agriculture publications as representative of their own products. In these cases, it will be apparent in the table that the data from the companies match exactly those from U.S.D.A. publications.

Analyses of foods to provide information on nutritive values are extremely expensive to conduct. Many small companies have not been able to afford to have their products analyzed and thus were unable to provide data for this book or were able to provide only the calories or only the carbohydrates. Other companies have simply never gotten around to having the analysis done. New requirements for labeling nutritive values of products may provide information on additional items in the future. Therefore, wherever data for carbohydrates were unavailable, blank spaces were left which may be filled in by the reader at a later time.

Bear in mind that small differences in calorie values on similar products of the same weight are not important in diet planning. They may be due to different methods of calculating the calories or to small differences in the nutritive values of the samples analyzed because no two foods ever have exactly the same composition. Some differences may also be due to the way the food was measured as noted in the case of green beans earlier.

Carbohydrates in this book are usually total carbohydrates by difference. A few manufacturers reported only "available carbohydrates." These values were omitted.

Foods Listed by Groups

Foods in the following classes are reported together rather than as individual items in the main alphabet. Baby Food, Bread; Cake, Cake Icing, Cake Icing Mix; Cake Mix; Candy; Cheese; Cookie; Cookie Mix; Cracker; Gravy; Salad Dressing; Sauce and Soft Drinks.

BARBARA KRAUS

Abbreviations and Symbols

(USDA)=United States Department
     of Agriculture
(HEW/FAO)=Health, Education
     and Welfare/Food
     and Agriculture
     Organization
*=prepared as package directs[1]
<=less than
&=and
"=inch
canned=bottles or jars
     as well as cans
dia.=diameter
fl.=fluid

liq.=liquid
lb.=pound
med.=medium
oz.=ounce
pkg.=package
pt.=pint
qt.=quart
sq.=square
T.=tablespoon
Tr.=trace
tsp.=teaspoon
wt.=weight

    italics or name in parentheses=registered trademark, ®
    Blank spaces indicate that no data are available.

Equivalents

By Weight
1 pound=16 ounces
1 ounce=28.35 grams
3.52 ounces=100 grams

By Volume
1 quart=4 cups
1 cup=8 fluid ounces
1 cup=½ pint
1 cup=16 tablespoons
2 tablespoons=1 fluid ounce
1 tablespoon=3 teaspoons

[1]If the package directions call for whole or skim milk, the data given here are for whole milk, unless otherwise stated.

Food and Description	Measure or Quantity	Calories	Carbo-hydrates (grams)

A

ABALONE (USDA):
Raw, meat only	4 oz.	111	3.9
Canned	4 oz.	91	2.6

ABISANTE LIQUEUR (Leroux)
100 proof	1 fl. oz.	87	1.0

AC'CENT
	¼ tsp. (1 gram)	3	0.

ACEROLA, fresh (USDA)
	½ lb. (weighed with seeds)	52	12.6

ALBACORE, raw, meat only (USDA)
	4 oz.	201	0.

ALCOHOLIC BEVERAGES (See individual listings)

ALE (See **BEER**)

ALEWIFE (USDA):
Raw, meat only	4 oz.	144	0.
Canned, solids & liq.	4 oz.	160	0.

ALEXANDER COCKTAIL
MIX (Holland House)	.6-oz. pkg.	69	16.0

ALLSPICE (French's)
	1 tsp.	6	1.3

ALMOND:
In shell:
(USDA)	10 nuts (2.5 grams)	60	2.0
(USDA)	1 cup (2.8 oz.)	187	6.1

(USDA): United States Department of Agriculture
(HEW/FAO): Health, Education and Welfare/Food and Agriculture Organization
* Prepared as Package Directs

Food and Description	Measure or Quantity	Calories	Carbo-hydrates (grams)
Shelled:			
Plain:			
(USDA) whole	½ cup (2.5 oz.)	425	13.8
(USDA) whole	1 oz.	170	5.5
(USDA) whole	13-15 almonds (.6 oz.)	105	3.4
(USDA) chopped	1 cup (4.5 oz.)	777	25.4
(Blue Diamond)	½ cup	504	19.4
Blanched (Blue Diamond) salted	½ cup	492	15.3
Chocolate-covered (See CANDY)			
Flavored (Blue Diamond)	1 oz.	180	9.5
Roasted:			
(USDA) salted	½ cup (2.8 oz.)	492	15.3
(Blue Diamond) diced	1 oz.	176	5.5
(Flavor House) dry	1 oz.	178	5.5
(Planters) dry	1 oz.	191	5.5
ALMOND EXTRACT:			
(Durkee)	1 tsp.	13	
(Ehlers)	1 tsp.	12	
(French's)	1 tsp.	12	
(Virginia Dare)	1 tsp. (4 grams)	10	0.
ALMOND MEAL, partially defatted (USDA)	1 oz.	116	8.2
ALPHABET SOUP MIX:			
*(Golden Grain)	1 cup	54	9.0
*(Goodman's)	8 oz.	43	
ALPHA-BITS, oat cereal (Post)	1 cup (1 oz.)	110	24.0
A.M., fruit juice drink (Mott's)	6 fl. oz.	90	22.0
AMARANTH, raw (USDA):			
Untrimmed	1 lb. (weighed untrimmed)	103	18.6
Trimmed	4 oz.	41	7.4

Food and Description	Measure or Quantity	Calories	Carbo-hydrates (grams)
AMBROSIA, chilled, bottled (Kraft)	4 oz.	85	14.7
ANCHOVY PASTE, canned (Crosse & Blackwell)	1 T.	20	1.0
ANCHOVY, PICKLED, canned, not heavily salted, drained (USDA)	2-oz. can	79	.1
ANESONE LIQUEUR (Leroux) 90 proof	1 fl. oz.	86	2.8
ANGEL FOOD CAKE (See **CAKE**)			
ANGEL FOOD CAKE MIX (See **CAKE MIX**)			
ANISE EXTRACT:			
(Durkee)	1 tsp.	16	
(Ehlers)	1 tsp.	26	
(French's)	1 tsp.	26	
(Virginia Dare)	1 tsp. (4 grams)	22	0.
ANISE SEED, dried (HEW/FAO)	½ oz.	58	6.3
ANISETTE LIQUEUR, red or white:			
(Bols) 50 proof	1 fl. oz.	111	13.9
(Dekuyper) 60 proof	1 fl. oz. (1.2 oz.)	95	11.4
(Garnier) 54 proof	1 fl. oz.	82	9.3
(Hiram Walker) 60 proof	1 fl. oz.	92	10.8
(Leroux) 60 proof	1 fl. oz.	89	9.9
APPLE, any variety: Fresh (USDA): Eaten with skin	1 lb. (weighed with skin & core)	242	60.5

(USDA): United States Department of Agriculture
(HEW/FAO): Health, Education and Welfare/Food and Agriculture
           Organization
* Prepared as Package Directs

Food and Description	Measure or Quantity	Calories	Carbo-hydrates (grams)
Eaten with skin	1 med., 2½" dia. (about 4 per lb.)	66	15.3
Eaten without skin	1 lb. (weighed without skin & core)	211	55.0
Eaten without skin	1 med., 2½" dia. (about 4 per lb.)	53	13.9
Pared, diced or sliced	1 cup (3.9 oz.)	59	15.5
Pared, quartered	1 cup (4.4 oz.)	68	17.6
Dehydrated (USDA):			
Uncooked	1 oz.	100	26.1
Cooked, sweetened	½ cup (4.2 oz.)	91	23.5
Dried:			
(USDA) uncooked	1 cup (3 oz.)	234	61.0
(USDA) cooked, unsweetened	½ cup (4.3 oz.)	94	24.6
(USDA) cooked, sweetened	½ cup (4.9 oz.)	157	40.9
(Del Monte) uncooked	1 cup (3 oz.)	151	37.2
Frozen, sweetened, slices, not thawed (USDA)	10-oz. pkg.	264	68.9
APPLE BROWN BETTY, home recipe (USDA)	1 cup (7.6 oz.)	325	63.9
APPLE BUTTER:			
(USDA)	1 T. (.6 oz.)	33	8.2
(Smucker's) cider	1 T. (.6 oz.)	37	9.2
(White House)	1 T.	28	7.6
APPLE CIDER:			
(USDA)	½ cup (4.4 oz.)	58	14.8
(Mott's) Sweet	½ cup	59	14.6
APPLE DRINK, canned:			
(Ann Page)	6 fl. oz. (6.5 oz.)	80	20.0
(H-C)	6 fl. oz.	92	23.0
(Wagner)	6 fl. oz.	90	22.5
APPLE FRITTERS, frozen			
(Mrs. Paul's)	½ of 8-oz. pkg.	235	31.7

Food and Description	Measure or Quantity	Calories	Carbo-hydrates (grams)
APPLE FRUIT ROLL, frozen			
(Chun King)	1 oz.	64	10.1
APPLE JACKS, cereal			
(Kellogg's)	1 cup (1 oz.)	110	26.0
APPLE JELLY:			
Sweetened:			
(Smucker's)	1 T. (.7 oz.)	52	13.3
(White House)	1 T. (.7 oz.)	46	13.0
Dietetic or low calorie:			
(Diet Delight)	1 T. (.6 oz.)	10	2.5
(Featherweight)	1 T.	14	4.0
(Kraft)	1 oz.	34	8.5
(Louis Sherry)	1 T. (.4 oz.)	6	1.5
(Slenderella)	1 T. (.7 oz.)	23	5.8
(Tillie Lewis) *Tasti-Diet*	1 T. (.6 oz.)	12	3.0
APPLE JUICE:			
Canned:			
(USDA)	½ cup (4.4 oz.)	58	14.8
(Ann Page)	½ cup (4.4 oz.)	79	20.0
(Mott's) regular or			
McIntosh	½ cup (4.4 oz.)	59	14.6
(Seneca)	½ cup (4.4 oz.)	61	14.8
(White House)	½ cup	58	15.0
*Frozen (Seneca)	½ cup (4.4 oz.)	61	14.8
APPLE PIE:			
(USDA) home recipe, 2			
crusts	⅛ of 9″ pie (5.6 oz.)	404	60.2
(Drake's)	2-oz. pie	204	25.5
(Hostess)	4½-oz. pie	409	53.7
(McDonald's) (See **McDONALD'S**)			
(Tastykake)	4-oz. pie	380	58.6
(Tastykake) French apple	4½-oz. pie	451	64.3

(USDA): United States Department of Agriculture
(HEW/FAO): Health, Education and Welfare/Food and Agriculture Organization
* Prepared as Package Directs

Food and Description	Measure or Quantity	Calories	Carbo-hydrates (grams)
Frozen:			
(USDA) baked	5 oz.	361	56.8
(Banquet)	⅕ of 20-oz. pie	288	42.6
(Morton)	⅙ of 24-oz. pie	295	40.9
(Morton) mini pie	½ of 8-oz. pie	299	44.3
Tart (Pepperidge Farm)	1 tart (3 oz.)	276	32.8
APPLE PIE FILLING:			
(Comstock)	⅙ of 8″ pie	115	28.5
(Lucky Leaf)	8 oz.	248	60.8
(Wilderness)	21-oz. can	709	163.7
APPLESAUCE, canned:			
Sweetened:			
(USDA)	½ cup (4.5 oz.)	116	30.5
(Del Monte)	½ cup (4.6 oz.)	111	27.2
(Mott's) cinnamon, country style	½ cup (4.5 oz.)	105	26.2
(Mott's) natural style	½ cup	107	26.2
(Seneca) cinnamon	½ cup (4.5 oz.)	134	30.2
(Seneca) 100% McIntosh	½ cup (4.5 oz.)	116	30.2
(Stokely-Van Camp)	½ cup (4.5 oz.)	90	22.5
(White House)	½ cup (4.5 oz.)	110	28.2
Unsweetened, dietetic or low calorie:			
(USDA)	½ cup (4.3 oz.)	50	13.2
(Blue Boy)	4 oz.	43	10.4
(Diet Delight)	½ cup (4.3 oz.)	50	13.0
(Featherweight)	½ cup	50	13.0
(Mott's) natural style	4-oz. serving	45	11.0
(S and W) *Nutradiet*	4 oz.	56	13.7
(Tillie Lewis) *Tasti-Diet*	½ cup (4.1 oz.)	61	15.2
APPLE TURNOVER:			
(Pepperidge Farm)	1 turnover (3.3 oz.)	315	30.2
(Pillsbury)	1 turnover	170	26.0
APRICOT:			
Fresh (USDA):			
Whole	1 lb. (weighed with pits)	217	54.6

Food and Description	Measure or Quantity	Calories	Carbohydrates (grams)
Whole	3 apricots (about 12 per lb.)	55	13.7
Halves	1 cup (5.5 oz.)	79	19.8
Canned, regular pack, solids & liq.:			
(USDA) juice pack	4 oz.	61	15.4
(USDA) light syrup	4 oz.	75	19.1
(USDA) heavy syrup, halves	½ cup (5.6 oz.)	111	28.4
(USDA) heavy syrup, halves	3 med. halves with 1¾ T. syrup (3.0 oz.)	73	18.7
(USDA) extra heavy syrup	4 oz.	115	29.5
(Del Monte) whole, peeled	½ cup	104	25.0
(Del Monte) halves, unpeeled	½ cup	101	24.4
(Hunt's) heavy syrup	½ cup (4.5 oz.)	103	26.9
(Libby's) heavy syrup, halves	½ cup	100	27.0
(Stokely-Van Camp)	½ cup (4.6 oz.)	110	27.0
Canned, unsweetened or dietetic:			
(USDA) water pack, halves, solids & liq.	½ cup (4.3 oz.)	46	11.8
(Cellu) water pack, solids & liq.	½ cup	35	9.0
(Diet Delight) juice pack, solids & liq.	½ cup (4.4 oz.)	63	15.0
(Diet Delight) water pack, solids & liq.	½ cup	35	9.0
(Featherweight) juice pack, solids & liq.	½ cup	50	13.0
(Libby's)	4 oz.	40	10.9
(S and W) *Nutradiet*, halves, solids & liq.	4 halves (3.5 oz.)	41	9.6

(USDA): United States Department of Agriculture
(HEW/FAO): Health, Education and Welfare/Food and Agriculture Organization
* Prepared as Package Directs

Food and Description	Measure or Quantity	Calories	Carbo-hydrates (grams)
(Tillie Lewis) *Tasti-Diet*, unpeeled, solids & liq.	½ cup (4.3 oz.)	54	13.4
Dehydrated:			
(USDA) uncooked, sulfured	4 oz.	376	95.9
(USDA) cooked, sugar added, solids & liq.	4 oz.	135	34.6
Dried:			
(USDA) uncooked	1 cup (4.6 oz.)	338	86.5
(USDA) uncooked	10 large halves (¼ cup or 1.7 oz.)	125	31.9
(USDA) cooked, sweetened	½ cup with liq. (4.7 oz.)	164	42.4
(USDA) cooked, unsweetened	½ cup with liq. (4.4 oz.)	106	27.0
(Del Monte)	½ cup (2.3 oz.)	145	39.9
Frozen, unthawed, sweetened (USDA)	10-oz. pkg.	278	71.2
APRICOT-APPLE JUICE & PRUNE (Sunsweet)	½ cup	63	16.0
APRICOT BRANDY (DeKuyper) 70 proof	1 fl. oz. (1.1 oz.)	85	6.9
APRICOT, CANDIED (USDA)	1 oz.	96	24.5
APRICOT LIQUEUR:			
(Bols) 60 proof	1 fl. oz.	96	8.9
(Hiram Walker) 60 proof	1 fl. oz.	82	8.2
(Leroux) 60 proof	1 fl. oz.	85	8.9
APRICOT NECTAR, canned:			
Sweetened:			
(USDA)	½ cup (4.4 oz.)	71	18.9
(Del Monte)	½ cup (4.4 oz.)	75	18.0
(Dewco)	½ cup	68	
(Sunsweet)	½ cup	75	18.0
Dietetic or low calorie (S and W) *Nutradiet*	4 oz. (by wt.)	35	8.2

Food and Description	Measure or Quantity	Calories	Carbo-hydrates (grams)
APRICOT PIE FILLING:			
(Comstock)	½ cup (5.2 oz.)	154	36.7
(Lucky Leaf)	8 oz.	316	77.6
(Wilderness)	21-oz. can	756	176.7
APRICOT & PINEAPPLE NECTAR, unsweetened (S and W) *Nutradiet*	4 oz. (by wt.)	35	8.5
APRICOT & PINEAPPLE PRESERVE:			
Sweetened:			
(Bama)	1 T. (.7 oz.)	54	13.5
(Smucker's)	1 T. (.7 oz.)	57	13.5
Low calorie or dietetic:			
(Diet Delight)	1 T. (.6 oz.)	10	2.3
(Tillie Lewis)	1 T. (.6 oz.)	12	3.0
APRICOT PRESERVE:			
Sweetened:			
(Bama)	1 T. (.7 oz.)	51	12.7
(Smucker's)	1 T. (.7 oz.)	50	12.9
Low calorie (Featherweight)	1 T.	16	4.0
APRICOT SOUR COCKTAIL:			
(Holland House) liquid mix	2 fl. oz.	86	24.0
(National Distillers) *Duet,* 12½% alcohol	2 fl. oz.	48	1.6
(Party Tyme) dry mix	½-oz. pkg.	50	11.6
(Party Tyme) liquid mix	2 fl. oz.	58	14.0
(Party Tyme) 12½% alcohol	2 fl. oz.	66	5.7
APRICOT SYRUP (Smucker's)	1 T. (.6 oz.)	45	11.6
AQUAVIT (Leroux) 90 proof	1 fl. oz.	75	Tr.

(USDA): United States Department of Agriculture
(HEW/FAO): Health, Education and Welfare/Food and Agriculture Organization
* Prepared as Package Directs

Food and Description	Measure or Quantity	Calories	Carbohydrates (grams)
ARTICHOKE, Globe or French (See also **JERUSALEM ARTICHOKE**):			
Raw, whole (USDA)	1 lb. (weighed untrimmed)	85	19.2
Boiled without salt, drained (USDA)	4 oz.	50	11.2
Canned, marinated, drained (Cara Mia)	6-oz. jar	179	7.2
Frozen (Birds Eye) deluxe hearts	⅓ of 9-oz. pkg.	20	5.0
ASPARAGUS:			
Raw (USDA) whole spears	1 lb. (weighed untrimmed	66	12.7
Boiled without salt, drained (USDA):			
Whole spears	4 spears (½″ at base, 2.1 oz.)	12	2.2
Cut spears, 1½″-2″ pieces	1 cup (5.1 oz.)	29	5.2
Canned, regular pack:			
(USDA) green, spears, solids & liq.	1 cup (8.6 oz.)	44	7.1
(USDA) green, spears only	1 cup (8.3 oz.)	49	8.0
(USDA) green, spears only	4 med. spears (2.8 oz.)	17	2.7
(USDA) green, liquid only	2 T.	3	.7
(USDA) white, spears, solids & liq.	1 cup (8.6 oz.)	44	8.1
(USDA) white, spears only	4 med. spears (2.8 oz.)	18	2.9
(USDA) white, liquid only	2 T.	3	.8
(Del Monte) green, spears, solids & liq.	1 cup (8.4 oz.)	45	3.0
(Del Monte) green, spears only	1 cup (8.5 oz.)	64.7	7.5
(Del Monte) white,			

Food and Description	Measure or Quantity	Calories	Carbo-hydrates (grams)
spears, solids & liq.	1 cup (8.6 oz.)	48	7.3
(Del Monte) white, spears only	1 cup (8.5 oz.)	55	8.0
(Green Giant) green, cut spears, solids & liq.	1 cup	40	5.0
(Le Sueur) green, spears, solids & liq.	1 cup	40	5.0
(Stokely-Van Camp) green, spears, solid & liq.	1 cup (8.4 oz.)	45	3.0
(Stokely-Van Camp) green, cut spears, solids & liq.	1 cup (8.4 oz.)	46	6.0
Canned, dietetic pack:			
(USDA) green, spears, solids & liq.	4 oz.	18	3.1
(USDA) green, spears only	4 oz.	23	3.5
(USDA) green, liquid only	4 oz.	10	2.3
(USDA) white, spears, solids & liq.	4 oz.	18	3.4
(Blue Boy) green, spears, solids & liq.	4 oz.	20	3.2
(Cellu) green, spears, solids & liq.	½ cup	18	3.0
(Cellu) green, cut spears, solid & liq.	½ cup	16	3.0
(Diet Delight) green, spears, solids & liq.	½ cup (4.2 oz.)	18	2.3
(Featherweight) green, spears, solids & liq.	½ cup	18	3.0
(Featherweight) green, cut spears, solids & liq.	½ cup	16	3.0
(Tillie Lewis) green	½ cup (4.3 oz.)	24	3.7
Frozen:			
(USDA) cuts & tips, unthawed	4 oz.	26	4.1
(USDA) cuts & tips, boiled, drained	½ cup (3.2 oz.)	20	3.2

(USDA): United States Department of Agriculture
(HEW/FAO): Health, Education and Welfare/Food and Agriculture Organization
* Prepared as Package Directs

Food and Description	Measure or Quantity	Calories	Carbo-hydrates (grams)
(USDA) spears, unthawed	4 oz.	27	4.4
(USDA) spears, boiled, drained	4 oz.	26	4.3
(Birds Eye) cuts, 5-minute style	½ of 10-oz. pkg.	25	3.0
(Birds Eye) spears, regular or jumbo	⅓ of 10-oz. pkg.	25	3.0
(Green Giant) cut spears, in butter sauce	1 cup	90	7.0
ASPARAGUS PUREE, canned, dietetic (Cellu)	½ cup	25	3.5
ASPARAGUS SOUP, cream of, canned:			
(USDA) condensed	8 oz. (by weight)	123	19.1
(USDA) prepared with equal volume water	1 cup (8.5 oz.)	65	10.1
(USDA) prepared with equal volume milk	1 cup (8.5 oz.)	144	16.3
*(Campbell) condensed	8-oz. serving	80	9.6
ASTI WINE (Gancia) 9% alcohol	3 fl. oz.	126	18.0
AUNT JEMIMA SYRUP	¼ cup	212	54.0
AVOCADO, peeled, pitted, all commercial varieties (USDA)			
Whole	1 fruit (10.7 oz., weighed with seed & skin)	378	14.3
Cubed	½ cup (5.3 oz.)	251	9.5
Puree	1 cup (8.1 oz.)	384	14.5
AWAKE (Birds Eye)	6 fl. oz.	90	21.0
AYDS, all flavors	1 piece (7 grams)	25	5.0

Food and Description	*Measure or Quantity*	*Calories*	*Carbo-hydrates (grams)*

B

BABY FOOD:			
Apple:			
& apricot, junior (Beech-Nut)	7¾ oz.	101	24.4
& apricot, strained (Beech-Nut)	4¾ oz.	61	15.2
& blueberry, junior (Gerber)	7¾ oz.	149	35.7
& blueberry, strained (Gerber)	4¾ oz.	87	20.5
& raspberry, junior (Gerber)	7¾ oz.	138	33.0
& raspberry, strained (Gerber)	4¾ oz.	87	20.5
Dutch dessert, junior (Gerber)	7¾ oz.	174	38.8
Dutch dessert, strained (Gerber)	4¾ oz.	106	23.8
Apple Betty (Beech-Nut):			
Junior	7¾ oz.	161	40.3
Strained	4¾ oz.	101	24.2
Apple-cherry juice, strained:			
(Beech-Nut)	4⅕ fl. oz. (4.4 oz.)	56	14.0
(Gerber)	4⅕ fl. oz. (4.6 oz.)	59	14.0
Apple-grape juice, strained:			
(Beech-Nut)	4⅕ fl. oz. (4.4 oz.)	64	16.0
(Gerber)	4⅕ fl. oz.	58	13.6
Apple juice, strained:			
(Beech-Nut)	4⅕ fl. oz. (4.4 oz.)	56	14.0
(Gerber)	4⅕ fl. oz. (4.2 oz.)	58	14.2
Apple-peach juice, strained:			
(Beech-Nut)	4⅕ fl. oz.	64	15.9
(Gerber)	4⅕ fl. oz.	55	13.1

(USDA): United States Department of Agriculture
(HEW/FAO): Health, Education and Welfare/Food and Agriculture Organization
* Prepared as Package Directs

Food and Description	*Measure or Quantity*	*Calories*	*Carbo-hydrates (grams)*
Apple-plum juice, strained, (Gerber)	4⅕ fl. oz.	60	14.7
Applesauce:			
Junior (Beech-Nut)	7¾ oz.	101	25.1
Junior (Gerber)	7¾ oz.	87	20.7
Strained (Beech-Nut)	4¾ oz.	60	15.0
Strained (Gerber)	4½ oz.	55	13.0
& apricots:			
Junior (Gerber)	7¾ oz.	186	44.3
Strained (Gerber)	4¾ oz.	112	27.4
& cherries, junior (Beech-Nut)	7¾ oz.	117	29.1
& cherries, strained (Beech-Nut)	4¾ oz.	69	17.3
& pineapple, junior (Gerber)	7½ oz.	87	20.5
& pineapple, strained (Gerber)	4½ oz.	52	12.1
& raspberries, junior (Beech-Nut)	7¾ oz.	101	25.1
& raspberries, strained (Beech-Nut)	4¾ oz.	88	15.8
Apricot with tapioca:			
Junior (Beech-Nut)	7¾ oz.	152	37.2
Junior (Gerber)	7¾ oz.	154	37.6
Strained (Beech-Nut)	4¾ oz.	88	22.0
Strained (Gerber)	4¾ oz.	94	23.1
Banana:			
& pineapple with tapioca:			
Junior (Beech-Nut)	7¾ oz.	103	26.0
Junior (Gerber)	7¾ oz.	162	39.4
Strained (Beech-Nut)	4¾ oz.	64	16.1
Strained (Gerber)	4¾ oz.	104	25.2
Dessert, junior (Beech-Nut)	7¾ oz.	161	39.0
With tapioca:			
Junior (Beech-Nut)	7¾ oz.	163	40.3
Junior (Gerber)	7¾ oz.	151	35.7
Strained (Beech-Nut)	4¾ oz.	96	24.0
Strained (Gerber)	4¾ oz.	91	21.9
Bean, green:			
Junior (Beech-Nut)	7¼ oz.	62	11.9

Food and Description	Measure or Quantity	Calories	Carbo-hydrates (grams)
Junior (Beech-Nut) in butter sauce	7¼ oz.	72	11.1
Junior (Gerber) creamed	7½ oz.	86	17.5
Strained (Beech-Nut)	4½ oz.	39	8.1
Strained (Beech-Nut) in butter sauce	4½ oz.	44	7.0
Strained (Gerber)	4½ oz.	31	5.9
With potatoes & ham, casserole, toddler (Gerber)	6¼ oz.	131	13.1
Beef:			
Junior (Gerber)	3½ oz.	88	.5
Strained (Gerber)	3½ oz.	96	0.
Beef & beef broth:			
Junior (Beech-Nut)	7½ oz.	228	1.3
Strained (Beech-Nut)	4½ oz.	136	.8
Beef & beef heart, strained (Gerber)	3½ oz.	87	.7
Beef dinner:			
Junior (Beech-Nut) high meat	4½ oz.	124	7.3
Strained (Beech-Nut) high meat	4½ oz.	125	7.3
& noodles:			
Junior (Beech-Nut)	7½ oz.	113	7.0
Junior (Gerber) with vegetables	7½ oz.	118	15.8
Strained (Beech-Nut)	4½ oz.	68	9.7
Strained (Gerber) with vegetables	4½ oz.	69	8.4
& rice, toddler (Gerber) with tomato sauce	6¼ oz.	143	16.7
With vegetables:			
Junior (Gerber)	4½ oz.	110	6.3
Strained (Gerber)	4½ oz.	109	6.1
Beef lasagna, toddler (Gerber)	6¼ oz.	133	16.7
Beef liver, strained (Gerber)	3½ oz.	96	2.4
Beef stew, toddler (Gerber)	6¼ oz.	100	11.5

(USDA): United States Department of Agriculture
(HEW/FAO): Health, Education and Welfare/Food and Agriculture Organization
* Prepared as Package Directs

Food and Description	Measure or Quantity	Calories	Carbo-hydrates (grams)
Beet, strained (Gerber)	4½ oz.	46	9.5
Caramel pudding (Beech-Nut):			
Junior	7¾ oz.	172	36.1
Strained	4¾ oz.	109	22.0
Carrot:			
Junior (Beech-Nut)	7½ oz.	62	12.1
Junior (Beech-Nut) in butter sauce	7½ oz.	81	14.1
Junior (Gerber)	7½ oz.	58	12.0
Strained (Beech-Nut)	4½ oz.	36	8.1
Strained (Beech-Nut) in butter sauce	4½ oz.	43	8.1
Cereal, dry:			
Barley (Beech-Nut)	1 oz.	111	19.9
Barley (Gerber)	6 T. (14.2 grams)	62	10.3
High protein (Gerber)	6 T. (14.2 grams)	53	5.9
High protein (Gerber) with apple & orange	6 T. (14.2 grams)	54	7.8
Hi-protein (Beech-Nut)	1 oz.	105	10.5
Mixed (Beech-Nut)	1 oz.	108	19.3
Mixed (Beech-Nut) honey	1 oz.	111	19.9
Mixed (Gerber)	6 T. (14.2 grams)	54	10.2
Mixed (Gerber) with banana	6 T. (14.2 grams)	55	10.7
Oatmeal (Beech-Nut)	1 oz.	102	19.3
Oatmeal (Beech-Nut) honey	1 oz.	114	19.9
Oatmeal (Gerber)	6 T. (14.2 grams)	56	9.3
Oatmeal (Gerber) with banana	6 T. (14.2 grams)	56	10.1
Rice (Beech-Nut)	1 oz.	108	22.7
Rice (Beech-Nut) honey	1 oz.	108	22.7
Rice (Gerber)	6 T. (14.2 grams)	54	10.8
Rice (Gerber) with banana	6 T. (14.2 grams)	54	10.9
Wheat (Beech-Nut) honey	1 oz.	105	21.9
Cereal or mixed cereal:			
With applesauce & banana:			
Junior (Gerber)	7¾ oz.	171	39.9
Strained (Beech-Nut)	4½ oz.	111	22.8
Strained (Gerber)	4¾ oz.	102	23.6

Food and Description	Measure or Quantity	Calories	Carbo-hydrates (grams)
With egg yolk:			
Junior (Gerber)	7½ oz.	110	14.7
Strained (Beech-Nut) & bacon	4½ oz.	111	8.9
Strained (Gerber)	4½ oz.	66	8.7
High protein with applesauce & banana, strained (Gerber)	4¾ oz.	115	20.2
Oatmeal with applesauce & banana:			
Junior (Gerber)	7¾ oz.	164	34.1
Strained (Beech-Nut)	4¾ oz.	100	20.0
Strained (Gerber)	4¾ oz.	88	19.7
Rice with applesauce & banana, strained:			
(Beech-Nut)	4¾ oz.	97	21.0
(Gerber)	4¾ oz.	111	25.8
Rice with mixed fruit, junior (Gerber)	7¾ oz.	176	40.3
Cheese:			
Cottage with pineapple, junior (Beech-Nut)	7¾ oz.	172	31.3
Cottage with pineapple juice, strained (Beech-Nut)	4¾ oz.	121	21.2
Cottage, dessert, with pineapple:			
Junior (Gerber)	7¾ oz.	203	40.3
Strained (Gerber)	4¾ oz.	120	23.4
Cherry vanilla pudding (Gerber):			
Junior	7¾ oz.	171	41.2
Strained	4¾ oz.	100	23.6
Chicken:			
Junior (Gerber)	3½ oz.	152	.3
Strained (Gerber)	3½ oz.	131	.2
Chicken & chicken broth:			
Junior (Beech-Nut)	7½ oz.	222	1.3

(USDA): United States Department of Agriculture
(HEW/FAO): Health, Education and Welfare/Food and Agriculture Organization
* Prepared as Package Directs

Food and Description	Measure or Quantity	Calories	Carbohydrates (grams)
Strained (Beech-Nut)	4½ oz.	136	.8
Chicken dinner:			
Junior (Beech-Nut) high meat	4½ oz.	91	8.3
Strained (Beech-Nut) high meat	4½ oz.	92	8.6
& noodle:			
Junior (Beech-Nut)	7½ oz.	85	16.2
Junior (Gerber)	7½ oz.	111	16.4
Strained (Beech-Nut)	4½ oz.	55	10.2
Strained (Gerber)	4½ oz.	66	8.6
& vegetables:			
Junior (Gerber)	4½ oz.	124	3.7
Strained (Gerber)	4½ oz.	111	6.5
Chicken soup, cream of, strained (Gerber)	4½ oz.	73	10.5
Chicken stew, toddler (Gerber)	6 oz.	143	10.4
Chicken sticks, junior (Gerber)	2½ oz.	134	.4
Cookie, animal-shaped (Gerber)	1 cookie (6.5 grams)	28	4.2
Cookie, Arrowroot (Gerber)	1 cookie (5.5 grams)	25	4.0
Corn, creamed:			
Junior (Beech-Nut)	7½ oz.	119	26.6
Strained (Beech-Nut)	4½ oz.	72	15.9
Strained (Gerber)	4½ oz.	73	14.9
Custard:			
Junior (Beech-Nut)	7¾ oz.	172	30.0
Strained (Beech-Nut)	4½ oz.	92	15.7
Chocolate, junior (Gerber)	7¾ oz.	201	37.4
Chocolate, strained (Beech-Nut)	4½ oz.	115	21.1
Chocolate, strained (Gerber)	4½ oz.	115	21.2
Vanilla, junior (Gerber)	7¾ oz.	206	35.4
Vanilla, strained (Gerber)	4½ oz.	118	20.2
Dutch apple dessert (See Apple, Dutch dessert)			

Food and Description	*Measure or Quantity*	*Calories*	*Carbohydrates (grams)*
Egg yolk, strained:			
(Beech-Nut)	3⅓ oz.	195	.6
(Gerber)	3⅓ oz.	184	1.0
Fruit dessert:			
Junior (Beech-Nut)	7¾ oz.	156	39.2
Junior (Gerber)	7¾ oz.	156	39.2
Strained (Beech-Nut)	4½ oz.	92	22.8
Strained (Gerber)	4¾ oz.	95	22.7
Tropical, junior (Beech-Nut)	7¾ oz.	132	33.2
Fruit juice, mixed, strained:			
(Beech-Nut)	4⅕ fl. oz. (4.4 oz.)	60	15.0
(Gerber)	4⅕ fl. oz. (4.2 oz.)	69	16.3
Grits with egg yolk, strained (Gerber)	4½ oz.	78	10.4
Ham:			
Junior (Gerber)	3½ oz.	121	.7
Strained (Gerber)	3½ oz.	106	.8
Ham dinner:			
Junior (Beech-Nut) high meat	4½ oz.	125	7.7
Strained (Beech-Nut) high meat	4½ oz.	130	6.6
With vegetables:			
Junior (Gerber)	4½ oz.	94	7.3
Strained (Gerber)	4½ oz.	94	7.0
Ham and ham broth, strained (Beech-Nut)	4½ oz.	121	.8
Hawaiian Delight (Gerber):			
Junior	7¾ oz.	206	46.0
Strained	4¾ oz.	126	28.3
Lamb:			
Junior (Gerber)	3½ oz.	98	0.
Strained (USDA)			
Strained (Gerber)	3½ oz.	96	.2
& noodles, junior (Beech-Nut)	7½ oz.	134	19.4

(USDA): United States Department of Agriculture
(HEW/FAO): Health, Education and Welfare/Food and Agriculture Organization

* Prepared as Package Directs

Food and Description	Measure or Quantity	Calories	Carbo-hydrates (grams)
Lamb & lamb broth (Beech-Nut):			
Junior	7½ oz.	254	1.3
Strained	4½ oz.	119	.8
Liver & bacon, strained (USDA)			
Macaroni:			
& bacon with vegetables, junior (Beech-Nut)	7½ oz.	160	17.7
& beef, junior (Beech-Nut)	7½ oz.	117	17.3
& cheese, junior (Gerber)	7½ oz.	132	17.5
& cheese, strained (Gerber)	4½ oz.	81	10.4
& ham, junior (Beech-Nut)	7½ oz.	121	17.7
With tomato and beef (Gerber):			
Junior	7½ oz.	108	16.8
Strained	4½ oz.	67	10.9
With tomato sauce and beef, strained (Beech-Nut)	4½ oz.	83	10.7
MBF, concentrate (Gerber)	2 T. (1.2 oz.)	43	3.2
MBF, diluted 1 to 1 (Gerber)	2 T. (1.1 oz.)	21	1.9
Meat sticks, junior (Gerber)	2½ oz.	126	.2
Orange-apple juice, strained:			
(Beech-Nut)	4⅛ fl. oz. (4.4 oz.)	56	14.0
(Gerber)	1 can (4.2 oz.)	63	14.3
Orange-apple-banana juice, strained (Gerber)	4-oz. can	58	13.6
Orange-apricot juice, strained (Gerber)	4-oz. can	58	12.9
Orange-banana juice, strained (Beech-Nut)	4⅛ fl. oz. (4.4 oz.)	64	16.1
Orange juice, strained:			
(Beech-Nut)	4⅛ fl. oz. (4.4 oz.)	60	15.0
(Gerber)	4-oz. can	54	12.0
Orange-pineapple dessert, strained (Beech-Nut)	4¾ oz.	100	25.1
Orange-pineapple juice, strained:			
(Beech-Nut)	4⅛ fl. oz. (4.4 oz.)	59	14.0

Food and Description	*Measure or Quantity*	*Calories*	*Carbohydrates (grams)*
(Gerber)	4⅕ fl. oz. (4.2 oz.)	61	14.1
Orange pudding, strained, (Gerber)	4¾ oz.	113	24.0
Pea:			
Junior (Beech-Nut)	7¼ oz.	97	15.2
Strained (Beech-Nut)	4½ oz.	65	15.0
Strained (Beech-Nut) in butter sauce	4½ oz.	78	10.0
Strained (Gerber)	4½ oz.	48	7.0
Pea, split (See Split pea)			
Peach:			
Junior (Beech-Nut)	7¾ oz.	110	26.0
Junior (Gerber)	7¾ oz.	176	41.6
Strained (Beech-Nut)	4¾ oz.	64	16.1
Strained (Gerber)	4¾ oz.	104	24.8
Peach cobbler:			
Junior (Gerber)	7¾ oz.	163	39.9
Strained (Gerber)	4¾ oz.	99	24.2
Peach Melba (Beech-Nut):			
Junior	7¾ oz.	112	28.0
Strained	4¾ oz.	69	17.1
Pear:			
Junior (Beech-Nut)	7½ oz.	96	24.1
Junior (Gerber)	7½ oz.	96	22.1
Strained (Beech-Nut)	4½ oz.	57	14.2
Strained (Gerber)	4½ oz.	55	12.7
Pear & pineapple:			
Junior (Beech-Nut)	7½ oz.	119	30.0
Junior (Gerber)	7½ oz.	98	22.2
Strained (Beech-Nut)	4½ oz.	72	18.2
Strained (Gerber)	4½ oz.	53	11.9
Pineapple dessert, strained (Beech-Nut)	4¾ oz.	100	25.1
Plum with tapioca:			
Junior (Beech-Nut)	7¾ oz.	161	40.3
Junior (Gerber)	7¾ oz.	191	46.0
Strained (Beech-Nut)	4¾ oz.	96	24.0
Strained (Gerber)	4¾ oz.	111	27.3

(USDA): United States Department of Agriculture
(HEW/FAO): Health, Education and Welfare/Food and Agriculture Organization
* Prepared as Package Directs

Food and Description	*Measure or Quantity*	*Calories*	*Carbo-hydrates (grams)*
Pork, strained (Gerber)	3½ oz.	115	.5
Pretzel (Gerber)	1 pretzel (6 grams)	23	4.8
Prune-orange juice, strained:			
(Beech-Nut)	4⅕ fl. oz. (4.4 oz.)	72	18.0
(Gerber)	4⅕ fl. oz. (4.2 oz.)	81	19.1
Prune with tapioca:			
Junior (Beech-Nut)	7¾ oz.	170	40.1
Junior (Gerber)	7¾ oz.	169	40.5
Strained (Beech-Nut)	4¾ oz.	92	22.1
Strained (Gerber)	4¾ oz.	103	24.3
Similac, ready-to-feed	1 fl. oz.	20	1.9
Spaghetti & meat balls, toddler (Gerber)	6¼ oz.	131	20.2
Spaghetti, tomato sauce & beef, junior:			
(Beech-Nut)	7½ oz.	132	19.6
(Gerber)	7½ oz.	140	22.4
Spinach, creamed:			
Junior (Gerber)	7½ oz.	101	12.8
Strained (Gerber)	4½ oz.	53	6.3
Split pea with ham, junior:			
(Beech-Nut)	7½ oz.	138	23.4
(Gerber)	7½ oz.	151	23.9
Squash:			
Junior (Beech-Nut)			
Junior (Beech-Nut) in butter sauce	7½ oz.	41	7.0
Strained (Beech-Nut)	4½ oz.	41	7.0
Strained (Gerber)	4½ oz.	34	6.8
Sweet potato:			
Junior (Beech-Nut)	7¾ oz.	110	23.1
Junior (Gerber)	7¾ oz.	132	29.3
Strained (Beech-Nut)	4½ oz.	72	14.2
Strained (Beech-Nut) in butter sauce	4½ oz.	67	14.2
Strained (Gerber)	4¾ oz.	94	21.5
Teething biscuit (Gerber)	1 piece	42	8.3
Tomato soup, strained (USDA)			
Turkey:			
Junior (Gerber)	3½ oz.	119	.1
Strained (Gerber)	3½ oz.	109	.4

Food and Description	Measure or Quantity	Calories	Carbo-hydrates (grams)
Turkey dinner:			
Junior (Beech-Nut) high meat	4½ oz.	107	8.3
Strained (Beech-Nut) high meat	4½ oz.	107	8.3
With rice:			
Junior (Beech-Nut)	7½ oz.	85	16.4
Strained (Beech-Nut)	4½ oz.	61	11.5
With rice & vegetables (Gerber):			
Junior	7½ oz.	112	14.9
Strained	4½ oz.	66	9.3
With vegetables:			
Junior (Gerber)	4½ oz.	115	6.8
Strained (Gerber)	4½ oz.	115	7.2
Turkey sticks, junior (Gerber)	2½ oz. jar	137	.6
Turkey & turkey broth, strained (Beech-Nut)	4½ oz.	138	.8
Veal:			
Junior (Gerber)	3½ oz.	95	0.
Strained (Gerber)	3½ oz.	89	0.
Veal dinner:			
Junior (Beech-Nut) high meat	4½ oz.	101	7.4
Strained (Beech-Nut) high meat	4½ oz.	101	7.3
With vegetables:			
Junior (Gerber)	4½ oz.	97	8.2
Strained (Gerber)	4½ oz.	91	7.7
Veal & veal broth, strained (Beech-Nut)	4½ oz.	127	.8
Vegetables:			
Strained (Beech-Nut) Garden	4½ oz.	58	11.1
Strained (Gerber) Garden	4½ oz.	37	5.8
Mixed, junior (Beech-Nut)	7½ oz.	77	16.6

(USDA): United States Department of Agriculture
(HEW/FAO): Health, Education and Welfare/Food and Agriculture Organization
* Prepared as Package Directs

Food and Description	Measure or Quantity	Calories	Carbo-hydrates (grams)
Mixed, junior (Gerber)	7½ oz.	80	15.1
Mixed, strained (Gerber)	4½ oz.	53	10.1
Vegetables & bacon:			
Junior (Beech-Nut)	7½ oz.	136	18.3
Junior (Gerber)	7½ oz.	147	16.8
Strained (Beech-Nut)	4½ oz.	82	10.0
Strained (Gerber)	4½ oz.	98	11.4
Vegetables & beef:			
Junior (Beech-Nut)	7½ oz.	115	17.5
Junior (Gerber)	7½ oz.	107	13.8
Strained (Beech-Nut)	4½ oz.	73	10.8
Strained (Gerber)	4½ oz.	59	7.5
Vegetables & chicken:			
Junior (Beech-Nut)	7½ oz.	87	16.0
Junior (Gerber)	7½ oz.	121	19.2
Strained (Beech-Nut)	4½ oz.	54	9.6
Strained (Gerber)	4½ oz.	55	8.3
Vegetable dinner, mixed,			
Strained (Beech-Nut)	4½ oz.	52	11.6
Vegetables & ham:			
Junior (Gerber)	7½ oz.	121	17.3
Strained (Beech-Nut)	4½ oz.	72	10.9
Strained (Gerber)	4½ oz.	66	9.0
Vegetables & lamb:			
Junior (Beech-Nut)	7½ oz.	113	16.6
Junior (Gerber)	7½ oz.	112	15.3
Strained (Beech-Nut)	4½ oz.	68	10.1
Strained (Gerber)	4½ oz.	70	8.7
Vegetables & liver:			
Junior (Beech-Nut)	7½ oz.	89	16.2
Junior (Gerber)	7½ oz.	95	16.6
Strained (Beech-Nut)	4½ oz.	54	9.7
Strained (Gerber)	4½ oz.	51	8.6
Vegetables & turkey:			
Junior (Gerber)	7½ oz.	107	16.8
Strained (Gerber)	4½ oz.	58	8.9
Toddler, casserole	6¼ oz.	148	15.4
BAC ONION (Lawry's)	1 tsp. (4 grams)	14	2.1
BACO NOIR BURGUNDY WINE (Great Western) 12% alcohol	3 fl. oz.	70	2.3

Food and Description	Measure or Quantity	Calories	Carbo- hydrates (grams)
BAC*Os (General Mills)	1 T.	40	2.0
BACON, cured:			
Raw:			
(USDA) slab	1 oz. (weighed with rind)	177	.3
(USDA) sliced	1 oz.	189	.3
(Hormel) *Black Label*	1 piece (.8 oz.)	125	.2
(Hormel) *Range Brand*	1 piece (1.6 oz.)	275	.5
(Wilson)	1 oz.	169	.3
Broiled or fried crisp:			
(USDA):			
Medium slice	1 slice (7.5 grams)	43	.2
Thick slice	1 slice (12 grams)	72	.4
Thin slice	1 slice (5 grams)	30	.2
(Lazy Maple)	3-4 slices (.8 oz.)	140	0.
(Oscar Mayer):			
Medium slice, drained	1 slice (6 grams)	36	.1
Thick slice, drained	1 slice (11 grams)	66	.2
(Swift)	3-4 slices (.8 oz.)	137	.7
Canned (USDA)	1 oz.	194	.3
BACON BITS:			
(Ann Page) imitation	1 tsp. (1.8 grams)	8	.5
(Durkee) imitation	1 tsp. (2 grams)	8	.5
(French's) imitation, crumbles	1 tsp. (2 grams)	6	<.5
(McCormick) imitation	1 tsp. (2 grams)	6	.5
BACON, CANADIAN:			
Unheated (Oscar Mayer)	1-oz. slice	38	.2
Broiled or fried (USDA), drained	1 oz.	79	Tr.
BACON, SIMULATED, cooked			
Sizzlean (Swift)	1 strip (.4 oz.)	50	0.

(USDA): United States Department of Agriculture
(HEW/FAO): Health, Education and Welfare/Food and Agriculture
          Organization
* Prepared as Package Directs

Food and Description	Measure or Quantity	Calories	Carbohydrates (grams)
BAGEL:			
Egg (USDA)	3" dia. (1.9 oz.)	161	28.3
Garlic, onion or poppyseed (Lender's)	2-oz. bagel	161	31.5
Water (USDA)	3" dia. (1.9 oz.)	165	30.0
BAKING POWDER:			
Phosphate (USDA)	1 tsp. (3.8 grams)	5	1.1
SAS (USDA)	1 tsp. (3 grams)	4	.9
Tartrate (USDA)	1 tsp. (2.8 grams)	2	.5
(Calumet)	1 tsp. (3.6 grams)	2	.5
BAKON DELITES (Wise):			
Regular	½-oz. bag	72	0.
Barbecue flavored	½-oz. bag	70	.3
BALSAMPEAR, fresh (HEW/FAO):			
Whole	1 lb. (weighed with cavity contents)	69	16.3
Flesh only	4 oz.	22	5.1
BAMBOO SHOOT:			
Raw (USDA) trimmed	4 oz.	31	5.9
Canned (Chun King) drained	1 cup	64	2.4
BANANA (USDA):			
Common, yellow:			
Fresh:			
Whole	1 lb. (weighed with skin)	262	68.5
Small size	4.9-oz. banana (7¾" x 1¹¹⁄₃₂")	81	21.1
Medium size	6.2-oz. banana (8¾" x 1¹³⁄₃₂")	101	26.4
Large size	7-oz. banana (9¾" x 1⁷⁄₁₆")	116	30.2
Mashed	1 cup (about 2 med.)	191	50.0
Sliced	1 cup (1¼ med.)	128	33.3
Dehydrated flakes	½ cup (1.8 oz.)	170	44.3
Red, fresh, whole	1 lb. (weighed with skin)	278	72.2

Food and Description	Measure or Quantity	Calories	Carbo-hydrates (grams)
BANANA, BAKING (See PLANTAIN)			
BANANA EXTRACT,			
imitation (Ehler's)	1 tsp.	20	
BANANA ICE CREAM			
(Breyer's) red raspberry and strawberry twirl	¼ pt.	150	21.0
BANANA PIE:			
(USDA) cream or custard, home recipe, unenriched or enriched	⅙ of 9″ pie	336	46.7
(Tastykake) cream	4-oz. pie	485	82.4
Frozen:			
(Banquet) cream	⅙ of 14-oz. pie	172	19.9
(Morton) cream	⅙ of 16-oz. pie	174	19.7
(Morton) cream, mini pie	3½-oz. pie	237	25.8
BANANA PIE FILLING,			
canned			
(Comstock) cream	⅙ of 21-oz. can	100	22.1
BANANA PUDDING or PIE FILLING:			
Canned:			
Regular pack (Del Monte)	5-oz. container	183	30.1
Dietetic or low calorie (Sego)	8 oz. container	250	39.0
Frozen (Rich's)	3-oz. container	142	19.3
Mix:			
(Ann Page) regular	¼ of 3½-oz. pkg.	84	21.0
*(Jell-O) regular, cream	⅙ of 8″ pie excluding crust	110	18.0
*(Jell-O) instant, cream	½ cup	180	30.0

(USDA): United States Department of Agriculture
(HEW/FAO): Health, Education and Welfare/Food and Agriculture Organization

* Prepared as Package Directs

Food and Description	Measure or Quantity	Calories	Carbo-hydrates (grams)
*(My-T-Fine) regular, cream	½ cup	175	32.6
*(Royal) regular	½ cup	163	26.4
*(Royal) instant	½ cup	176	28.7
BARBADOS CHERRY (See **ACEROLA**)			
BARBECUE SEASONING (French's)	1 tsp. (2.5 grams)	6	1.0
BARDOLINO WINE, Italian red (Antinori) 12% alcohol	3 fl. oz.	84	6.3
BARLEY, pearled, dry: Light:			
(USDA)	¼ cup (1.8 oz.)	174	39.4
(Quaker-Scotch)	¼ cup (1.7 oz.)	173	37.4
Pot or Scotch (USDA)	2 oz.	197	43.8
BASIL: (HEW/FAO) Sweet, fresh leaves	½ oz.	6	1.0
(French's) dried leaves	1 tsp. (1.1 grams)	3	.7
BASS (USDA): Black Sea: Raw, whole	1 lb. (weighed whole)	165	0.
Baked, stuffed, home recipe	4 oz.	294	12.9
Smallmouth & largemouth, raw: Whole	1 lb. (weighed whole)	146	0.
Meat only	4 oz.	118	0.
Striped: Raw, whole	1 lb. (weighed whole)	205	0.
Raw, meat only	4 oz.	119	0.
Oven-fried	4 oz.	222	7.6
White, raw, meat only	4 oz.	111	0.

Food and Description	Measure or Quantity	Calories	Carbo-hydrates (grams)
BAVARIAN PIE FILLING (Lucky Leaf)	8 oz.	306	51.8
***BAVARIAN PIE** or **PUDDNG MIX,** custard, *Rice-A-Roni*	4 oz.	143	24.6
BAY LEAF (French's)	1 tsp. (1.3 grams)	5	1.0
B AND B LIQUEUR (Julius Wile) 86 proof	1 fl. oz.	94	5.7
B.B.Q. SAUCE & BEEF, frozen (Banquet) sliced, cooking bag	5-oz. bag	126	12.5
BEAN, BAKED: Canned:			
(USDA) with pork & molasses sauce	1 cup (9 oz.)	383	53.8
(USDA) with pork & tomato sauce	1 cup (9 oz.)	311	48.5
(USDA) with tomato sauce	1 cup (9 oz.)	306	58.7
(Ann Page) with pork & molasses sauce, Boston style	½ of 16-oz. can	287	49.8
(Ann Page) with pork & tomato sauce	½ of 16-oz. can	235	41.6
(Ann Page) vegetarian in tomato sauce	½ of 16-oz. can	236	44.1
(B & M) pea bean with pork in brown sugar sauce	8-oz can	336	51.2
(B & M) yellow eye bean in brown sugar sauce	½ of 16-oz. can	360	50.4

(USDA): United States Department of Agriculture
(HEW/FAO): Health, Education and Welfare/Food and Agriculture
 Organization
* Prepared as Package Directs

Food and Description	Measure or Quantity	Calories	Carbo-hydrates (grams)
(B & M) red kidney in brown sugar sauce	½ of 16-oz. can	360	49.6
(Campbell) home style	½ of 16-oz. can	300	52.0
(Campbell) old fashioned in molasses & brown sugar sauce	½ of 16-oz. can	290	49.0
(Campbell) with pork and tomato sauce)	8-oz. can	260	44.0
(Libby's) with pork in molasses sauce	½ of 14-oz can	223	33.6
(Libby's) with pork in tomato sauce	½ of 14-oz. can	217	40.2
(Libby's) vegetarian in tomato sauce	½ of 14-oz. can	211	40.8
(Morton House) with tomato sauce	½ of 16-oz. can	270	45.0
(Sultana) with pork in tomato sauce	½ of 16-oz. can	232	41.8
(Van Camp) with brown sugar sauce	1 cup	350	61.0
(Van Camp) with pork	1 cup	260	47.0
(Van Camp) vegetarian style	1 cup	260	48.0
Frozen (Holloway House)	4 oz.	280	33.0
BEAN, BARBECUE (Campbell)	½ of 15¾-oz. can	277	45.4
BEAN, BAYO, black or brown, dry (USDA)	4 oz.	384	69.4
BEAN & BEEF PATTIES frozen (Swanson)	11-oz. TV dinner	500	16.0
BEAN, CALICO, dry (USDA)	4 oz.	396	72.2
BEAN, CHILI (See CHILI)			
BEAN & FRANKFURTER, canned: (USDA)	1 cup (9 oz.)	367	32.1

Food and Description	Measure or Quantity	Calories	Carbohydrates (grams)
(Campbell) in tomato & molasses sauce	8-oz. can	370	16.0
BEAN & FRANKFURTER DINNER, frozen:			
(Banquet)	10¾-oz. dinner	591	63.1
(Morton)	10¾-oz. dinner	528	79.4
(Swanson)	11½-oz. dinner	550	75.0
BEAN, GREEN or SNAP:			
Fresh (USDA):			
Whole	1 lb. (weighed untrimmed)	128	28.3
French style	½ cup (1.4 oz.)	13	2.8
Boiled, drained, whole (USDA)	½ cup (2.2 oz.)	16	3.3
Boiled, drained, 1½ to 2" pieces (USDA)	½ cup (2.4 oz.)	17	3.7
Canned, regular pack:			
(USDA) solids & liq.	½ cup (4.2 oz.)	22	5.0
(USDA) drained solids, whole	4 oz.	27	5.9
(USDA) drained solids, cut	½ cup (2.5 oz.)	17	3.6
(USDA) drained liquid	4 oz.	11	2.7
(Comstock) cut, drained	½ cup (2.1 oz.)	13	2.4
(Comstock) French-style, drained	½ cup (2.1 oz.)	13	2.4
(Del Monte) cut, solids & liq.	½ cup	21	3.8
(Del Monte) cut, drained solids	½ cup	30	5.3
(Del Monte) French-style, solids & liq.	½ cup	18	3.4
(Del Monte) French-style, drained solids	½ cup	27	4.9
(Del Monte) seasoned, solids & liq.	½ cup	22	4.1

(USDA): United States Department of Agriculture
(HEW/FAO): Health, Education and Welfare/Food and Agriculture
          Organization
* Prepared as Package Directs

Food and Description	Measure or Quantity	Calories	Carbo-hydrates (grams)
(Del Monte) seasoned, drained solids	½ cup	30	5.5
(Del Monte) whole, solids & liq.	½ cup	17	2.9
(Green Giant) whole, cut or French-style, solids & liq.	½ cup	15	3.0
(Libby's) cut, Blue Lake, solids & liq.	½ cup (4.2 oz.)	18	4.1
(Libby's) French-style, Blue Lake, sol. & liq.	½ cup (4.2 oz.)	18	4.2
(Stokely-Van Camp) cut, sliced or whole, solids & liq.	½ cup (4.2 oz.)	20	4.0
Canned, dietetic pack:			
(USDA) solids & liq.	4 oz.	18	4.1
(USDA) drained solids	4 oz.	25	5.4
(Cellu) cut, solids & liq.; low sodium	½ cup	20	5.0
(Diet Delight) solids & liq.	½ cup (4.2 oz.)	17	3.4
(Featherweight) cut, solids & liq.	½ cup	20	5.0
(Tillie Lewis)	½ cup	19	3.6
Frozen:			
(USDA):			
Cut or French-style, unthawed	10-oz. pkg.	74	17.0
Cut or French-style, boiled, drained	½ cup (2.8 oz.)	20	4.6
(Birds Eye):			
Cut, 5-minute	⅓ of 9-oz. pkg.	25	5.0
French-style, 5-minute	⅓ of 9-oz. pkg.	30	6.0
French-style, with sliced mushrooms	⅓ of 9-oz. pkg.	30	6.0
French-style, with toasted almonds	½ of 9-oz. pkg.	52	6.0
With pearl onions	⅓ of 9-oz. pkg.	30	6.0
Whole, deluxe	⅓ of 9-oz. pkg.	25	5.0
(Green Giant):			
Cut, French-style, in butter sauce	½ cup	35	3.5

Food and Description	Measure or Quantity	Calories	Carbo-hydrates (grams)
(Green Giant) with onions & bacon bits	½ cup	40	4.5
BEAN, ITALIAN:			
Canned (Del Monte):			
Solids & liq.	1 cup	57	10.9
Drained solids	½ cup	43	8.2
Frozen (Birds Eye)			
5-Minute	⅓ of 9-oz. pkg.	30	6.0
BEAN, KIDNEY or RED:			
Dry:			
(USDA)	1 lb.	1556	280.8
(USDA)	½ cup (3.3 oz.)	319	57.6
(Sinsheimer)	1 oz.	99	17.6
Cooked (USDA)	½ cup (3.3 oz.)	109	19.8
Canned, regular pack:			
(USDA) solids & liq.	½ cup (4.5 oz.)	115	21.0
(Ann Page)	¼ of 15½-oz. can	104	19.3
(Ann Page) in chili gravy	½ of 15-oz. can	208	33.7
(Van Camp) red	1 cup	230	43.0
(Van Camp) New Orleans-style	1 cup	210	38.0
BEAN, LIMA:			
Raw (USDA):			
Young, whole	1 lb. (weighed in pod)	223	40.1
Mature, dry	½ cup (3.4 oz.)	331	61.4
Young, without shell	1 lb. (weighed shelled)	558	100.2
Boiled, drained (USDA) mature	½ cup (3.4 oz.)	131	24.3
Canned, regular pack:			
(USDA) solids & liq.	½ cup (4.4 oz.)	88	16.6
(USDA) drained solids	½ cup (3 oz.)	81	15.5
(Del Monte) solids & liq.	½ cup	76	4.1

(USDA): United States Department of Agriculture
(HEW/FAO): Health, Education and Welfare/Food and Agriculture Organization
* Prepared as Package Directs

Food and Description	Measure or Quantity	Calories	Carbohydrates (grams)
(Del Monte) drained solids	½ cup (3.1 oz.)	89	17.0
(Libby's) solids & liq.	½ cup (4.3 oz.)	86	15.9
(Stokely-Van Camp) green, solids & liq.	½ cup (4.4 oz.)	90	16.5
(Sultana) baby, solids & liq.	¼ of 15-oz. can	93	17.0
(Sultana) butter bean, solids & liq.	¼ of 15-oz. can	82	14.6
Canned, dietetic pack:			
(USDA) solids & liq., low sodium	4 oz.	79	14.6
(USDA) drained solids, low sodium	4 oz.	108	20.1
(Featherweight) solids & liq.	½ cup	73	16.0
Frozen:			
(USDA):			
Baby, unthawed	4 oz.	138	26.1
Fordhooks, unthawed	4 oz.	112	21.7
Boiled, drained solids	½ cup (3.1 oz.)	106	20.0
Fordhooks, boiled, drained	½ cup (3 oz.)	83	16.0
(Birds Eye):			
Baby butter	½ of 10-oz. pkg.	130	24.0
Baby, 5-minute	⅓ of pkg.	120	22.0
Fordhooks, 5-minute	⅓ pkg.	100	18.0
Tiny deluxe	⅓ of 10-oz. pkg.	120	20.0
(Green Giant) in butter sauce, Boil-in-Bag	½ cup	110	16.0
BEAN, MUNG, dry (USDA)	½ cup (3.7 oz.)	357	63.3
BEAN, PINTO, dry:			
(USDA)	½ cup (3.4 oz.)	335	61.2
(Sinsheimer)	4 oz.	397	70.3
BEAN, RED (See **BEAN, KIDNEY** or **BEAN, RED MEXICAN**)			
BEAN, RED MEXICAN:			
	4 oz.	396	72.2

Food and Description	Measure or Quantity	Calories	Carbo-hydrates (grams)
Canned (Green Giant) solids & liq.	¼ of 15½-oz. can	97	17.5
BEAN, REFRIED, canned (Ortega)	½ cup (4.8 oz.)	170	25.0
BEAN SALAD, MIXED, canned (Green Giant)	1 cup	190	42.0
BEAN SOUP, canned:			
(USDA) with pork, condensed	8 oz. (by wt.)	304	39.3
*(USDA) with pork, prepared with equal volume water	1 cup (8.8 oz.)	168	21.8
*(Ann Page) with bacon	1 cup	141	19.0
(Campbell) *Chunky* with ham	11-oz. can	300	35.0
*(Campbell) condensed with bacon	10-oz. serving	100	12.0
(Campbell) *Soup For One,* old fashioned	7¾-oz. can	210	28
BEAN SOUP, BLACK, canned:			
*(Campbell) condensed (Crosse & Blackwell)	10-oz. serving 6½-oz. (½ can)	96	15.5
BEAN SOUP, LIMA, canned (Manischewitz)	8 oz. (by wt.)	93	15.3
BEAN SOUP, NAVY, dehydrated (USDA)	1 oz.	93	17.8
BEAN SPROUT:			
Mung (USDA):			
Raw	½ lb.	80	15.0
Raw	½ cup (1.4 oz.)	19	3.5
Boiled, drained	½ cup (2.2 oz.)	17	3.2

(USDA): United States Department of Agriculture
(HEW/FAO): Health, Education and Welfare/Food and Agriculture
        Organization
* Prepared as Package Directs

Food and Description	Measure or Quantity	Calories	Carbo-hydrates (grams)
Soy (USDA):			
Raw	½ lb.	104	12.0
Raw	½ cup (1.9 oz.)	25	2.9
Boiled, drained	4 oz.	43	4.2
Canned (Chun King)	1 cup	39	2.5
BEAN, WAX (See BEAN, YELLOW)			
BEAN, WHITE:			
Raw:			
(USDA) Great Northern	½ cup (3.1 oz.)	303	54.6
(USDA) navy or pea	½ cup (3.7 oz.)	354	63.8
(USDA) white	1 oz.	96	17.4
(Sinsheimer) navy or pea	1 oz.	99	17.6
Cooked:			
(USDA) Great Northern	½ cup (3 oz.)	100	18.0
(USDA) navy or pea	½ cup (3.4 oz.)	113	20.4
(USDA) all other white	4 oz.	134	24.0
BEAN, YELLOW or WAX:			
Raw, whole (USDA)	1 lb. (weighed untrimmed)	108	24.0
Boiled, drained, 1″ pieces (USDA)	½ cup (2.9 oz.)	18	3.7
Canned, regular pack:			
(USDA) solids & liq.	½ cup (4.2 oz.)	23	5.0
(USDA) drained solids	½ cup (2.2 oz.)	15	3.2
(USDA) drained liq.	4 oz.	12	2.8
(Del Monte) cut, solids & liq.	½ cup (4 oz.)	19	3.4
(Del Monte) French-style, solids & liq.	½ cup (4 oz.)	10	1.8
(Libby's) solids & liq.	½ of 8-oz. can	21	4.4
(Stokely-Van Camp) cut, solids & liq.	½ cup (4.3 oz.)	23	4.0
Canned, dietetic pack:			
(USDA) solids & liq.	4 oz.	17	3.9
(USDA) drained solids	4 oz.	24	5.3
(Blue Boy) solids & liq.	4 oz.	24	5.0
(Cellu) cut, solids & liq., low sodium	½ cup	20	5.0
(Featherweight), cut, solids & liq.	½ cup	20	5.0

Food and Description	Measure or Quantity	Calories	Carbo-hydrates (grams)
Frozen:			
(USDA) cut, unthawed	4 oz.	32	7.4
(USDA) boiled, drained	4 oz.	31	7.0
(Birds Eye) cut, 5-minute	⅛ of 9-oz. pkg.	30	4.0
BEAUJOLAIS WINE, French Burgundy, (Barton & Guestier) St. Louis, 11% alcohol	3 fl. oz.	60	.1
BEAUNE WINE:			
Clos de Feves, French Burgundy, (Chanson) 12% alcohol	3 fl. oz.	84	6.3
St. Vincent, French Burgundy (Chanson) 12% alcohol	3 fl. oz.	84	6.3
BEAVER, roasted (USDA)	4 oz.	281	0.
BEECHNUT (USDA):			
Whole	4 oz. (weighed in shell)	393	14.0
Shelled	4 oz. (weighed shelled)	644	23.0

BEEF. Values for beef cuts are given below for "lean and fat" and for "lean only." Beef purchased by the consumer at the retail store usually is trimmed to about one-half inch layer of fat. This is the meat described as "lean and fat." If all the fat that can be cut off with a knife is removed, the remainder is the "lean only."

(USDA): United States Department of Agriculture
(HEW/FAO): Health, Education and Welfare/Food and Agriculture Organization
* Prepared as Package Directs

Food and Description	Measure or Quantity	Calories	Carbo-hydrates (grams)
These cuts still contain flecks of fat known as "marbling" distributed through the meat. Cooked meats are medium done. Choice grade cuts (USDA):			
Brisket:			
Raw	1 lb. (weighed with bone)	1284	0.
Braised:			
Lean & fat	4 oz.	467	0.
Lean only	4 oz.	252	0.
Chuck:			
Raw	1 lb. (weighed with bone)	984	0.
Braised or pot-roasted:			
Lean & fat	4 oz.	371	0.
Lean only	4 oz.	243	0.
Dried (See BEEF CHIPPED)			
Fat, separable, cooked	1 oz.	207	0.
Filet mignon. There are no data available on its composition. For dietary estimates, the data for sirloin steak, lean only, afford the closest approximation.			
Flank:			
Raw	1 lb.	653	0.
Braised	4 oz.	222	0.
Foreshank:			
Raw	1 lb. (weighed with bone)	531	0.
Simmered:			
Lean & fat	4 oz.	310	0.
Lean only	4 oz.	209	0.
Ground:			
Lean:			
Raw	1 lb.	812	0.
Raw	1 cup (8 oz.)	405	0.
Broiled	4 oz.	248	0.

Food and Description	Measure or Quantity	Calories	Carbo- hydrates (grams)
Regular:			
Raw	1 lb.	1216	0.
Raw	1 cup (8 oz.)	606	0.
Broiled	4 oz.	324	0.
Heel of round:			
Raw	1 lb.	966	0.
Roasted:			
Lean & fat	4 oz.	296	0.
Lean only	4 oz.	204	0.
Hindshank:			
Raw	1 lb. (weighed with bone)	604	0.
Simmered:			
Lean & fat	4 oz.	409	0.
Lean only	4 oz.	209	0.
Neck:			
Raw	1 lb. (weighed with bone)	820	0.
Pot-roasted:			
Lean & fat	4 oz.	332	0.
Lean only	4 oz.	222	0.
Plate:			
Raw	1 lb. (weighed with bone)	1615	0.
Simmered:			
Lean & fat	4 oz.	538	0.
Lean only	4 oz.	252	0.
Rib roast:			
Raw	1 lb. (weighed with bone)	1673	0.
Roasted:			
Lean & fat	4 oz.	499	0.
Lean only	4 oz.	273	0.
Round:			
Raw	1 lb. (weighed with bone)	863	0.

(USDA): United States Department of Agriculture
(HEW/FAO): Health, Education and Welfare/Food and Agriculture Organization
* Prepared as Package Directs

Food and Description	Measure or Quantity	Calories	Carbo-hydrates (grams)
Broiled:			
Lean & fat	4 oz.	296	0.
Lean only	4 oz.	214	0.
Rump:			
Raw	1 lb. (weighed with bone)	1167	0.
Roasted:			
Lean & fat	4 oz.	393	0.
Lean only	4 oz.	236	0.
Steak, club:			
Raw	1 lb. (weighed without bone)	1724	0.
Broiled:			
Lean & fat	4 oz.	515	0.
Lean only	4 oz.	277	0.
One 8-oz. steak (weighed without bone before cooking) will give you:			
Lean & fat	5.9 oz.	754	0.
Lean only	3.4 oz.	234	0.
Steak, porterhouse:			
Raw	1 lb. (weighed with bone)	1603	0.
Broiled:			
Lean & fat	4 oz.	527	0.
Lean only	4 oz.	254	0.
One 16-oz. steak (weighed with bone before cooking) will give you:			
Lean & fat	10. 2 oz.	1339	0.
Lean only	5.9 oz.	372	0.
Steak, ribeye, broiled:			
One 10-oz. steak (weighed before cooking without bone) will give you:			
Lean & fat	7.3 oz.	911	0.
Lean only	3.8 oz.	258	0.
Steak, sirloin, double-bone:			
Raw	1 lb. (weighed with bone)	1240	0.

Food and Description	Measure or Quantity	Calories	Carbo- hydrates (grams)
Broiled:			
Lean & fat	4 oz.	463	0.
Lean only	4 oz.	245	0.
One 16-oz. steak (weighed before cooking with bone) will give you:			
Lean & fat	8.9 oz.	1028	0.
Lean only	5.9 oz.	359	0.
One 12-oz. steak (weighed before cooking with bone) will give you:			
Lean & fat	6.6 oz.	767	0.
Lean only	4.4 oz.	268	0.
Steak, sirloin, hipbone:			
Raw	1 lb. (weighed with bone)	1585	0.
Broiled:			
Lean & fat	4 oz.	552	0.
Lean only	4 oz.	272	0.
Steak, sirloin, wedge & round-bone:			
Raw	1 lb. (weighed with bone)	1316	0.
Broiled:			
Lean & fat	4 oz.	439	0.
Lean only	4 oz.	235	0.
Steak, T-bone:			
Raw	1 lb. (weighed with bone)	1596	0.
Broiled:			
Lean & fat	4 oz.	536	0.
Lean only	4 oz.	253	0.
One 16 oz. steak (weighed before cooking with bone) will give you:			

(USDA): United States Department of Agriculture
(HEW/FAO): Health, Education and Welfare/Food and Agriculture
　　　　　Organization
* Prepared as Package Directs

Food and Description	Measure or Quantity	Calories	Carbo-hydrates (grams)
Lean & fat	9.8 oz.	1315	0.
Lean only	5.5 oz.	348	0.
BEEFAMATO COCKTAIL			
(Mott's)	½ cup	49	10.7
BEEFARONI, canned			
(Chef-Boy-Ar-Dee)	⅛ of 40-oz. can	206	27.9
BEEF & BEEF STOCK			
(Bunker Hill)	15-oz. can	920	0.
BEEF BOUILLON, cubes or powder:			
(Croyden House)	1 tsp. (5 grams)	12	2.2
(Herb-Ox)	1 cube (4 grams)	6	.5
(Herb-Ox)	1 packet (4 grams)	8	.8
(Maggi)	1 cube (3.5 grams)	6	0.
MBT	1 packet (5.5 grams)	14	2.0
(Steero)	1 cube	6	.5
(Wyler's)	1 envelope (5 grams)	11	1.4
(Wyler's) no salt	1 cube (4 grams)	10	1.6
BEEF BROTH:			
Canned:			
*(Campbell) condensed	10-oz. serving	35	3.0
(College Inn)	1 cup	19	5.2
(Swanson)	½ of 13¾-oz. can	20	1.0
Mix (Weight Watchers)	.2-oz. packet	10	1.0
BEEF, CHIPPED:			
Uncooked:			
(USDA)	½ cup (2.9 oz.)	166	0.
(Armour Star)	1 oz.	48	0.
Cooked, creamed, home recipe (USDA)	½ cup (4.3 oz.)	188	8.7
Frozen, creamed (Banquet)	5 oz.	124	10.5
(Armour Star)	12-oz. can	1042	4.4
(Hormel)	12-oz. can	867	2.0
BEEF, CORNED (See CORNED BEEF)			

Food and Description	Measure or Quantity	Calories	Carbo-hydrates (grams)
BEEF DINNER, frozen:			
(Banquet)	11-oz. dinner	312	20.9
(Banquet) chopped	11-oz. dinner	443	32.8
(Morton)	10-oz. dinner	261	20.0
(Morton) chopped	11-oz. dinner	334	18.9
(Morton) chopped sirloin, *Steak House*	9½-oz. dinner	748	43.2
(Morton) rib eye, *Steak House*	9-oz. dinner	816	38.4
(Morton) sirloin strip, *Steak House*	9½-oz. dinner	923	48.9
(Morton) sliced, *Country Table*	14-oz. dinner	545	63.7
(Morton) tenderloin, *Steak House*	9½-oz. dinner	907	45.9
(Swanson)	11½-oz. TV dinner	370	34.0
(Swanson) chopped, *Hungry Man*	18-oz. dinner	730	70.0
(Swanson) sliced, *Hungry Man*	17-oz. dinner	540	51.0
(Swanson) 3-course	15-oz. dinner	490	58.0
(Weight Watchers) beefsteak with peppers & mushrooms	10-oz. meal	387	11.1
(Weight Watchers) sirloin, 3-compartment	16-oz. meal	516	10.0
BEEF, DRIED (Swift)	¾-oz. serving	35	0.
BEEF ENTREE, frozen (Swanson):			
Sliced with gravy & whipped potatoes	8-oz. entree	190	23.0
Sliced, *Hungry Man*	12¼-oz. entree	330	23.0
BEEF GOULASH:			
Canned (Bounty)	7½-oz. can	203	16.3
Seasoning mix (Lawry's)	1 pkg. (1.7 oz.)	127	24.1

(USDA): United States Department of Agriculture
(HEW/FAO): Health, Education and Welfare/Food and Agriculture
          Organization
* Prepared as Package Directs

Food and Description	Measure or Quantity	Calories	Carbo-hydrates (grams)
BEEF GROUND (See BEEF, Ground)			
BEEF, GROUND, SEASONING MIX:			
(Durkee)	1.1-oz. pkg.	91	18.0
*(Durkee)	1 cup	654	9.0
(Durkee) with onion	1.1-oz. pkg.	102	13.0
*(Durkee) with onion	1 cup	659	6.5
(French's) with onion	1⅛-oz. pkg.	100	24.0
BEEF HASH, ROAST:			
Canned (Hormel)	7½-oz.	390	9.0
Frozen (Stouffer's)	11½-oz. pkg.	460	21.7
BEEF JERKY (Lowrey's)	¼-oz. piece	24	<.1
BEEF PIE:			
Home recipe, baked (USDA)	4¼″ pie (8 oz. before baking)	558	42.7
Frozen:			
(Banquet)	8-oz. pie	409	40.9
(Morton)	8-oz. pie	316	31.8
(Swanson)	8-oz. pie	430	43.0
(Swanson) *Hungry Man*	16-oz. pie	770	65.0
(Swanson) *Hungry Man,* sirloin burger	16-oz. pie	800	55.0
BEEF, POTTED (USDA)	1 oz.	70	0.
BEEF PUFFS, frozen (Durkee)	1 piece	47	3.0
BEEF ROAST, canned:			
(USDA)	4 oz.	254	0.
(Wilson) *Tender Made*	4 oz.	134	0.
BEEF, SLICED, with barbecue sauce (Banquet)	5-oz. bag	152	13.0
BEEF SOUP Canned:			
(USDA) bouillon, condensed	8 oz. (by weight)		

Food and Description	Measure or Quantity	Calories	Carbo-hydrates (grams)
*(USDA) bouillon, prepared with equal volume water	1 cup (8.5 oz.)	31	2.6
(USDA) consomme, condensed	8 oz. (by wt.)	59	5.0
*(USDA) consomme, condensed, prepared with equal volume water	1 cup (8.5 oz.)	31	2.6
(USDA) & noodle, condensed	8 oz. (by wt.)	129	13.2
*(USDA) & noodle, condensed, prepared with equal volume water	1 cup (8.5 oz.)	67	7.0
*(Ann Page) & vegetable	1 cup	71	9.5
(Campbell) *Chunky*	10¾-oz. can	220	22.0
(Campbell) *Chunky,* low sodium	7½-oz. can	170	16.0
(Campbell) *Chunky* sirloin burger	10¾-oz. can	230	24.0
*(Campbell) condensed	8-oz. serving	80	11.2
*(Campbell) consomme, condensed, gelatin added	8-oz. serving	36	3.2
*(Campbell) & noodle, condensed	8-oz. serving	72	8.0
*(Campbell) & noodle with ground beef, condensed	8-oz. serving	88	11.2
*(Manischewitz) barley	1 cup (8 oz. by wt.)	83	11.2
*(Manischewitz) noodle	1 cup (8 oz.)	64	8.0
Dietetic (Dia-Mel) & noodle	8-oz. serving	70	5.0
Mix:			
*(USDA)	1 cup (8.1 oz.)	64	11.0
*(Lipton) & noodle, *Cup-a-Soup*	6 fl. oz.	35	6.0

(USDA): United States Department of Agriculture
(HEW/FAO): Health, Education and Welfare/Food and Agriculture
           Organization
* Prepared as Package Directs

Food and Description	Measure or Quantity	Calories	Carbo-hydrates (grams)
*(Nestlé) *Souptime*	6 fl. oz.	30	4.0
*(Wyler's) & noodle	6 fl. oz.	37	7.0
*BEEF STEAK, freeze dry (Wilson)	4 oz.	199	0.
BEEF STEW:			
Home recipe (USDA)			
Canned, regular pack:			
(USDA)	15-oz. can	336	30.2
(Armour Star)	24-oz. can	590	38.8
(Bounty)	7½-oz. can	185	19.2
(Hormel) *Dinty Moore*	8 oz.	190	13.6
(Libby's)	8 oz.	154	15.2
(Morton House)	⅓ of 24-oz. can	240	17.0
(Swanson)	½ of 15¼-oz. can	192	18.2
Canned, dietetic or low calorie:			
(Dia-Mel)	8-oz. can	200	19.0
(Featherweight)	7¼-oz. can	210	24.0
*Freeze dry (Wilson)	8 oz.	268	17.9
Frozen:			
(Banquet) buffet	2-lb. pkg.	700	90.9
(Green Giant) & biscuits, *Bake n' Serve*	7-oz. pkg.	190	21.0
BEEF STEW SEASONING MIX:			
(Durkee)	1.8-oz. pkg.	99	22.0
*(Durkee)	1 cup	379	16.8
(Lawry's)	1¾-oz. pkg.	131	24.2
BEEF STOCK BASE			
(French's)	1 tsp. (4 grams)	8	2.0
BEEF STROGANOFF:			
Canned (Hormel)	1 lb. can	645	9.5
Mix (Chef-Boy-Ar-Dee)	6⅔-oz. pkg.	232	30.6
Seasoning mix (Durkee)	1¼-oz. pkg.	90	18.0
BEER, canned:			
Regular:			
Black Horse Ale, 5% alcohol	12 fl. oz. (12.7 oz.)	162	13.8

Food and Description	Measure or Quantity	Calories	Carbo-hydrates (grams)
Black Label, 4.9% alcohol	12 fl. oz.	140	11.3
Buckeye, 4.6% alcohol	12 fl. oz.	144	11.0
Budweiser, 4.9% alcohol	12 fl. oz.	156	12.3
Budweiser, 3.9% alcohol	12 fl. oz.	137	11.9
Busch Bavarian:			
4.9% alcohol	12 fl. oz.	156	12.3
3.9% alcohol	12 fl. oz.	137	11.9
Eastside Lager	12 fl. oz.	145	
Hamm's	12 fl. oz.	151	13.3
Heidelberg, 4.6% alcohol	12 fl. oz.	133	10.7
Knickerbocker, 4.6% alcohol	12 fl. oz.	160	13.7
Meister Brau Premium, 4.6% alcohol	12 fl. oz.	144	11.0
Meister Brau Premium Draft, 4.6% alcohol	12 fl. oz.	144	11.0
Michelob, 4.9% alcohol	12 fl. oz.	160	12.8
Narraganset, 4.7% alcohol	12 fl. oz.	155	14.4
North Star, regular, 4.8% alcohol	12 fl. oz.	165	14.9
North Star, 3.2 low gravity	12 fl. oz.	142	13.6
Old Milwaukee	12 fl. oz.	145	13.7
Pabst Blue Ribbon	12 fl. oz.	150	
Pfeifer, regular, 4.8% alcohol	12 fl. oz.	165	14.9
Pfeifer, 3.2 low gravity	12 fl. oz.	141	13.6
Red Cap Ale, 5.6% alcohol	12 fl. oz.	153	10.8
Rheingold, 4.6% alcohol	12 fl. oz.	160	13.7
Schlitz, 4.8% alcohol	12 fl. oz.	157	13.6
Schmidt, regular or extra special, 4.8% alcohol	12 fl. oz.	165	14.9
Schmidt, 3.2 low gravity	12 fl. oz. (12.7 oz.)	142	13.6
Tuborg USA, 4.8% alcohol	12 fl. oz.	140	12.1
Yuengling Premium	12 fl. oz.	144	15.1
Low carbohydrate:			
Dia-beer	12 fl. oz.	145	4.2
Dia-beer	7 fl. oz.	85	2.8

(USDA): United States Department of Agriculture
(HEW/FAO): Health, Education and Welfare/Food and Agriculture Organization
* Prepared as Package Directs

Food and Description	Measure or Quantity	Calories	Carbo-hydrates (grams)
Gablinger's, 4.5% alcohol	12 fl. oz.	99	.2
Meister Brau Lite, 4.6% alcohol	12 fl. oz.	96	1.4
Schlitz Light	12 fl. oz.	97	5.1
BEER, NEAR:			
Kingsbury, 0.4% alcohol	12 fl. oz.	62	15.0
Metbrew, 0.4% alcohol	12 fl. oz.	73	13.7
BEET:			
Raw (USDA)	1 lb. (weighed with skins, without tops)	137	31.4
Raw, diced (USDA)	½ cup (2.4 oz.)	29	6.6
Boiled, drained (USDA):			
Whole	2 beets (2″ dia., 3.5 oz.)	31	7.2
Diced	½ cup (3 oz.)	27	6.1
Slices	½ cup (3.6 oz.)	33	7.3
Canned, regular pack:			
(USDA) solids & liq.	½ cup (4.3 oz.)	42	9.7
(USDA) whole, drained solids	½ cup (2.8 oz.)	30	7.0
(USDA) diced, drained solids	½ cup (2.9 oz.)	30	7.2
(USDA) sliced, drained solids	½ cup (3.1 oz.)	33	7.7
(Del Monte) pickled, sliced, solids & liq.	½ cup	77	18.1
(Del Monte) pickled, sliced, drained solids	½ cup	81	18.9
(Del Monte) sliced, solids & liq.	½ cup	29	7.0
(Del Monte) sliced, drained solids	½ cup	36	3.6
(Del Monte) whole, tiny, solids & liq.	½ cup	42	9.1
(Libby's) Harvard, diced, solids & liq.	½ cup (4.2 oz.)	84	19.8
(Libby's) pickled, sliced, solids & liq.	¼ of 16-oz. jar	74	18.5
(Stokely-Van Camp) Harvard, solids & liq.	½ cup (4.5 oz.)	80	18.0

Food and Description	Measure or Quantity	Calories	Carbo-hydrates (grams)
(Stokely-Van Camp) pickled, solids & liq.	½ cup (4.3 oz.)	95	22.5
(Stokely-Van Camp) whole, solids & liq.	½ cup (4.3 oz.)	45	10.0
Canned, dietetic pack:			
(USDA) solids & liq.	4 oz.	36	8.8
(USDA) drained solids	4 oz.	42	9.9
(Cellu) sliced, solids & liq., low sodium	½ cup	40	10.0
(Featherweight) sliced, solids & liq.	½ cup	40	10.0
(Tillie Lewis)	½ cup (4.3 oz.)	39	8.6
BEET GREENS (USDA)			
Raw, whole	1 lb. (weighed untrimmed	61	11.7
Boiled, leaves & stems, drained	½ cup (2.6 oz.)	13	2.4
BENEDICTINE LIQUEUR			
(Julius Wile) 86 proof	1 fl. oz.	112	10.3
BERRY PIE (Hostess)	4½-oz. pie	404	51.1
BEVERAGE (See individual listings)			
BIG MAC (See **McDONALD'S**)			
BIG WHEEL (Hostess)	1.3-oz. cake	175	21.5
BISCUIT:			
Home recipe (USDA) baking powder	1-oz. biscuit (2" dia.)	103	12.8

(USDA): United States Department of Agriculture
(HEW/FAO): Health, Education and Welfare/Food and Agriculture Organization
* Prepared as Package Directs

Food and Description	Measure or Quantity	Calories	Carbo-hydrates (grams)
(Stella D'oro) egg:			
Regular	1 piece (.4 oz.)	42	6.9
Dietetic	1 piece (.4 oz.)	42	6.6
BISCUIT DOUGH, refrigerated:			
(Borden):			
Big 10's	1 biscuit (.9 oz.)	82	11.2
Buttered Up	1 biscuit (.9 oz.)	90	11.8
Gem	1 biscuit (.9 oz.)	82	11.2
(Pillsbury):			
Ballard, Oven-Ready	1 biscuit	60	11.0
Buttermilk	1 biscuit	105	10.5
Buttermilk, extra light	1 biscuit	60	10.5
Cornbread	1 biscuit	95	12.5
Country-style	1 biscuit	55	10.5
1869 Brand, baking powder	1 biscuit	100	12.0
1869 Brand, pre-baked	1 biscuit	100	12.0
Hungry Jack, buttermilk or regular	1 biscuit	90	11.5
Hungry Jack, buttermilk, extra light	1 biscuit	60	10.5
BISCUIT MIX:			
(USDA) dry, with enriched flour	1 oz.	120	19.5
*(USDA) baked from mix, with added milk	1-oz. biscuit	91	14.6
BI-SICLE (Popsicle Industries)	2½ fl. oz.	112	21.4
BITTER LEMON (See SOFT DRINKS)			
BITTERS (Angostura)	½ tsp. (5 grams)	7	1.0
BLACKBERRY:			
Fresh (includes boysenberry, dewberry, youngsberry):			
With hulls (USDA)	1 lb. (weighed untrimmed)	250	55.6
Hulled (USDA)	½ cup (2.6 oz.)	41	9.4

Food and Description	Measure or Quantity	Calories	Carbohydrates (grams)
Canned, regular pack, solids & liq. (USDA):			
Juice pack	4 oz.	61	13.7
Light syrup	4 oz.	82	19.6
Heavy syrup	½ cup (4.6 oz.)	118	28.9
Extra heavy syrup	4 oz.	125	30.7
Canned, low calorie, solids & liq. (S and W) *Nutradiet*	4 oz.	50	11.2
Frozen (USDA):			
Sweetened, unthawed	4 oz.	109	27.7
Unsweetened, unthawed	4 oz.	55	12.9
BLACKBERRY BRANDY			
(DeKuyper) 70 proof	1 fl. oz. (1.1 oz.)	85	6.9
BLACKBERRY JELLY:			
Sweetened (Smucker's)	1 T. (.7 oz.)	53	13.5
Dietetic (Featherweight)	1 T.	16	4.0
BLACKBERRY LIQUEUR:			
(Bols) 60 proof	1 fl. oz.	96	8.9
(Hiram Walker) 60 proof	1 fl. oz.	100	12.8
BLACKBERRY PIE:			
Home recipe (USDA)	⅙ of 9″ pie (5.6 oz.)	384	54.4
(Tastykake)	4-oz. pie	386	60.0
Frozen (Banquet)	4-oz. serving	376	55.5
BLACKBERRY PIE FILLING:			
(Comstock)	1 cup (10¾-oz.)	438	108.5
(Lucky Leaf)	8 oz.	258	62.4
BLACKBERRY PRESERVE or JAM:			
Sweetened (Smucker's)	1 T. (.7 oz.)	54	13.7

(USDA): United States Department of Agriculture
(HEW/FAO): Health, Education and Welfare/Food and Agriculture
         Organization
❂ Prepared as Package Directs

Food and Description	Measure or Quantity	Calories	Carbo-hydrates (grams)
Dietetic:			
(Diet Delight)	1 T. (.6 oz.)	14	3.4
(Featherweight)	1 T.	16	4.0
BLACKBERRY SOUR COCKTAIL, liquid mix (Holland House)	1½ fl. oz.	75	18.0
BLACKBERRY SYRUP (Smucker's)	1 T. (.6 oz.)	45	11.6
BLACKBERRY WINE (Mogen David) 12% alcohol	3 fl. oz.	135	18.7
BLACK-EYED PEA (See also COWPEA):			
Boiled, drained (USDA)	½ cup (3 oz.)	111	20.1
Canned (Sultana) with pork	½ of 15-oz. can	204	33.9
Frozen:			
(Birds Eye)	⅛ of 10-oz. pkg.	120	21.0
(Green Giant)	½ cup	140	16.0
BLACK RUSSIAN COCKTAIL, liquid mix (Holland House)	1½ fl. oz.	138	34.5
BLANCMANGE (See VANILLA PUDDING)			
BLOOD PUDDING or SAUSAGE (USDA)	1 oz.	112	.1
BLOODY MARY MIX:			
Dry (Holland House)	1 serving (.5 oz.)	56	14.0
Liquid mix (Sacramento)	5½-fl.-oz. can	39	9.1
BLUEBERRY:			
Fresh (USDA):			
Whole	1 lb. (weighed untrimmed)	259	63.8
Trimmed	½ cup (2.6 oz.)	45	11.2
Canned, regular pack, solids & liq. (USDA)			
Syrup pack, extra heavy	½ cup (4.4 oz.)	126	32.5

Food and Description	Measure or Quantity	Calories	Carbo-hydrates (grams)
Water pack	½ cup (4.3 oz.)	47	11.9
Canned, dietetic pack (Featherweight) water pack, solids & liq.	½ cup	41	10.7
Frozen: (USDA)			
Sweetened, solids & liq.	½ cup (4 oz.)	120	30.2
Unsweetened, solids & liq.	½ cup (2.9 oz.)	45	11.2
BLUEBERRY PIE:			
(USDA) home recipe	⅛ of 9″ pie (5.6 oz.)	382	55.1
(Hostess)	4½-oz. pie	394	49.9
Frozen:			
(Banquet)	⅛ of 20-oz. pie	253	37.5
(Morton)	⅛ of 24-oz. pie	286	38.6
(Morton) mini pie	½ of 8-oz. pie	294	43.2
Tart (Pepperidge Farm)	3-oz. tart	277	34.5
BLUEBERRY PIE FILLING			
(Wilderness)	¼ of 32-oz. can	275	65.8
BLUEBERRY PRESERVE or JAM:			
Sweetened (Smucker's)	1 T.	52	13.7
Dietetic (Featherweight)	1 T.	16	4.0
BLUEBERRY SYRUP:			
Sweetened (Smucker's)	1 T. (.6 oz.)	45	11.6
Dietetic (Featherweight)	1 T.	14	3.0
BLUEBERRY TURNOVER			
frozen (Pepperidge Farm)	1 turnover (3.3 oz.)	321	32.0
BLUEFISH (USDA):			
Raw:			
Whole	1 lb. (weighed whole)	271	0.

(USDA): United States Department of Agriculture
(HEW/FAO): Health, Education and Welfare/Food and Agriculture Organization
⊕ Prepared as Package Directs

Food and Description	Measure or Quantity	Calories	Carbo-hydrates (grams)
Meat only	4 oz.	133	0.
Baked or broiled	4.4-oz. piece (3½″ x 3″ x ½″)	199	0.
Fried	5.3-oz. piece (3½″ x 3″ x ½″)	308	7.0
BOLOGNA:			
(Armour Star) all meat	1 oz.	99	0.
(Hormel):			
All meat	1 oz.	85	.5
Coarse ground	1 oz.	75	.9
(Oscar Mayer):			
Beef	.8-oz. slice	73	.7
Thin	1 slice	16	.4
(Swift)	1 slice (1 oz.)	95	1.5
(Wilson)	1 oz.	87	.5
BONITO:			
Raw (USDA):			
Whole	1 lb. (weighed whole)	442	0.
Meat only	4 oz.	191	0.
Canned (Star-Kist) chunk, in oil	6½-oz. can	590	0.
BOO*BERRY cereal	1 cup (1 oz.)	110	24.0
BORDEAUX WINE (See also individual regional, vineyard or brand names or **CLARET WINE**):			
Rouge (Cruse) 10½ alcohol	3 fl. oz.	63	
BORSCHT:			
(Manischewitz)	8 oz. (by wt.)	72	17.5
Egg (Mother's)	8 fl. oz.	48	
BOSCO (Best Foods)	1 T. (.7 oz.)	56	12.7
*BOSTON CREAM PIE, mix (Betty Crocker)	⅛ of pie	270	48.0
BOUILLON CUBE (See individual flavors)			

Food and Description	Measure or Quantity	Calories	Carbo-hydrates (grams)
BOURBON WHISKY, unflavored (See **DISTILLED LIQUOR**)			
BOYSENBERRY:			
Fresh (See **BLACKBERRY**)			
Canned, dietetic (S and W)			
Nutradiet	4 oz.	36	9.8
Frozen, sweetened (USDA)	10-oz. pkg.	273	69.3
BOYSENBERRY JELLY (Smucker's)	1 T. (.7 oz.)	54	13.7
BOYSENBERRY PIE, frozen (Banquet)	5-oz. serving	374	55.8
BOYSENBERRY PRESERVE or **JAM:**			
Sweetened (Smucker's)	1 T. (.7 oz.)	54	13.7
Dietetic or low calorie:			
(S and W)	1 T. (.5 oz.)	11	2.5
(Slenderella)	1 T. (.7 oz.)	25	6.4
BRAINS, all animals, raw (USDA)	4 oz.	142	.9
BRAN, crude (USDA)	1 oz.	60	17.5
BRAN BREAKFAST CEREAL:			
(Kellogg's):			
All-Bran	½ cup (1 oz.)	60	20.0
Bran-Buds, 40% bran flakes	⅓ cup (1 oz.)	70	21.0
Cracklin' Bran	½ cup (1 oz.)	110	19.0
40% bran flakes	¾ cup (1 oz.)	70	22.0
With raisins	¾ cup (1⅛ oz.)	110	28.0
(Post) 40% bran flakes	⅔ cup (1 oz.)	90	22.0
(Nabisco) 100% bran	½ cup (1 oz.)	70	21.0

(USDA): United States Department of Agriculture
(HEW/FAO): Health, Education and Welfare/Food and Agriculture
　　　　　　　Organization
* Prepared as Package Directs

Food and Description	Measure or Quantity	Calories	Carbohydrates (grams)
(Post)	½ cup (1 oz.)	90	22.0
(Ralston Purina):			
Bran Chex	⅔ cup (1 oz.)	110	20.0
Raisin	½ cup (1 oz.)	100	22.0

BRANDY, unflavored (See DISTILLED LIQUOR)

BRANDY EXTRACT:

(Ehlers) pure	1 tsp.	16	
(French's) imitation	1 tsp.	16	

BRANDY, FLAVORED:

Apricot:			
(Bols) 70 proof	1 fl. oz.	100	7.4
(Garnier) 70 proof	1 fl. oz.	86	7.1
(Hiram Walker) 70 proof	1 fl. oz.	88	7.5
(Leroux) 70 proof	1 fl. oz.	92	8.6
(Mr. Boston's) apricot & brandy, 42 proof	1 fl. oz.	75	8.0
Blackberry:			
(Bols) 70 proof	1 fl. oz.	100	7.4
(Garnier) 79 proof	1 fl. oz.	86	7.1
(Hiram Walker) 70 proof	1 fl. oz.	86	7.0
(Leroux) 70 proof	1 fl. oz.	91	8.3
(Leroux) Polish, 70 proof	1 fl. oz.	92	8.6
(Mr. Boston's) blackberry & brandy, 42 proof	1 fl. oz.	75	8.0
Cherry:			
(Bols) 70 proof	1 fl. oz.	100	7.4
(Garnier) 70 proof	1 fl. oz.	86	7.1
(Hiram Walker) 70 proof	1 fl. oz.	86	7.0
(Leroux) 70 proof	1 fl. oz.	91	8.3
Coffee:			
(Garnier) 70 proof	1 fl. oz.	86	7.1
(Leroux) coffee & brandy, 70 proof	1 fl. oz.	91	8.3
Ginger:			
(Garnier) 70 proof	1 fl. oz.	74	4.0
(Hiram Walker) 70 proof	1 fl. oz.	72	3.5
(Leroux) 70 proof	1 fl. oz.	76	4.4
(Leroux) sharp, 70 proof	1 fl. oz.	77	4.7

Food and Description	Measure or Quantity	Calories	Carbo-hydrates (grams)
Peach:			
(Garnier) 70 proof	1 fl. oz.	86	— 7.1
(Hiram Walker) 70 proof	1 fl. oz.	87	7.2
(Leroux) 70 proof	1 fl. oz.	93	8.9
BRAUNSCHWEIGER:			
(Oscar Mayer):			
8-oz. chub	1 oz.	94	.7
Sliced	.9-oz. slice	95	.4
(Swift) 8-oz. chub	1 oz.	109	1.4
(Wilson)	1 oz.	90	.7
BRAZIL NUT (USDA)			
Whole, in shell	1 cup (4.3 oz.)	383	6.4
Shelled	½ cup (2.5 oz.)	458	7.6
Shelled	4 nuts (.6 oz.)	114	1.9
BREAD (listed by type or brand name):			
American Granary (Arnold)	.9-oz. slice	70	12.5
Banana nut loaf (Van de Kamp's)	14-oz. loaf	1288	
Boston brown (USDA)	1.7-oz. slice (3″ x ¾″)	101	21.9
Bran'nola (Arnold)	1.2-oz. slice	90	15.5
Cinnamon raisin (Thomas')	.8-oz. slice	60	11.7
Cracked-wheat:			
(USDA) 20 slices to 1 lb.	.8-oz. slice	69	12.0
(Wonder)	1-oz. slice	75	13.5
Datenut loaf:			
(Mannafood)	.9-oz. slice	71	
(Thomas') cake	1.1-oz. slice	92	18.4
Dutch Crunch, 1-lb. loaf (Van de Kamp's)	.8-oz. slice	63	
Egg sesame, 1-lb. loaf (Van de Kamp's)	.9-oz. slice	77	
French:			
(USDA) 20 slices to 1 lb.	.8-oz. slice	67	12.7

(USDA): United States Department of Agriculture
(HEW/FAO): Health, Education and Welfare/Food and Agriculture Organization
* Prepared as Package Directs

Food and Description	Measure or Quantity	Calories	Carbo- hydrates (grams)
(Pepperidge Farm)	⅛ of 1-lb. loaf	150	28.0
(Wonder)	1-oz. slice	75	13.5
Glutogen Gluten (Thomas')	1 slice (.4 oz.)	32	5.9
Hillbilly (Wonder)	1-oz. slice	70	12.5
Hollywood, dark or light	1-oz. slice	70	12.5
Honey bran (Pepperidge Farm)	1 slice	58	11.0
Honey Wheatberry (Arnold)	1.2-oz. slice	90	16.0
Ideal Flatbrod:			
Caraway or whole grain	1 slice (5 grams)	19	4.0
Ultra thin	1 slice (3 grams)	12	2.5
Italian:			
(USDA) 20 slices to 1 lb.	.8-oz. slice	63	13.0
(Pepperidge Farm)	⅛ of 1-lb. loaf	150	28.0
Low sodium (Wonder)	1-oz. slice	70	13.5
Naturel (Arnold)	.9-oz. slice	65	12.0
Profile (Wonder) dark or light	.8-oz. slice	75	12.5
Protogen protein (Thomas')	.7-oz. slice	45	8.3
Protogen protein (Thomas') frozen	.9-oz. slice	55	10.2
Pumpernickel:			
(Arnold)	1-oz. slice	75	14.0
(Levy's)	1.1-oz. slice	70	12.4
(Pepperidge Farm)	1 slice	75	15.0
Raisin:			
Cinnamon (See Cinnamon raisin)			
Tea (Arnold)	.9-oz. slice	70	13.0
Roman Meal	1-oz. slice	70	13.5
Rye:			
(Arnold) Jewish	1.1-oz. slice	75	14.0
(Arnold) melba thin	.7-oz. slice	50	9.5
(Arnold) soft	1.1-oz. slice	75	15.0
(Pepperidge Farm) family	1 slice	80	14.5
Wasa Crisp:			
Brown	.4-oz. slice	43	9.1
Golden	1 slice	37	7.8
Hearty	1 slice	37	7.8
Lite	.3-oz. slice	30	6.3
Seasoned	1 slice	34	7.1
(Wonder)	1-oz. slice	75	13.5
Salt rising (USDA)	.9-oz. slice	67	13.0

Food and Description	Measure or Quantity	Calories	Carbo-hydrates (grams)
Sesame, *Wasa Crisp*	1 slice (14 grams)	60	9.0
Sourdough, *DiCarlo*	1-oz. slice	70	13.5
Sourdough toast, *Wasa Crisp*	1 slice (12 grams)	46	9.5
Toaster cake (See **TOASTER CAKE**)			
Wheat:			
Fresh Horizons	1-oz. slice	50	9.5
Home Pride	1-oz. slice	75	13.0
(Pepperidge Farm)	1 slice	90	17.0
Proclaim	1-oz. slice	70	11.0
(Wonder)	1-oz. slice	75	13.5
Wheatberry, *Home Pride*	1-oz. slice	70	12.5
Wheat germ (Pepperidge Farm)	1 slice	65	12.5
White:			
(USDA):			
Prepared with 1-4% non-fat dry milk	.8-oz. slice	62	11.6
Prepared with 5-6% non-fat dry milk	.8-oz. slice	63	11.5
(Arnold):			
Brick Oven	.8-oz. slice	65	11.0
Brick Oven	1.1-oz. slice	85	14.6
Hearthstone, 2-lb. loaf	1.1-oz. slice	85	15.0
Hearthstone, country	.9-oz. slice	70	12.5
Melba thin	.5-oz. slice	50	7.0
(Pepperidge Farm):			
Large loaf	1 slice	75	13.5
Sandwich	1 slice	65	12.0
Sliced	.8-oz. slice	75	13.0
Toasting	1.2-oz. slice	85	16.0
Very thin slice	1 slice	40	8.0
(Wonder):			
Regular and with buttermilk	1-oz. slice	75	13.5
Fresh Horizons	1-oz. slice	60	9.5
Home Pride	1-oz. slice	75	13.0
Proclaim	1-oz. slice	70	11.0

(USDA): United States Department of Agriculture
(HEW/FAO): Health, Education and Welfare/Food and Agriculture Organization
* Prepared as Package Directs

Food and Description	Measure or Quantity	Calories	Carbo-hydrates (grams)
Whole-wheat:			
(USDA):			
Prepared with 2% non-fat dry milk	.9-oz. slice	61	11.9
Prepared with 2% non-fat dry milk	.8-oz. slice	56	11.0
Prepared with water	.9-oz. slice	60	12.3
(Arnold):			
Brick Oven	.8-oz. slice	60	9.5
Brick Oven	1.1-oz. slice	80	13.0
Melba thin	.5-oz. slice	40	6.5
(Pepperidge Farm) thin sliced	1 slice	70	12.0
(Thomas')	.8-oz. slice	56	10.1
BREAD, CANNED (B&M):			
Brown, plain	1-oz. slice	52	11.4
Brown with raisins	1-oz. slice	52	11.1
BREAD CRUMBS:			
(Buitoni)	1 oz.	104	18.5
(Contadina) seasoned	1 cup (4.1 oz.)	411	79.9
(Old London)	1 cup (4½ oz.)	458	97.2
*****BREAD DOUGH,** frozen (Rich's):			
French	1/20 of loaf	59	11.0
Italian	1/20 of loaf	60	11.0
Raisin	1/20 of loaf	66	12.3
*****BREAD MIX** (Pillsbury):			
Applesauce	1/16 of loaf	120	21.0
Apricot nut, banana, blueberry nut	1/16 of loaf	110	20.0
Cranberry	1/16 of loaf	120	22.0
Date	1/12 of loaf	120	23.0
BREAD PUDDING with raisins, home recipe (USDA)	1 cup (9.3 oz.)	496	75.3
BREAD STICK:			
(Keebler):			
Cheese	1 piece (3 grams)	10	1.8

Food and Description	Measure or Quantity	Calories	Carbo-hydrates (grams)
Garlic (Stella D'oro):	1 piece (3 grams)	11	1.9
Dietetic	1 piece (9 grams)	39	6.3
Regular	1 piece (10 grams)	40	6.6
Sesame	1 piece (9 grams)	41	5.9
BREADFRUIT, fresh (USDA):			
Whole	1 lb. (weighed untrimmed)	360	91.5
Peeled & trimmed	4 oz.	117	29.7
BREAKFAST BAR (Carnation):			
Almond crunch	1 piece	210	20.0
Chocolate chip	1 piece	210	24.0
Chocolate crunch	1 piece	210	23.0
Granola with peanut butter	1 piece	200	21.0
Granola with raisins	1 piece	190	19.0
Peanut butter crunch	1 piece	200	22.0
BREAKFAST DRINK, instant:			
(Ann Page)	2 tsps. (.6 oz.)	63	15.9
(Pillsbury):			
Chocolate or chocolate malt	1 pouch	130	26.0
Strawberry or vanilla	1 pouch	130	27.0
BREAKFAST SQUARES (General Mills), all flavors	2 bars (3 oz.)	380	45.0
BRIGHT & EARLY	6 fl. oz. (6.6 oz.)	90	21.6
BROCCOLI: Raw (USDA):			
Whole	1 lb. (weighed untrimmed)	89	16.3

(USDA): United States Department of Agriculture
(HEW/FAO): Health, Education and Welfare/Food and Agriculture Organization

Food and Description	Measure or Quantity	Calories	Carbo-hydrates (grams)
Large leaves removed	1 lb. (weighed partially trimmed)	113	20.9
Boiled (USDA):			
½" pieces, drained	½ cup (2.8 oz.)	20	3.5
Drained	1 med. stalk (6.3 oz.)	47	8.1
Frozen:			
(Birds Eye) in cheese sauce	⅓ of 10-oz. pkg.	110	7.0
(Birds Eye) chopped, spears or baby deluxe spears	⅓ of 10-oz. pkg.	25	4.0
(Birds Eye) in Hollandaise sauce	⅓ of 10-oz. pkg.	100	4.0
(Green Giant) spears in butter sauce	½ cup	45	4.0
(Green Giant) in cream sauce	½ cup	65	6.5
(Green Giant) cheese sauce, *Bake 'n Serve*	½ cup	130	8.5
(Mrs. Paul's) & cheese, batter fried	⅓ of 7¾-oz. pkg.	163	18.8
BROTH & SEASONING (See also individual kinds):			
Maggi	1 T. (.6 oz.)	22	.1
(George Washington) Golden	1 packet (4 grams)	5	1.0
(George Washington) Rich Brown	1 packet (4 grams)	5	1.2
BROWNIE (See **COOKIE**)			
BRUSSELS SPROUTS:			
Raw (USDA)	1 lb.	188	34.6
Boiled, drained (USDA) 1¼"-1½" dia.	1 cup (7-8 sprouts, 5.5 oz.)	56	9.9
Frozen:			
Boiled, drained (USDA)	4 oz.	37	7.4
(Birds Eye)	⅓ of 10-oz. pkg.	30	5.0
(Birds Eye) baby sprouts	½ of pkg.	35	6.0
(Green Giant) in butter sauce	½ cup	55	5.0

Food and Description	Measure or Quantity	Calories	Carbohydrates (grams)
(Green Giant) halves in cheese sauce	½ cup	85	9.5
BUCKWHEAT:			
Flour (See **FLOUR**)			
Groats:			
(Birkett) *Wolff's Kasha*	1 oz.	108	23.3
(Pocono) whole, brown	1 oz.	104	19.4
(Pocono) whole, white	1 oz.	102	20.1
BUC WHEATS, cereal (General Mills)	1 cup	110	23.0
BULGAR (from hard red winter wheat) (USDA):			
Dry	1 lb.	1605	343.4
Canned:			
Unseasoned	4 oz.	191	39.7
Seasoned	4 oz.	206	37.2
BULLOCK'S-HEART (See **CUSTARD APPLE**)			
BUN (See **ROLL**)			
BURGER KING:			
Cheeseburger	1 burger	310	26.0
Cheeseburger, double meat	1 burger	420	26.0
French fries	1 small order	200	28.0
Hamburger	1 burger	240	25.0
Hamburger, double meat	1 burger	370	25.0
Hot dog	1 frankfurter	290	24.0
Onion rings	1 small order	150	20.0
Whaler	1 sandwich	720	66.0
Whaler with cheese	1 sandwich	820	66.0
Whopper:			
Regular	1 burger	650	50.0

(USDA): United States Department of Agriculture
(HEW/FAO): Health, Education and Welfare/Food and Agriculture Organization
* Prepared as Package Directs

Food and Description	Measure or Quantity	Calories	Carbo-hydrates (grams)
With cheese	1 burger	760	51.0
Double meat	1 burger	870	50.0
Double meat with cheese	1 burger	980	51.0
Junior	1 burger	300	26.0
Junior with cheese	1 burger	360	26.0
Junior, double meat	1 burger	410	26.0
Junior, double meat with cheese	1 burger	460	26.0
Yumbo	1 sandwich	410	31.0
BURGUNDY WINE (See also individual regional, vineyard, grape or brand names):			
(Gallo) 13% alcohol	3 fl. oz.	52	.9
(Gallo) hearty, 14% alcohol	3 fl. oz.	48	1.2
(Gold Seal) 12% alcohol	3 fl. oz.	82	.4
(Great Western) 12% alcohol	3 fl. oz.	70	2.3
(Inglenook) Navalle, 12% alcohol	3 fl. oz. (2.9 oz.)	64	1.7
(Inglenook) Vintage, 12% alcohol	3 fl. oz. (2.9 oz.)	59	.3
(Italian Swiss Colony) 13% alcohol	3 fl. oz. (2.9 oz.)	61	.9
(Italian Swiss Colony-Gold Medal) 12.3% alcohol	3 fl. oz.	63	.7
(Louis M. Martini) 12½% alcohol	3 fl. oz.	90	.2
(Mogen David) American, 12% alcohol	3 fl. oz.	24	1.8
(Petri) 13% alcohol	3 fl. oz. (2.9 oz.)	63	1.3
(Taylor) 12.5% alcohol	3 fl. oz.	75	3.3
BURGUNDY WINE, SPARKLING:			
(Barton & Guestier) French red, 12% alcohol	3 fl. oz.	69	2.2
(Chanson) French red	3 fl. oz.	72	3.6
(Gold Seal) 12% alcohol	3 fl. oz.	87	2.6
(Great Western) 12% alcohol	3 fl. oz.	82	5.1
(Lejon) 12% alcohol	3 fl. oz.	67	2.3
(Taylor) 12.5% alcohol	3 fl. oz.	78	4.2

Food and Description	Measure or Quantity	Calories	Carbo-hydrates (grams)
BUTTER, salted or unsalted:			
(USDA)	¼ lb. (1 stick, ½ cup)	812	.5
(USDA)	1 T. (⅛ stick, .5 oz.)	100	.1
(Breakstone)	1 T. (.5 oz.)	100	<.1
(Breakstone) whipped	1 T. (9 grams)	67	.1
(Meadow Gold)	1 tsp.	35	0
BUTTER BEAN (See **BEAN, LIMA**)			
BUTTERFISH, raw (USDA):			
Gulf:			
Whole	1 lb. (weighed whole)	220	0.
Meat only	4 oz.	180	0.
Northern:			
Whole	1 lb. (weighed whole)	391	0.
Meat only	4 oz.	192	0.
BUTTER FLAVORING, imitation (Ehlers)	1 tsp.	8	
BUTTERMILK (See **MILK**)			
BUTTERNUT (USDA):			
Whole	1 lb. (weighed in shell)	399	5.3
Shelled	4 oz.	713	9.5
BUTTER PECAN ICE CREAM (Breyer's)	¼ pt.	180	15.0
***BUTTER PECAN PUDDING or PIE FILLING**, mix, sweetened (Jell-O) instant	½ cup	180	29.0

(USDA): United States Department of Agriculture
(HEW/FAO): Health, Education and Welfare/Food and Agriculture
Organization
* Prepared as Package Directs

Food and Description	Measure or Quantity	Calories	Carbo-hydrates (grams)
BUTTERSCOTCH PIE:			
Home recipe (USDA)	⅙ of 9″ pie (5.4 oz.)	406	58.2
Frozen (Banquet) cream	2½-oz. serving	187	27.0
BUTTERSCOTCH PUDDING:			
Canned, sweetened:			
(Del Monte)	5-oz. container	186	30.8
(Hunt's) Snack Pack	5-oz. can	190	26.0
Canned, dietetic or low calorie, *Sego*	½ of 8-oz. can	125	18.5
Frozen (Rich's)	4½-oz. container	199	27.4
Mix, sweetened:			
(Ann Page) regular	¼ of 3⅝-oz. pkg.	96	24.1
(Ann Page) instant	¼ of 3¼-oz. pkg.	85	21.3
*(Jell-O) regular & instant	½ cup	180	30.0
*(My-T-Fine) regular	½ cup	143	28.0
Mix, dietetic or low calorie (D-Zerta)	½ cup (4.6 oz.)	70	13.0

C

CABBAGE:			
White (USDA):			
Raw:			
Whole	1 lb. (weighed untrimmed)	86	19.3
Finely shredded or chopped	1 cup (3.2 oz.)	22	4.9
Coarsely shredded or sliced	1 cup (2.5 oz.)	17	3.8
Wedge	3½″ x 4½″	24	5.4
Boiled:			
Shredded, in small amount of water, short time, drained	½ cup (2.6 oz.)	15	3.1
Wedges, in large amount of water, long time, drained	½ cup (3.2 oz.)	16	3.7
Dehydrated	1 oz.	87	20.9

Food and Description	Measure or Quantity	Calories	Carbohydrates (grams)
Red, raw, whole (USDA)	1 lb. (weighed untrimmed)	111	24.7
Red, canned, sweet & sour (Greenwood's) solids & llq.	½ cup (3.9 oz.)	62	13.6
Savory, raw, whole (USDA)	1 lb. (weighed untrimmed	86	16.5
CABBAGE, CHINESE or CELERY, raw (USDA):			
Whole	1 lb. (weighed untrimmed	62	13.2
1" pieces, leaves with stalk	½ cup (1.3 oz.)	5	1.1
CABBAGE, STUFFED, frozen (Green Giant) with beef in tomato sauce	7-oz. entree	220	17.0
CABERNET SAUVIGNON WINE:			
(Inglenook) Estate, 12% alcohol	3 fl. oz. (2.9 oz.)	58	.3
(Louis M. Martini) 12½% alcohol	3 fl. oz.	90	.2
CAFE COMFORT, 55 proof	1 fl. oz.	79	8.8
CAKE:			
Plain:			
Home recipe, with butter, with boiled white icing	⅑ of 9" square	401	70.5
Home recipe, with butter, with chocolate icing	⅑ of 9" square	453	73.1
Angel food, home recipe	1/12 of 8" cake	108	24.1
Banana, frozen (Sara Lee)	⅛ of cake	175	26.8
Banana, frozen (Sara Lee) *Light 'n Luscious*	⅛ of cake	105	19.1

(USDA): United States Department of Agriculture
(HEW/FAO): Health, Education and Welfare/Food and Agriculture Organization
* Prepared as Package Directs

Food and Description	*Measure or Quantity*	*Calories*	*Carbo-hydrates (grams)*
Banana nut layer, frozen (Sara Lee)	⅛ of cake	233	26.5
Black forest, frozen (Sara Lee)	⅛ of cake	203	27.9
Caramel:			
Home recipe, without icing	⅑ of 9″ square	331	46.2
Home recipe, with caramel icing	⅑ of 9″ square	322	50.2
Cheesecake, frozen:			
(Rich's)	1/16 of cake	212	19.6
(Sara Lee):			
Cherry cream cheese	⅙ of cake	214	30.3
Cream cheese, small	⅓ of cake	287	28.3
Cream cheese, large	⅙ of cake	240	23.0
Strawberry cream cheese	⅙ of cake	214	30.0
Chocolate:			
Home recipe, with chocolate icing, 2-layer	1/12 of 9″ cake	365	55.2
Frozen:			
(Pepperidge Farm) fudge	⅙ of cake	315	43.4
(Pepperidge Farm) golden	⅙ of cake	320	43.6
(Sara Lee)	⅛ of cake	185	24.3
(Sara Lee) *Light 'n Luscious*	⅛ of cake	120	19.6
(Sara Lee) 'n cream, layer	⅛ of cake	209	23.8
(Sara Lee) double chocolate, layer	⅛ of cake	214	24.0
(Sara Lee) German	⅛ of cake	170	17.3
Coffee:			
(Drake's):			
Junior	1 cake (1.1 oz.)	126	18.4
Lemon ring	13-oz. ring	1028	217.3
Pecan ring	13-oz. ring	1109	210.8
Raisin snack	2¼-oz. cake	222	36.4
Raspberry ring	13-oz. ring	1028	199.6
Small	1 cake (2.4 oz.)	280	40.3

Food and Description	*Measure or Quantity*	*Calories*	*Carbo-hydrates (grams)*
Frozen:			
(Pepperidge Farm) cinnamon twist	1/6 of cake (1.8 oz.)	156	21.3
(Pepperidge Farm) pecan	1 bun (1.7 oz.)	195	20.5
(Sara Lee):			
Almond	1/8 of cake	169	19.3
Almond ring	1/8 of cake	141	16.0
Apple *Fruit 'n Danish*	1/8 of cake	147	18.8
Blueberry *Fruit 'n Danish*	1/8 of cake	142	18.1
Blueberry ring	1/8 of cake	133	17.6
Cherry *Fruit 'n Danish*	1/8 of cake	140	18.4
Cinnamon	1/8 of cake	154	18.1
Maple crunch ring	1/8 of cake	146	15.6
Pecan, large	1/8 of cake	165	18.0
Pecan, small	1/4 of cake	191	20.8
Raspberry ring	1/8 of cake	140	18.2
Streusel, large	1/8 of cake	160	16.6
Crumb, frozen (Sara Lee):			
Blueberry	1 cake	155	23.9
French	1 cake	172	27.0
Devil's food:			
Home recipe, without icing	3" x 2" x 1½" piece	201	28.6
Home recipe, with chocolate icing, 2-layer	1/16 of 9" cake	277	41.8
Frozen:			
(Pepperidge Farm)	1/6 of cake	326	47.0
(Sara Lee)	1/8 of cake	189	25.1
Fruit:			
Home recipe, dark	1/30 of 8" loaf	57	9.0
Home recipe, light, made with butter	1/30 of 8" loaf	58	8.6

(USDA): United States Department of Agriculture
(HEW/FAO): Health, Education and Welfare/Food and Agriculture Organization
* Prepared as Package Directs

Food and Description	Measure or Quantity	Calories	Carbo-hydrates (grams)
Honey (Holland Honey cake), low sodium:			
Fruit and raisin	½" slice (.9 oz.)	80	19.0
Orange and premium unsalted	½" slice (.9 oz.)	70	17.0
Orange, frozen (Sara Lee)	⅛ of cake	175	25.3
Pound:			
Home recipe, equal weights flour, sugar, butter & eggs	3½" x 3½" slice (1.1 oz.)	142	14.1
Home recipe, traditional, made with butter	3½" x 3½" slice (1.1 oz.)	123	16.4
(Drake's):			
Plain	1 slice (1.6 oz.)	153	25.1
All butter, junior	1 slice (1.2 oz.)	110	19.2
Raisin	1½-oz. slice	210	34.0
Frozen (Sara Lee):			
Regular	⅒ of cake	124	14.4
Banana nut	⅒ of cake	117	15.1
Chocolate	⅒ of cake	122	13.0
Chocolate swirl	⅒ of cake	130	17.9
Family size	⅟₁₅ of cake	127	14.8
Home style	⅒ of cake	109	12.7
Raisin	⅒ of cake	127	19.3
Sponge, home recipe	⅟₁₂ of 10" cake	196	35.7
Strawberry 'n Cream, frozen (Sara Lee)	⅛ of cake	213	27.4
Strawberry shortcake, frozen (Sara Lee)	⅛ of cake	193	25.9
Walnut, frozen (Sara Lee) layer	⅛ of cake	211	22.3
White:			
Home recipe, made with butter, without icing, 2-layer	⅑ of 9" wide, 3" high cake	353	50.8
Home recipe, made with butter, with coconut icing, 2-layer	⅟₁₂ of 9" wide, 3" high cake	386	63.1

Food and Description	Measure or Quantity	Calories	Carbo-hydrates (grams)
Yellow:			
Home recipe, made with butter, without icing, 2-layer	1/19 of cake	351	56.3
(Sara Lee) frozen, *Light 'n Luscious*	1/8 of cake	122	21.7
CAKE ICING:			
Butter pecan (Betty Crocker) ready to spread	1/12 of can	170	27.0
Caramel, home recipe (USDA)	4 oz.	408	86.8
Cherry (Betty Crocker) ready to spread	1/12 of can	160	26.0
Chocolate:			
Home recipe (USDA)	4 oz.	426	76.4
(Betty Crocker) ready to spread	1/12 of can	170	25.0
(Betty Crocker) milk, ready to spread	1/12 of can	160	25.0
(Betty Crocker) nut, ready to spread	1/12 of can	160	24.0
(Pillsbury) fudge, ready to spread	1/12 pkg.	160	24.0
(Pillsbury) milk, ready to spread	1/12 pkg.	160	24.0
Coconut, home recipe (USDA)	4 oz.	413	84.9
Dark dutch (Betty Crocker) ready to spread	1/12 of can	160	24.0
Double Dutch (Pillsbury) ready to spread	1/12 pkg.	160	24.0
Lemon (Betty Crocker) *Sunkist,* ready to spread	1/12 of can	160	36.0
Lemon (Pillsbury) ready to spread	1/12 pkg.	160	27.0
Orange (Betty Crocker) ready to spread	1/12 of can	160	26.0

(USDA): United States Department of Agriculture
(HEW/FAO): Health, Education and Welfare/Food and Agriculture Organization
* Prepared as Package Directs

Food and Description	Measure or Quantity	Calories	Carbo-hydrates (grams)
Sour cream chocolate (Betty Crocker) ready to spread	⅟₁₂ of can	170	25.0
Sour cream white (Betty Crocker) ready to spread	⅟₁₂ of can	160	26.0
Strawberry (Pillsbury) ready to spread	⅟₁₂ pkg.	160	27.0
Vanilla (Betty Crocker) ready to spread	⅟₁₂ of can	160	26.0
Vanilla (Pillsbury), ready to spread	⅟₁₂ pkg.	160	27.0
White:			
Home recipe, boiled (USDA)	4 oz.	358	91.1
Home recipe, uncooked (USDA)	4 oz.	426	92.5
*CAKE ICING MIX:			
Banana (Betty Crocker) *Chiquita,* creamy	⅟₁₂ of cake's icing	170	30.0
Butter Brickle (Betty Crocker) creamy	⅟₁₂ of cake's icing	170	30.0
Butter pecan (Betty Crocker) creamy	⅟₁₂ of cake's icing	170	30.0
Caramel, golden (Betty Crocker)	⅟₁₂ of cake's icing	170	30.0
Caramel (Pillsbury) *Rich 'n Easy*	⅟₁₂ of cake's icing	170	29.0
Cherry, creamy (Betty Crocker)	⅟₁₂ of cake's icing	170	30.0
Cherry fluff (Betty Crocker)	⅟₁₂ of cake's icing	60	16.0
Chocolate chip (Betty Crocker) creamy	⅟₁₂ of cake's icing	180	32.0
Chocolate:			
Fudge:			
Home recipe (USDA)	4 oz.	429	76.0
(Betty Crocker) creamy	⅟₁₂ of cake's icing	180	32.0
(Pillsbury) *Rich 'n Easy*	⅟₁₂ of cake's icing	170	30.0
Malt (Betty Crocker) creamy	⅟₁₂ of cake's icing	170	30.0
Milk (Betty Crocker) creamy	⅟₁₂ of cake's icing	170	30.0

Food and Description	Measure or Quantity	Calories	Carbo-hydrates (grams)
Milk (Pillsbury) *Rich 'n Easy*	¹⁄₁₂ of cake's icing	170	29.0
Whipped (Betty Crocker)	¹⁄₁₂ of cake's icing	130	18.0
Coconut almond (Pillsbury)	¹⁄₁₂ of cake's icing	170	17.0
Coconut pecan (Betty Crocker) creamy	¹⁄₁₂ of cake's icing	140	18.0
Coconut pecan (Pillsbury)	¹⁄₁₂ of cake's icing	150	20.0
Double Dutch (Pillsbury) *Rich 'n Easy*	¹⁄₁₂ of cake's icing	170	30.0
Fudge:			
Home recipe, prepared with water, creamy (USDA)	4 oz.	384	84.6
(Betty Crocker) dark chocolate	¹⁄₁₂ of cake's icing	170	30.0
Lemon:			
(Betty Crocker) *Sunkist*, creamy	¹⁄₁₂ of cake's icing	170	30.0
(Betty Crocker) whipped	¹⁄₁₂ of cake's icing	130	18.0
(Pillsbury) *Rich 'n Easy*	¹⁄₁₂ of cake's icing	170	30.0
Orange (Betty Crocker) creamy	¹⁄₁₂ of cake's icing	170	30.0
Rocky road (Betty Crocker) creamy	¹⁄₁₂ of cake's icing	170	27.0
Spice (Betty Crocker) creamy	¹⁄₁₂ of cake's icing	170	30.0
Sour cream chocolate fudge (Betty Crocker) creamy	¹⁄₁₂ of cake's icing	170	30.0
Sour cream white (Betty Crocker) creamy	¹⁄₁₂ of cake's icing	170	30.0
Strawberry (Pillsbury) *Rich 'n Easy*	¹⁄₁₂ of cake's icing	170	29.0
Strawberry cream (Betty Crocker) whipped	¹⁄₁₂ of cake's icing	130	18.0
Vanilla (Betty Crocker) whipped	¹⁄₁₂ of cake's icing	100	18.0
Vanilla (Pillsbury) *Rich 'n Easy*	¹⁄₁₂ of cake's icing	170	29.0

(USDA): United States Department of Agriculture
(HEW/FAO): Health, Education and Welfare/Food and Agriculture Organization
* Prepared as Package Directs

Food and Description	Measure or Quantity	Calories	Carbohydrates (grams)
White (Betty Crocker) creamy	1/12 of cake's icing	190	33.0
White (Betty Crocker) fluffy	1/12 of cake's icing	60	16.0
White (Pillsbury) fluffy	1/12 of cake's icing	70	17.0
CAKE MIX:			
Angel food:			
*(USDA)	1/12 of 10" cake	137	31.5
(Betty Crocker):			
Chocolate	1/12 pkg.	140	32.0
Confetti	1/12 pkg.	150	34.0
Lemon custard	1/12 pkg.	140	32.0
One-step	1/12 pkg.	140	32.0
Strawberry	1/12 pkg.	150	34.0
Traditional	1/12 pkg.	130	30.0
(Duncan Hines)	1/12 pkg.	131	28.9
*(Pillsbury) raspberry	1/12 of cake	140	33.0
*(Pillsbury) white	1/12 of cake	140	33.0
*(Swans Down)	1/12 of cake	132	29.7
Applesauce (Betty Crocker) raisin, *Snackin' Cake*	1/9 pkg.	200	34.0
*Banana (Betty Crocker) *Chiquita*, layer	1/12 of cake	200	34.0
Banana nut (Duncan Hines) *Moist & Easy*	1/9 pkg.	196	31.0
Banana walnut (Betty Crocker) *Snackin' Cake*	1/9 pkg.	200	33.0
*Butter Brickle (Betty Crocker) layer	1/12 of cake	200	34.0
*Butter pecan (Betty Crocker) layer	1/12 of cake	200	34.0
Cheesecake:			
*(Jell-O)	1/8 of 8" cake	250	33.0
*(Pillsbury) no bake	1/8 of cake	260	34.0
*Cherry chip (Betty Crocker) layer	1/12 of cake	200	36.0
*Cherry fudge (Betty Crocker)	1/12 of cake	200	34.0
Chocolate:			
(Betty Crocker):			
Almond, *Snackin' Cake*	1/9 pkg.	210	33.0
Chip, *Snackin' Cake*	1/9 pkg.	220	35.0
Fudge, *Snackin' Cake*	1/9 pkg.	220	34.0

Food and Description	Measure or Quantity	Calories	Carbo-hydrates (grams)
*Fudge supreme, layer	1/12 of cake	200	34.0
*German chocolate, layer	1/12 of cake	200	34.0
*Malt, layer	1/12 of cake	200	34.0
*Milk, layer	1/12 of cake	200	34.0
*Pudding	1/6 of cake	230	45.0
(Duncan Hines):			
Chip, *Moist & Easy*	1/9 pkg.	185	32.7
Chip, golden, *Moist & Easy*	1/9 pkg.	187	32.7
*(Pillsbury):			
Dark, *Pillsbury Plus*	1/12 of cake	260	33.0
German, *Bundt Basic*	1/12 of cake	260	35.0
German, *Pillsbury Plus*	1/12 of cake	260	33.0
German, *Streusel Swirl*	1/12 of cake	350	50.0
Macaroon, *Bundt* ring	1/12 of cake	320	47.0
*(Swans Down) German chocolate	1/12 of cake	187	35.8
*Cinnamon (Pillsbury), *Streusel Swirl*	1/12 of cake	330	51.0
Coffee cake:			
*(Aunt Jemima)	1/8 of cake	170	29.0
*(Pillsbury):			
Apple cinnamon	1/8 of cake	230	40.0
Blueberry	1/8 of cake	230	39.0
Butter pecan	1/8 of cake	310	39.0
Cinnamon streusel	1/8 of cake	250	41.0
Sour cream	1/8 of cake	270	35.0
Date nut (Betty Crocker) *Snackin' Cake*	1/9 pkg.	200	33.0
Devil's food:			
*(USDA) with chocolate icing	1/16 of 9" cake	234	40.2
*(Betty Crocker) layer	1/12 of cake	200	34.0
*(Betty Crocker) layer, butter recipe	1/12 of cake	280	35.0
(Duncan Hines)	1/12 pkg.	189	33.0

(USDA): United States Department of Agriculture
(HEW/FAO): Health, Education and Welfare/Food and Agriculture
        Organization
* Prepared as Package Directs

Food and Description	Measure or Quantity	Calories	Carbohydrates (grams)
(Duncan Hines) pudding recipe	½₂ pkg.	187	34.8
*(Pillsbury):			
Bundt Basic	½₂ of cake	260	34.0
Pillsbury Plus	½₂ of cake	260	33.0
Streusel Swirl	½₂ of cake	330	50.0
*(Swans Down)	½₂ of cake	184	35.3
*French vanilla (Betty Crocker) layer	½₂ of cake	200	34.0
*Fudge (Pillsbury):			
Bundt ring, nut crown	½₂ of cake	290	41.0
Bundt ring, triple fudge	½₂ of cake	300	42.0
Pillsbury Plus, marble	½₂ of cake	270	36.0
Streusel Swirl, marble	½₂ of cake	340	51.0
Lemon:			
*(Betty Crocker) chiffon, Sunkist lemon	½₂ of cake	190	35.0
*(Betty Crocker) pudding	⅙ of cake	230	45.0
(Duncan Hines) pudding recipe	½₂ pkg.	183	36.1
*(Pillsbury):			
Bundt Basic	½₂ of cake	260	35.0
Bundt ring, blueberry	½₂ of cake	280	42.0
Pillsbury Plus	½₂ of cake	260	33.0
Streusel Swirl	½₂ of cake	340	51.0
Marble:			
*(Betty Crocker) layer	½₂ of cake	210	36.0
*(Pillsbury) supreme, Bundt ring	½₂ of cake	330	51.0
*Orange (Betty Crocker) layer, Sunkist Orange	½₂ of cake	200	34.0
*Pineapple (Betty Crocker) layer, Dole Pineapple	½₂ of cake	200	34.0
Pound:			
*(Betty Crocker) golden	½₂ of cake	190	27.0
*(Dromedary)	1″ slice	320	46.0
*(Pillsbury) Bundt ring	½₂ of cake	310	45.0
*Sour cream chocolate supreme (Betty Crocker) layer	½₂ of cake	200	34.0
*Sour cream white (Betty Crocker) layer	½₂ of cake	200	34.0

Food and Description	Measure or Quantity	Calories	Carbohydrates (grams)
Spice (Betty Crocker):			
*'n Apple with raisin, layer	1/12 of cake	210	37.0
Raisin, Snackin' Cake	1/9 pkg.	200	34.0
*Sour cream, layer	1/12 of cake	200	34.0
*Strawberry 'n Cream (Betty Crocker)	1/12 of cake	190	34.0
*Upside down cake (Betty Crocker) pineapple	1/9 of cake	270	42.0
White:			
*(USDA) made with egg whites and water with chocolate icing, 2-layer	1/16 of 9" cake	249	44.6
(Duncan Hines)	1/12 pkg.	187	34.8
(Duncan Hines) pudding recipe	1/12 pkg.	183	36.5
*(Pillsbury) Pillsbury Plus	1/12 of cake	250	36.0
*(Swans Down)	1/12 of cake	177	36.2
Yellow:			
*(USDA) made with eggs and water with chocolate icing, 2-layer	1/16 of 9" cake	253	43.2
*(Betty Crocker) layer	1/12 of cake	200	35.0
(Duncan Hines)	1/12 pkg.	185	35.7
(Duncan Hines) pudding recipe	1/12 pkg.	183	37.0
*(Pillsbury) Bundt Basic	1/12 of cake	260	36.0
*(Pillsbury) Pillsbury Plus	1/12 of cake	260	33.0
*(Pillsbury) Pillsbury Plus, butter recipe	1/12 of cake	240	33.0
*(Swans Down)	1/12 of cake	186	36.1
CAMPARI, 45 proof	1 fl. oz. (1.1 oz.)	66	7.1

CANADIAN WHISKY (See DISTILLED LIQUOR)

(USDA): United States Department of Agriculture
(HEW/FAO): Health, Education and Welfare/Food and Agriculture Organization
* Prepared as Package Directs

Food and Description	Measure or Quantity	Calories	Carbohydrates (grams)
CANDIED FRUIT (See individual kinds)			
CANDY. The following values of candies from the U.S. Department of Agriculture are representative of the types sold commercially. These values may be useful when individual brands or sizes are not known. (See also CANDY, COMMERCIAL):			
Almond:			
Chocolate-coated	1 cup (6.3 oz.)	1024	71.3
Chocolate-coated	1 oz.	161	11.2
Sugar-coated or Jordan	1 oz.	129	19.9
Butterscotch	1 oz.	113	26.9
Candy corn	1 oz.	103	25.4
Caramel:			
Plain	1 oz.	113	21.7
Plain with nuts	1 oz.	121	20.0
Chocolate	1 oz.	113	21.7
Chocolate with nuts	1 oz.	121	20.0
Chocolate-flavored roll	1 oz.	112	23.4
Chocolate:			
Bittersweet	1 oz.	135	13.3
Milk:			
Plain	1 oz.	147	16.1
With almonds	1 oz.	151	14.5
With peanuts	1 oz.	154	12.6
Semisweet	1 oz.	144	16.2
Sweet	1 oz.	150	16.4
Chocolate discs, sugar-coated	1 oz.	132	20.6
Coconut center, chocolate-coated	1 oz.	124	20.4
Fondant, plain	1 oz.	103	25.4
Fondant, chocolate-covered	1 oz.	116	23.0
Fudge:			
Chocolate fudge	1 oz.	113	21.3
Chocolate fudge, chocolate-coated	1 oz.	122	20.7

Food and Description	Measure or Quantity	Calories	Carbo-hydrates (grams)
Chocolate fudge with nuts	1 oz.	121	19.6
Chocolate fudge with nuts, chocolate-coated	1 oz.	128	19.1
Vanilla fudge	1 oz.	113	21.2
Vanilla fudge with nuts	1 oz.	120	19.5
With peanuts & caramel, chocolate-coated	1 oz.	130	16.6
Gum drops	1 oz.	98	24.8
Hard	1 oz.	109	27.6
Honeycombed hard candy, with peanut butter, chocolate-covered	1 oz.	131	20.0
Jelly beans	1 oz.	104	26.4
Marshmallows	1 oz.	90	22.8
Mints, uncoated	1 oz.	103	25.4
Nougat & caramel, chocolate-covered	1 oz.	118	20.6
Peanut bar	1 oz.	146	13.4
Peanut brittle	1 oz.	119	23.0
Peanuts, chocolate-covered	1 oz.	159	11.1
Raisins, chocolate-covered	1 oz.	120	20.0
Vanilla creams, chocolate-covered	1 oz.	123	19.9

CANDY, COMMERCIAL:
Regular:

Food and Description	Measure or Quantity	Calories	Carbo-hydrates (grams)
Air Bon (Whitman's)	1 piece	10	
Almond cluster (Kraft)	1 piece (.4 oz.)	63	5.0
Almonds, chocolate-covered (Kraft)	1 piece (3 grams)	14	1.0
Almond toffee bar (Kraft)	1-oz. bar	142	17.9
Babies, chocolate flavor (Heide)	1 oz.	101	
Baby Ruth (Curtiss):			
Bar	1-oz. bar	123	18.0
Fun size	.5 oz.	61	10.0
Nugget	.4 oz.	48	7.0
Baffle Bar (Cardinet's)	1 bar (1¾-oz.)	189	10.9

(USDA): United States Department of Agriculture
(HEW/FAO): Health, Education and Welfare/Food and Agriculture Organization

* Prepared as Package Directs

Food and Description	Measure or Quantity	Calories	Carbohydrates (grams)
Berries (Mason)	1 oz.	100	
Black-Crows (Mason)	1 oz.	100	
Brazil nuts, chocolate-covered (Kraft)	1 piece (6 grams)	32	1.7
Breath Saver (Life Savers)	1 piece (1.6 grams)	7	1.7
Bridge mix:			
(Kraft):			
Almond	1 piece (4 grams)	22	1.6
Caramelette	1 piece (3 grams)	12	1.9
Jelly	1 piece (3 grams)	12	1.9
Malted milk ball	1 piece (2 grams)	11	1.4
Mintette	1 piece (3 grams)	12	1.8
Peanut	1 piece (1 gram)	8	.5
Peanut crunch	1 piece (5 grams)	23	3.4
Raisin	1 piece (1 gram)	5	.8
(Nabisco)	1 piece (2 grams)	8	1.4
Bun Bars (Wayne), vanilla or maple	1 oz.	133	17.0
Butterfinger (Curtiss):			
Bar	1 oz.	134	21.0
Fun size	.5 oz.	60	9.0
Chips	6.5 grams	30	5.0
Butternut (Hollywood)	1 bar (1¼ oz.)	168	20.6
Butterscotch Skimmers (Nabisco)	1 piece (6 grams)	25	5.7
Candy corn:			
(Brach's)	1 piece (2 grams)	7	1.8
(Curtiss)	1 piece (2 grams)	4	1.0
Caramel:			
(Brach's) *Milk Maid*	1 piece (9 grams)	34	6.3
(Curtiss)	1 oz.	119	24.1
(Curtiss) chocolate	1 piece (7 grams)	29	5.0
(Curtiss) vanilla	1 piece (8 grams)	34	6.0
(Holloway) *Milk Duds*	1 oz.	111	
(Kraft):			
Carametette	1 piece (3 grams)	12	1.9
Chocolate	1 piece (8 grams)	33	6.2
Chocolate, bar	1 piece (6 grams)	26	4.9
Coconut	1 piece (8 grams)	32	5.5
Vanilla, bar	1 piece (6 grams)	26	4.9

Food and Description	Measure or Quantity	Calories	Carbohydrates (grams)
Vanilla, chocolate-covered	1 piece (9 grams)	39	6.2
Vanilla, plain	1 piece (8 grams)	33	6.2
(Pearson) *Caramel Nip*	1 piece (6.5 grams)	27	5.0
(Pearson) Vanilla nut	1 piece (8 grams)	34	6.0
(Wayne) *Caramel Flipper*	1 oz.	128	19.0
Cashew cluster (Kraft)	1 piece (.4 oz.)	58	4.9
Charleston Chew, bar	1½-oz. bar	179	32.6
Cherry, chocolate-covered:			
(Brach's)	1 piece (.6 oz.)	66	13.2
(Nabisco) dark	1 piece (.6 oz.)	67	13.0
(Nabisco) milk	1 piece (.6 oz.)	66	13.1
Cherry-A-Let (Hoffman)	1 piece	215	
Chewees (Curtiss)	1 oz.	116	24.1
Chocolate bar:			
Choco'Lite (Nestlé)	1 oz.	150	18.0
Milk chocolate:			
(Ghirardelli)	1.1-oz. bar	169	18.9
(Hershey's)	1.05-oz. bar	164	17.0
(Hershey's) miniature	.5-oz. bar	78	8.1
(Nestlé)	1 oz.	150	17.0
Mint chocolate (Ghirardelli)	1.0-oz. bar	171	18.7
Special dark (Hershey's)	1.05-oz. bar	161	18.4
Chocolate bar with almonds:			
(Hershey's)	1.05-oz. bar	164	16.1
(Hershey's)	.5-oz. bar	78	7.7
(Nestlé)	1 oz.	150	17.0
Chocolate blocks, milk (Ghirardelli)	1 sq. (1 oz.)	147	16.2
Chocolate crisp bar:			
(Ghirardelli)	1-oz. bar	161	17.6
(Kraft)	1 oz.	132	18.6
Chocolate crunch bar (Nestlé)	1 oz.	150	18.0

(USDA): United States Department of Agriculture
(HEW/FAO): Health, Education and Welfare/Food and Agriculture Organization
* Prepared as Package Directs

Food and Description	Measure or Quantity	Calories	Carbohydrates (grams)
Chocolate Parfait (Pearson's)	1 piece	28	5.0
Choc-Shop (Hoffman)	1 piece	241	
Chuckles	1 oz.	92	23.0
Chunky	1 oz.	131	
Cinnamon Hearts (Curtiss)	10 pieces (3.1 grams)	12	3.0
Circlets (Curtiss)	1 oz.	108	26.1
Circus peanuts (Curtiss)	1 piece (6 grams)	19	6.0
Cluster:			
(Nabisco) crispy	1 piece (.6 oz.)	65	14.0
Peanut, chocolate-covered:			
(Hoffman)	1 cluster	204	
(Kraft)	1 piece (.4 oz.)	59	4.1
Royal Clusters (Nabisco)	1 piece (.6 ōz.)	78	7.5
Coco-Mello (Nabisco)	1 piece (.7 oz.)	91	13.8
Coconut:			
(Brach's) Neapolitan	1 piece (.4 oz.)	48	8.0
(Curtiss) bar	1 oz.	124	20.0
(Curtiss) squares	1 piece (.4 oz.)	53	9.0
(Hershey's) cream egg	1 oz.	142	20.4
(Nabisco) bar, *Welch's*	1 piece (1.1 oz.)	132	21.8
Coffee-ets (Saylor's)	1 piece	13	
Coffee Nips (Pearson's)	1 piece	25	5.0
Coffioca (Pearson)	1 piece (6.5 grams)	25	5.0
Cup-O-Gold (Hoffman)	1 piece	210	
Dots (Mason)	1 oz.	100	
Eggs (Nabisco) *Chuckles*	1 piece (2 grams)	10	2.3
Expresso Discs (Curtiss)	1 piece (5.5 grams)	21	5.0
Fall Festival Mix (Curtiss)	1 piece (5.5 grams)	20	5.0
Fiddle Faddle	1½-oz. packet	177	34.7
5th Avenue Bar (Luden's):			
5¢ size	1 bar	71	
10¢ size	1 bar	129	
15¢ size	1 bar	179	
Frappe (Welch's)	1 piece (1.1 oz.)	132	23.5
Fruit 'n Nut chocolate bar (Nestlés)	1 oz.	140	16.5

Food and Description	Measure or Quantity	Calories	Carbohydrates (grams)
Fruit roll (Sahadi):			
Apple, cherry or plain	1-oz. piece	90	20.0
Apricot, grape, raspberry	1-oz. piece	90	21.0
Strawberry	1 oz. piece	100	22.0
Fudge:			
(Kraft) *Fudgies,* chocolate	1 piece (8.1 grams)	35	6.2
(Nabisco) bar, *Welch's*	1 piece (1.1 oz.)	144	20.5
(Nabisco) nut, bar or squares	1 piece (.5 oz.)	71	10.2
Golden Almond (Hershey's)	1 oz.	163	12.4
Good & Fruity	1 oz.	106	16.3
Good & Plenty	1 oz.	100	24.8
Hard candy:			
(Bonomo)	1 oz.	112	
(H-B)	1 piece	12	2.9
(Peerless Maid)	1 piece	22	5.6
Butterscotch:			
(Brach's) disks	1 piece (6 grams)	23	5.7
(Reed's)	1 piece	17	
Cinnamon (Reed's)	1 piece	17	
Cinnamon balls (Curtiss)	1 piece (7 grams)	27	7.0
Fruit drops (Curtiss)	1 piece (5.5 grams)	21	5.0
Grape suckers (Pearson)	1 piece (.7 oz.)	82	21.0
Lemon drops (Curtiss)	1 piece (4 grams)	15	4.8
Lemon sour (Pearson)	1 piece (6.5 oz.)	28	6.0
Peppermint (Reed's)	1 piece	17	
Root Beer Barrels	1 piece (6.5 grams)	25	5.0
Sherbit (F&F)	1 piece	9	2.2
Sour apples (Curtiss)	1 piece (7.0 grams)	27	7.0
Spearmint (Reed's)	1 piece	17	
Stix Bars (Jolly Rancher)	1 oz.	102	25.5
Stix Kisses (Jolly Rancher)	1 piece	27	7.0

(USDA): United States Department of Agriculture
(HEW/FAO): Health, Education and Welfare/Food and Agriculture Organization
* Prepared as Package Directs

Food and Description	Measure or Quantity	Calories	Carbohydrates (grams)
Stix Pak (Jolly Rancher)	1 piece	18	4.0
Washington cherries (Curtiss)	1 piece (7 grams)	27	7.0
Wintergreen (Reed's)	1 piece	17	
Hershey-Ets, candy-coated	1 piece (.9 grams)	5	.6
Hollywood	1½-oz. bar	185	28.9
Jelly (See also individual flavors and brand names in this section):			
Beans:			
(Curtiss)	1 piece (3.5 grams)	12	3.0
(Heide)	1 oz.	90	
(Brach's) *Big Ben Jellies*	1 piece (8 grams)	26	6.8
(Brach's) *Iced Jelly Cones*	1 piece (4 grams)	15	3.4
(Brach's) nougats	1 piece (.4 oz.)	43	10.0
(Curtiss) bar	1 piece (.6 oz.)	59	15.0
(Curtiss) fruit slices	1 piece (.4 oz.)	34	9.0
(Curtiss) strings	1 piece (3.5 grams)	12	3.0
(Nabisco) rings, *Chuckles*	1 piece (.4 oz.)	37	9.0
Jube Jels (Brach's)	1 piece (3 grams)	11	2.7
Jujubes, assorted (Nabisco)	1 piece	13	3.3
Ju Jus, assorted (Curtiss)	1 piece (2 grams)	7	2.0
Ju Jus, coins or raspberries (Curtiss)	1 piece (4.3 grams)	15	4.0
Jujyfruits (Heide)	1 oz.	94	
Kisses, milk chocolate (Hershey's)	1 piece (5 grams)	28	2.8
Kit Kat (Hershey's)	1⅛-oz. bar	161	18.9
Krackel Bar (Hershey's)	1.05-oz. bar	157	17.8
Licorice:			
(Curtiss) black	1 piece (.4 oz.)	27	6.0
(Heide) *Diamond Drops*	1 oz.	94	
(Heide) *Pastilles*	1 oz.	96	
(Nabisco) *Chuckles*	1 piece (.4 oz.)	36	9.0
(Pearson) *Licorice Nip*	1 piece (6.5 oz.)	26	5.0
(Switzer) red or black	1 oz.	100	24.0

Food and Description	Measure or Quantity	Calories	Carbohydrates (grams)
Life Savers (Beech-Nut):			
Drop	1 piece (3 grams)	10	2.4
Mint	1 piece (2 grams)	7	1.7
Log Rolls (Curtiss)	1 piece (7 grams)	29	5.0
Lollipop (Life Savers)	1 piece (.9 oz.)	99	24.0
Lollipop (Life Savers)	1 piece (.6 oz.)	69	-16.7
Lozenges, mint or wintergreen (Brach's)	1 piece (3 grams)	11	2.9
Mallo Cup (Boyer):			
5¢ size	¾-oz. cup	104	14.8
10¢ size	1¼-oz. cup	173	24.6
15¢ size	1⅝-oz. cup	225	32.5
Malted milk balls, milk chocolate-covered (Brach's)	1 piece (2 grams)	9	1.6
Malted milk crunch (Welch's)	1 piece (2 grams)	9	.9
Maple Nut Goodies (Brach's)	1 piece (6 grams)	29	4.0
Mars Almond Bar (M&M/Mars)	1 oz.	130	16.9
Marshmallow:			
(Campfire)	1 oz.	111	24.9
(Curtiss) egg	1 oz.	133	35.0
(Kraft):			
Chocolate	1 piece (7 grams)	24	5.4
Coconut	1 piece (.4 oz.)	40	7.5
Flavored, regular	1 piece (7 grams)	23	5.8
Flavored, miniature	1 piece (<1 gram)	2	.5
White, miniature	1 piece (.6 grams)	2	.5
White, regular	1 piece (7 grams)	23	5.8
Mary Jane (Miller):			
2¢ size	1 piece (¼ oz.)	18	3.3
15¢ size	1 piece (1.5 oz.)	108	19.5
Milk Shake (Hollywood)	1¼ oz.	150	26.8
Milky Way, milk or dark chocolate (M&M/Mars)	1 oz.	120	17.7

(USDA): United States Department of Agriculture
(HEW/FAO): Health, Education and Welfare/Food and Agriculture Organization
* Prepared as Package Directs

Food and Description	Measure or Quantity	Calories	Carbo-hydrates (grams)
Mint or peppermint:			
Afterdinner (Richardson):			
Butter	1 oz.	109	27.0
Colored, pastel	1 oz.	109	28.0
Jelly center	1 oz.	104	26.0
Midget	1 oz.	109	27.0
Striped	1 oz.	109	28.0
Buttermint (Kraft)	1 piece (2 grams)	8	2.0
Chocolate-covered bar (Brach's)	1 piece (.6 oz.)	74	13.8
Chocolate-covered (Richardson)	1 oz.	106	27.0
Cool Mint (Curtiss)	1 piece (5.5 grams)	21	5.0
Encore (Kraft)	1 piece (2 grams)	6	1.7
Jamaica Mints (Nabisco)	1 piece (6 grams)	24	5.8
Liberty Mints (Nabisco)	1 piece (6 grams)	24	5.8
Merri-mints (Delson)	1 piece	30	
Mighty Mint (Life Savers)	1 piece (.4 grams)	2	.4
Mini-mint (Kraft)	1 piece (3 grams)	12	1.9
Mint Parfait (Pearson's)	1 piece	26	5.0
Party (Kraft)	1 piece (2 grams)	8	2.0
Pattie, chocolate-covered:			
(Hoffman)	1 piece	120	
Mason Mints (Nabisco) *Junior*	1 oz.	200	
Mint Pattie (Nabisco) peppermint	1 piece (.5 oz.)	64	12.5
pattie	1 piece (.5 oz.)	64	12.5
Sherbit, pressed mints (F&F)	1 piece	7	1.8
Starlight Mints (Brach's)	1 piece (5 grams)	19	4.8
Swedish (Brach's)	1 piece (2 grams)	8	1.9
Thin (Delson)	1 piece	45	
Thin (Nabisco)	1 piece (.4 oz.)	42	8.1
Wafers (Nabisco)	1 piece (2 grams)	10	1.0

Food and Description	Measure or Quantity	Calories	Carbo-hydrates (grams)
M&M's (M&M/Mars):			
Chocolate	1 oz.	140	18.1
Peanut	1 oz.	140	16.8
Mr. Goodbar (Hershey's)	1.3-oz. bar	203	18.1
Necco:			
Canada Mints	1 piece	13	
Necco Mints	1 piece	7	
Wintergreen	1 piece	13	
Nib Nax, all flavors (Y&S)	1 piece	10	2.5
Nibs, all flavors (Y&S)	1 piece	6	1.5
North Pole (F&F)	1 bar (1⅜ oz.)	150	31.0
Nougat centers (Nabisco)			
Chuckles	1 piece (1.0 grams)	35	9.0
$100,000 Bar (Nestlés)	1 oz.	140	19.0
Orange slices (Curtiss)	1 piece (.6 oz.)	55	14.4
Orange slices (Nabisco)			
Chuckles	1 piece (8 grams)	29	7.2
Payday (Hollywood)	1¼ oz.	154	22.3
Peaks (Mason)	1 oz.	175	
Peanut:			
Chocolate-covered:			
(BB)	1 oz.	158	6.5
(Curtiss)	1 piece	5	1.0
(Kraft)	1 piece (2 grams)	12	.9
(Nabisco)	1 piece (4 grams)	24	1.6
(Tom Houston)	1 oz.	157	10.9
French burnt (Curtiss)	1 piece (2 grams)	4	1.0
Peanut brittle:			
(Bonomo)	1 oz.	132	
(Kraft)	1 oz.	126	19.8
(Kraft) coconut	1 oz.	125	21.7
(Planters) *Jumbo Peanut Block Bar,* regular size	1-oz. bar	119	23.0
(Planters) *Jumbo Peanut Block Bar,* fun size	1 piece (.4 oz.)	61	12.0

(USDA): United States Department of Agriculture
(HEW/FAO): Health, Education and Welfare/Food and Agriculture Organization
* Prepared as Package Directs

Food and Description	Measure or Quantity	Calories	Carbo-hydrates (grams)
Peanut butter cup:			
(Boyer)			
5¢ size	.6-oz. cup	69	8.1
10¢ size	1½-oz. cup	148	17.4
Smoothie	.6-oz. cup	69	6.8
Smoothie	1½-oz. cup	148	14.5
(Reese's)	.6-oz. cup	92	8.7
Peanut butter parfait			
(Pearson)	1 oz.	56	6.0
Peanut Plank (Tom Houston)	1½-oz. bar	202	21.1
P-Nut Butter Crunch			
(Pearson's)	1 piece	35	
Pom Poms (Nabisco)	1 piece (3 grams)	14	2.3
Poppycock	1 oz.	147	22.0
Raisin, chocolate-covered:			
(B&B) *Raisinets*	5¢ box	140	15.4
(Curtiss)	1 oz.	120	20.0
(Ghirardelli)	1.1-oz. bar	160	19.4
(Nabisco)	1 piece (<1 gram)	4	.6
Rally (Hershey's)	1.5-oz. bar	217	22.7
Red Hot Dollars (Heide)	1 oz.	94	
Saf-T-Pops (Curtiss)	1 piece	37	9.0
Sesame crunch (Sahadi)	¾-oz. bar	120	9.0
Sesame crunch (Sahadi)	10 pieces from 6-oz. jar	90	6.5
Snickers (M&M/Mars)	1 oz.	130	15.0
Spearmint leaves (Curtiss)	1 piece (.7 oz.)	32	8.0
Spearmint leaves (Nabisco) *Chuckles*	1 piece (8 grams)	27	6.6
Sprint, chocolate wafer bar (M&M/Mars)	1 oz.	150	16.2
Stark Wafer Roll	1¼-oz. piece	132	32.9
Stars, chocolate:			
(Brach's)	1 piece (3 grams)	16	1.7
(Nabisco)	1 piece (3 grams)	15	1.6
Sugar Babies (Nabisco)	1 piece (2 grams)	6	1.3
Sugar Daddy (Nabisco):			
Giant sucker	1 piece (1 lb.)	1809	398.6
Junior sucker	1 piece (.4 oz.)	50	11.1
Junior sucker, chocolate flavored	1 piece (.4 oz.)	51	10.6
Nugget	1 piece (7 grams)	27	6.0

Food and Description	Measure or Quantity	Calories	Carbo-hydrates (grams)
Sucker, caramel	1 piece (1.1 oz.)	121	26.4
Sugar Mama (Nabisco)	1 piece (.8 oz.)	101	18.6
Sugar Wafer (F&F)	1¼-oz. pkg.	180	26.0
Taffy:			
Salt water (Brach's)	1 piece (8 grams)	31	6.8
Turkish (Bonomo):			
Bar	1⅛ oz.	115	29.3
Bite-size	1 piece	19	4.6
Miniatures	1 piece	21	5.6
Nibbles,			
chocolate-covered	1 piece	9	1.7
Pop	1 piece	45	11.3
Roll	1¢ size	21	5.6
3 Musketeers Bar			
(M&M/Mars)	1 oz.	120	19.6
Toffee:			
(Brach's) assorted	1 piece (7 grams)	28	5.2
(Kraft) all flavors	1 piece (7 grams)	29	5.2
Tootsie Roll:			
Regular:			
1¢ size of midgee	1 piece (7 grams)	26	5.0
2¢ size	1 piece (.4 oz.)	43	8.1
5¢ size	1 piece (¾ oz.)	87	16.2
10¢ size	1 piece (1.5 oz.)	174	32.3
Twin-Pak, 10¢ size	1 piece (1¼ oz.)	137	26.9
Twin-Pack 15¢ size	1 piece (2 oz.)	219	43.1
Vending-machine size	1 piece (.18 oz.)	21	3.9
Pop, 2 for 5¢ size	1 piece (.5 oz.)	55	13.2
Pop, 5¢ size	1 piece (1 oz.)	110	26.4
Pop-drop	1 piece (5 grams)	18	4.4
Triple decker bar			
(Nestlés)	1 oz.	148	16.8
Twizzler (Y&S):			
Chocolate	1 oz.	100	24.0
Grape	1 oz.	110	23.0
Licorice & strawberry			
bars	1¼ oz.	125	30.0

(USDA): United States Department of Agriculture
(HEW/FAO): Health, Education and Welfare/Food and Agriculture Organization
✳ Prepared as Package Directs

Food and Description	Measure or Quantity	Calories	Carbo-hydrates (grams)
Licorice & strawberry bars	1¾ oz.	175	42.0
Licorice & strawberry bars	2⅛ oz.	212	51
Strawberry	1¾ oz.	178	24.0
U-No (Cardinet's)	1 bar (⅞ oz.)	161	9.3
Virginia Nut Roll (Queen Anne)	10¢ size	250	
Walnut Hill (F&F)	1 bar (1⅜ oz.)	177	29.0
Wetem & Wearem (Heide)	1 oz.	94	
Whirligigs (Nabisco)	1 piece (6 grams)	26	5.1
World Series Bar	1 oz.	128	21.3
Dietetic or low calorie:			
Assorted, *Sug'r Like*	1 piece	12	3.0
Chocolate, assorted:			
(Estee) Milk	1 piece (8 grams)	49	3.3
Slimtreats	1 piece (2 grams)	9	0.
Chocolate bar with almonds:			
(Estee)	¾-oz. bar	120	9.0
(Estee)	1 section of 3-oz. bar	40	2.9
Chocolate bar, bittersweet:			
(Estee)	1 section of 3-oz. bar	38	3.3
(Estee)	3-oz. bar	460	40.0
Chocolate bar, crunch:			
(Estee)	⅝-oz. bar	96	8.5
(Estee)	1 section of 2½-oz. bar	32	2.8
Chocolate bar, fruit-nut			
(Estee)	1 section of 3-oz. bar	57	3.3
Chocolate bar, milk:			
(Estee)	¾-oz. bar	116	9.9
(Estee)	1 section of 3-oz. bar	39	3.3
Gum drops:			
(Estee) fruit	1 piece (2 grams)	3	.8
Sug'r Like, all flavors	1 piece	6	2.0
Hard candy:			
(Estee) all flavors	1 piece (3 grams)	13	3.0
Slimtreats	1 piece	9	0.

Food and Description	Measure or Quantity	Calories	Carbohydrates (grams)
Mint:			
(Estee) all flavors	1 piece	4	1.0
Sug'r Like, all flavors	1 piece	6	
Peanut butter cup (Estee)	1 cup (8 grams)	45	2.9
Raisin, chocolate-covered			
(Estee)	1 piece (1 gram)	6	.7
TV mix (Estee)	1 piece (2 grams)	10	.7
CANE SYRUP (USDA)	1 T. (.7 oz.)	55	14.0
CANNELLONI FLORENTINE, frozen (Weight Watchers) casserole	13-oz. meal	448	45.8
CANTALOUPE, fresh (USDA):			
Whole, medium	1 lb. (weighed with skin & cavity contents)	68	17.0
Cubed	½ cup (2.9 oz.)	24	6.1
CAPERS (Crosse & Blackwell)	1 T. (.6 oz.)	6	1.0
CAPICOLA or CAPACOLA SAUSAGE (USDA)	1 oz.	141	0.
CAP'N CRUNCH, cereal (Quaker):			
Crunchberries	¾ cup (1 oz.)	120	22.9
Peanut butter	¾ cup (1 oz.)	127	20.9
Regular	¾ cup (1 oz.)	121	22.9
CAPPELLA WINE (Italian Swiss Colony) 13% alcohol	3 fl. oz. (2.8 oz.)	64	1.5
CARAMBOLA, raw (USDA):			
Whole	1 lb. (weighed whole)	149	34.1
Flesh only	4 oz.	40	9.1

(USDA): United States Department of Agriculture
(HEW/FAO): Health, Education and Welfare/Food and Agriculture Organization
* Prepared as Package Directs

Food and Description	Measure or Quantity	Calories	Carbo- hydrates (grams)
*CARAMEL NUT PUDDING, instant (Royal)	½ cup (5.1 oz.)	194	30.3
CARAWAY SEED (French's)	1 tsp.	8	.8
CARISSA or NATAL PLUM, raw (USDA):			
Whole	1 lb. (weighed whole)	273	62.4
Flesh only	4 oz.	79	18.1
CARNATION INSTANT BREAKFAST:			
Chocolate-fudge or malt	1 pkg. (1.3 oz.)	130	23.0
Coffee and vanilla	1 pkg.	130	24.0
CAROUSEL WINE (Gold Seal):			
Pink or white, 13-14% alcohol	3 fl. oz. (3.3 oz.)	125	9.8
Red, 13-14% alcohol	3 fl. oz. (3.2 oz.)	104	5.2
CARP, raw (USDA):			
Whole	1 lb. (weighed whole)	156	0.
Meat only	4 oz.	130	0.
CARROT:			
Raw (USDA)			
Whole	1 lb. (weighed with full tops)	112	26.0
Partially trimmed	1 lb. (weighed without tops, with skins)	156	36.1
Trimmed	5½″ x 1″ carrot (1.8 oz.)	21	4.8
Trimmed	25 thin strips (1.8 oz.)	21	4.8
Chunks	½ cup (2.4 oz.)	29	6.7
Diced	½ cup (2.5 oz.)	30	7.0
Grated or shredded	½ cup (1.9 oz.)	23	5.3
Slices	½ cup (2.2 oz.)	27	6.2
Strips	½ cup (2 oz.)	24	5.6
Boiled (USDA):			
Chunks, drained	½ cup (2.8 oz.)	25	5.8

Food and Description	Measure or Quantity	Calories	Carbohydrates (grams)
Diced, drained	½ cup (2.4 oz.)	22	5.0
Slices, drained	½ cup (2.6 oz.)	24	5.4
Canned, regular pack:			
(USDA) diced, solids & liq.	½ cup (4.3 oz.)	34	8.0
(Del Monte) diced, drained	½ cup	35	6.8
(Del Monte) sliced, drained	½ cup	37	7.4
(Libby's) sliced, solids & liq.	½ cup	23	5.3
(Stokely-Van Camp) diced, solids & liq.	½ cup (4.3 oz.)	30	6.0
(Stokely-Van Camp) sliced, solids & liq.	½ cup (4.3 oz.)	25	5.0
Canned dietetic pack:			
(USDA) low sodium, solids & liq.	4 oz.	25	5.7
(USDA) low sodium, drained	½ cup (2.8 oz.)	20	4.5
(Cellu) low sodium, sliced, solids & liq.	½ cup	25	6.0
(Tillie Lewis)	½ cup (4.3 oz.)	30	6.2
Dehydrated (USDA)	1 oz.	97	23.0
Frozen:			
(Birds Eye) with brown sugar glaze	⅓ pkg.	80	15.0
(Green Giant) nuggets in butter sauce	½ cup	50	6.0
CARROT PUREE, canned, dietetic (Cellu)	½ cup	35	7.5
CASABA MELON, fresh (USDA):			
Whole	1 lb. (weighed whole)	61	14.7
Flesh only	4 oz.	31	7.4

(USDA): United States Department of Agriculture
(HEW/FAO): Health, Education and Welfare/Food and Agriculture Organization
* Prepared as Package Directs

Food and Description	Measure or Quantity	Calories	Carbohydrates (grams)
CASHEW NUT:			
(USDA)	1 oz.	159	8.3
(USDA)	½ cup (2.5 oz.)	393	20.5
(USDA)	5 large or 8 med.	60	3.1
(A&P) dry roasted	1 oz.	173	7.3
(Planters) dry roasted	1 oz.	171	7.9
(Planters) oil roasted	15¢ bag (.9 oz.)	159	7.0
(Skippy) dry roasted	1 oz.	174	8.0
(Tom Houston)	15 nuts (1.1 oz.)	168	8.8
CATAWBA WINE:			
(Great Western) pink, 12% alcohol	3 fl. oz.	111	11.3
(Mogen David) New York State, 12% alcohol	3 fl. oz.	75	11.6
(Taylor) 12% alcohol	3 fl. oz.	96	9.0
CATFISH, freshwater, raw, fillet (USDA)	4 oz.	117	0.
CATSUP:			
Regular pack:			
(USDA)	1 T. (.6 oz.)	19	4.6
(USDA)	1 cup (5 oz.)	149	35.8
(Del Monte)	1 T. (.7 oz.)	24	5.5
(Hunt's)	1 T. (.6 oz.)	18	5.8
(Nalley's)	1 oz.	31	6.9
(Smucker's)	1 T. (.6 oz.)	19	4.6
Dietetic pack:			
(Dia-Mel)	1 T. (14 grams)	7	1.5
(Featherweight)	1 T. (.6 oz.)	7	1.2
CAULIFLOWER:			
Raw (USDA):			
Whole	1 lb. (weighed untrimmed)	48	9.2
Flowerbuds	½ cup (1.8 oz.)	14	2.6
Slices	½ cup (1.5 oz.)	11	2.2
Boiled, flowerbuds, drained (USDA)	½ cup (2.2 oz.)	14	2.5
Frozen:			
(USDA) unthawed	10-oz. pkg.	62	12.2

Food and Description	Measure or Quantity	Calories	Carbohydrates (grams)
(USDA) boiled, drained	½ cup (3.4 oz.)	16	3.0
(Birds Eye)	⅓ of 10-oz. pkg.	25	4.0
(Birds Eye) in cheese sauce	⅓ of 10-oz. pkg.	110	8.0
(Green Giant) in cheese sauce, *Bake 'n Serve*	1 cup	220	17.0
(Kounty Kist)	1 cup	25	4.0
(Mrs. Paul's) & cheese, batter fried	⅓ of 8-oz. pkg.	126	15.5

CAVIER, STURGEON
(USDA):

Pressed	1 oz.	90	1.4
Whole eggs	1 T. (.6 oz.)	42	.5

CELERIAC ROOT, raw
(USDA):

Whole	1 lb. (weighed unpared)	156	33.2
Pared	4 oz.	45	9.6

CELERY, all varieties
(USDA):
Fresh:

whole	1 lb. (weighed untrimmed)	58	13.3
1 large outer stalk	8″ x 1½″ at root end (1.4 oz.)	7	1.6
Diced, chopped or cut in chunks	½ cup (2.1 oz.)	10	2.3
Slices	½ cup (1.8 oz.)	9	2.1
Boiled, drained solids:			
Diced or cut in chunks	½ cup (2.7 oz.)	10	2.4
Slices	½ cup (3 oz.)	12	2.6

CELERY CABBAGE (See CABBAGE, CHINESE)

(USDA): United States Department of Agriculture
(HEW/FAO): Health, Education and Welfare/Food and Agriculture Organization
* Prepared as Package Directs

Food and Description	Measure or Quantity	Calories	Carbo-hydrates (grams)
CELERY SALT (French's)	1 tsp. (4.6 oz.)	22	<.5
CELERY SEED (French's)	1 tsp. (2.4 grams)	11	1.1
CELERY SOUP, cream of:			
(USDA) Condensed	8 oz. (by wt.)	163	16.8
*(USDA) prepared with equal volume water	1 cup (8.5 oz.)	86	8.9
*(USDA) prepared with equal volume milk	1 cup (8.4 oz.)	169	15.2
*(Ann Page) condensed	1 cup	63	8.3
*(Campbell) condensed	1 cup (8 oz. by wt.)	88	8.0
CEREAL (See kind of cereal, such as **CORN FLAKES**, or brand name such as **KIX**)			
CERTS (Warner-Lambert)	1 piece	6	1.5
CERVELAT (USDA):			
Dry	1 oz.	128	.5
Soft	1 oz.	87	.5
CHABLIS WINE:			
(Barton & Guestier) 12% alcohol	3 fl. oz.	60	.1
(Chanson) St. Vincent, 11½% alcohol	3 fl. oz.	81	6.3
(Cruse) 11% alcohol	3 fl. oz.	66	
(Gallo) 12% alcohol	3 fl. oz.	50	.9
(Gallo) pink, 13% alcohol	3 fl. oz.	61	3.0
(Gold Seal) 12% alcohol	3 fl. oz.	82	.4
(Great Western) 12% alcohol	3 fl. oz.	70	2.3
(Great Western) Diamond, 12% alcohol	3 fl. oz.	69	2.0
(Inglenook) Navalle, 12% alcohol	3 fl. oz.	59	.5
(Inglenook) Vintage, 12% alcohol	3 fl. oz. (2.9 oz.)	56	.2
(Italian Swiss Colony) Gold, 12% alcohol	3 fl. oz. (2.9 oz.)	66	3.0
(Italian Swiss Colony) pink, 12% alcohol	3 fl. oz. (2.9 oz.)	67	3.2

Food and Description	Measure or Quantity	Calories	Carbo-hydrates (grams)
(Louis M. Martini) 12½ % alcohol	3 fl. oz.	90	.2
(Taylor) 12% alcohol	3 fl. oz.	72	1.3
CHAMPAGNE:			
(Bollinger)	3 fl. oz.	72	3.6
(Gold Seal) brut, 12% alcohol	3 fl. oz.	85	1.4
(Gold Seal) brut C.F., 12% alcohol	3 fl. oz.	82	.7
(Gold Seal) pink, extra dry, 12% alcohol	3 fl. oz.	87	2.6
(Great Western) 12% alcohol	3 fl. oz.	71	2.4
(Great Western) brut, 12% alcohol	3 fl. oz.	74	3.4
(Great Western) extra dry, 12.5% alcohol	3 fl. oz.	78	4.3
(Great Western) pink, 12% alcohol	3 fl. oz.	81	4.9
(Lejon) 12% alcohol	3 fl. oz. (2.9 oz.)	66	2.5
(Mogen David) American Concord red, 12% alcohol	3 fl. oz.	90	8.9
(Mogen David) American dry, 12% alcohol	3 fl. oz.	36	4.4
(Mumm's) Cordon Rouge brut, 12% alcohol	3 fl. oz.	65	1.4
(Mumm's) extra dry, 12% alcohol	3 fl. oz.	82	5.6
(Taylor) brut, 12.5% alcohol	3 fl. oz.	75	3.3
(Taylor) dry, 12.5% alcohol	3 fl. oz.	78	3.9
(Taylor) pink, 12.5% alcohol	3 fl. oz.	81	4.8
(Veuve Clicquot) 12.5% alcohol	3 fl. oz.	78	.6
CHARD, Swiss (USDA):			
Raw, whole	1 lb. (weighed untrimmed)	104	19.2
Raw, trimmed	4 oz.	28	5.2
Boiled, drained solids	½ cup (3.4 oz.)	17	3.2

(USDA): United States Department of Agriculture
(HEW/FAO): Health, Education and Welfare/Food and Agriculture Organization
* Prepared as Package Directs

Food and Description	Measure or Quantity	Calories	Carbohydrates (grams)
CHARLOTTE RUSSE, with ladyfingers, whipped cream filling, home recipe (USDA)	4 oz.	324	38.0
CHATEAU LA GARDE CLARET, French red Bordeaux (Chanson) 11½% alcohol	3 fl. oz.	60	6.3
CHATEAUNEUF-DU-PAPE, French red Rhone: (Barton & Guestier) 13.5% alcohol	3 fl. oz.	70	.5
(Chanson) 13% alcohol	3 fl. oz.	90	6.3
(Cruse) 12% alcohol	3 fl. oz.	72	
CHATEAU OLIVIER BLANC, French white Graves (Chanson) 11½% alcohol	3 fl. oz.	60	6.3
CHATEAU OLIVIER ROUGE, French red Graves (Chanson) 11½% alcohol	3 fl. oz.	60	6.3
CHATEAU PONTET CANET (Cruse) 12% alcohol	3 fl. oz.	72	
CHATEAU RAUSAN SEGLA, French red Bordeaux (Chanson) 11½% alcohol	3 fl. oz.	60	6.3
CHATEAU ST. GERMAIN, French red Bordeaux (Chanson) 11½% alcohol	3 fl. oz.	60	6.3
CHATEAU VOIGNY, French Sauternes (Chanson) 13% alcohol	3 fl. oz.	96	7.5

Food and Description	Measure or Quantity	Calories	Carbo-hydrates (grams)
CHAYOTE, raw (USDA):			
Whole	1 lb. (weighed unpared)	108	27.4
Pared	4 oz.	32	8.1
*CHEDDAR CHEESE SOUP (Campbell) condensed	1 cup (8 oz. by wt.)	144	9.6
*CHEERI-AID mix (Ann Page) all flavors	1 serving (.8 oz.)	85	21.1
CHEERIOS (General Mills)	1¼ cups (1 oz.)	110	20.0
CHEESE:			
American or cheddar:			
(USDA) natural	1″ cube (.6 oz.)	68	.4
(USDA) process	1″ cube (.6 oz.)	67	.3
(USDA) natural, diced	1 cup (5.6 oz.)	521	2.8
(USDA) natural, grated or shredded	1 cup (3.9 oz.)	442	2.3
(USDA) natural, grated or shredded	1 T. (.7 grams)	27	.1
(Borden) process	¾-oz. slice	83	1.2
(Borden) *Miracle Melt*, process	1 T. (.5 oz.)	38	.6
(Borden) *Vera Sharp*, process	1 oz.	104	.6
(Cellu) natural, low sodium	1 oz.	110	0.0
(Fisher) process	1 oz.	110	1.0
(Kraft) natural	1 oz.	113	.6
(Kraft) *Cracker Barrel*	1 oz.	116	.5
(Kraft) process, loaf or slice	1 oz.	105	.5
(Sealtest) natural, cheddar	1 oz.	115	.6
(Sealtest) process	1 oz.	105	.5

(USDA): United States Department of Agriculture
(HEW/FAO): Health, Education and Welfare/Food and Agriculture Organization
* Prepared as Package Directs

Food and Description	Measure or Quantity	Calories	Carbohydrates (grams)
Wispride, natural, sharp cheddar	1 T. (.5 oz.)	50	1.5
American blue, process			
(Borden) *Miracle Melt*	1 T. (.5 oz.)	38	.5
Asiago (Frigo)	1 oz.	113	.6
Bleu or blue:			
(USDA) natural	1″ cube (.6 oz.)	63	.3
(Borden) *Blufort*	1¼-oz. pkg.	131	.7
(Borden) Danish	1 oz.	105	.6
(Borden) *Flora Danica*	1 oz.	105	.6
(Foremost Blue Moon)	1 T.	52	Tr.
(Frigo)	1 oz.	99	.5
(Kraft) cold pack and natural	1 oz.	99	.5
(Stella)	1 oz.	112	.6
Wispride	1 T. (.5 oz.)	49	1.6
Bondost, natural (Kraft)	1 oz.	103	.4
Brick:			
(USDA) natural	1 oz.	105	.5
(Kraft) natural	1 oz.	103	.3
(Kraft) process, slices	1 oz.	101	.4
Camembert, domestic:			
(USDA) natural	1 oz.	85	.5
(Borden)	1 oz.	86	.5
(Kraft) natural	1 oz.	85	.5
Caraway, natural (Kraft)	1 oz.	111	.6
Chantelle, natural (Kraft)	1 oz.	90	.3
Cheddar (See American)			
Colby:			
(Cellu) low sodium	1 oz.	110	0.
(Fisher)	1 oz.	110	1.0
(Kraft) natural	1 oz.	111	.6
(Pauly) low sodium	1 oz.	115	.6
Cottage:			
Creamed, unflavored:			
(USDA) large or small curd	1 T. (.5 oz.)	16	.4
(Borden)	8-oz. container	240	6.6
(Borden) *Lite Line*, low fat	1 cup	189	7.0
(Breakstone) *California*	8-oz. container	216	4.8
Breakstone) tangy small curd	8-oz. container	216	4.8

Food and Description	Measure or Quantity	Calories	Carbo-hydrates (grams)
(Breakstone) tiny soft curd	8-oz. container	216	4.8
(Dean)	8-oz. container	218	5.4
(Foremost Blue Moon)	1 oz.	27	.9
(Kraft)	1 oz.	27	.9
(Sealtest)	½ cup	120	4.0
(Sealtest) extra creamy, 6% fat	½ cup	120	3.0
(Sealtest) *Light n' Lively*	1 cup (7.9 oz.)	155	5.6
(Sealtest) low fat, 2% fat	1 cup (7.9 oz.)	193	7.4
(Viva) low fat, 2% fat	1 cup	200	8.0
Creamed, flavored:			
(Breakstone) chive	8-oz. container	216	4.8
(Breakstone) peach, low fat	8-oz. container	232	24.9
(Breakstone) pineapple	1 T. (.6 oz.)	19	2.4
(Breakstone) pineapple, low fat	8-oz. container	268	34.2
(Sealtest) chive-pepper	1 cup (8 oz.)	206	5.4
(Sealtest) *Garden Salad*	½ cup	120	5.0
(Sealtest) *Garden Salad Light n' Lively*	½ cup	90	5.0
(Sealtest) peach-pineapple	1 cup (7.9 oz.)	228	17.9
(Sealtest) peach-pineapple, *Light n' Lively*	½ cup	100	11.0
(Sealtest) pineapple	1 cup (7.9 oz.)	222	16.1
Uncreamed:			
(Borden) pot-style	8-oz. container	195	6.1
(Breakstone) pot-style	1 T. (.6 oz.)	12	.3
(Breakstone) skim milk, no added salt	8-oz. container	182	1.6
(Dean)	8-oz. container	191	3.6
(Kraft)	1 oz.	26	.6
(Sealtest)	1 cup (7.9 oz.)	179	1.6

(USDA): United States Department of Agriculture
(HEW/FAO): Health, Education and Welfare/Food and Agriculture Organization
* Prepared as Package Directs

Food and Description	Measure or Quantity	Calories	Carbo-hydrates (grams)
Cream cheese:			
Plain, unwhipped:			
(Borden)	1 oz.	101	1.5
(Breakstone)	1 oz.	98	.6
(Kraft) *Hostess*	1 oz.	98	.6
(Kraft) *Philadelphia Brand*	1 oz.	104	.9
(Kraft) imitation, *Philadelphia Brand*	1 oz.	52	1.9
Plain, whipped:			
(Breakstone) *Temp-Tee*	1 oz.	98	.6
(Breakstone) *Temp-Tee*	1 T. (9 grams)	32	.2
(Kraft) *Philadelphia Brand*	1 oz.	99	1.1
Flavored, unwhipped:			
(Borden) chive	1 oz.	96	.6
(Borden) pimiento	1 oz.	76	.6
Flavored, whipped:			
(Kraft) *Philadelphia Brand*:			
With bacon & horseradish	1 oz.	93	1.3
With chive	1 oz.	93	1.3
With onion	1 oz.	86	1.9
With pimiento	1 oz.	86	1.8
With smoked salmon	1 oz.	92	1.1
Edam:			
(House of Gold)	1 oz.	105	.3
(Kraft) natural	1 oz.	104	.3
Farmer:			
(Breakstone) midget	1 oz.	40	.6
(Dean)	1 oz.	46	.7
Fontina:			
(Kraft) natural	1 oz.	113	.6
(Stella)	1 oz.	112	.6
Frankenmuth, natural (Kraft)	1 oz.	113	.7
Gjetost, natural (Kraft)	1 oz.	134	13.0
Gorgonzola (Foremost Blue Moon)	1 oz.	110	Tr.
Gouda:			
(Borden) Dutch Maid	1 oz.	86	.5

Food and Description	Measure or Quantity	Calories	Carbo- hydrates (grams)
(Foremost Blue Moon) baby	1 oz.	120	Tr.
(Kraft) natural	1 oz.	107	.5
Gruyère:			
(Borden) process	1 oz.	93	1.4
(Kraft) natural	1 oz.	110	.6
Swiss Knight	1 oz.	101	.5
Jack-dry, natural (Kraft)	1 oz.	101	.4
Jack-fresh, natural (Kraft)	1 oz.	95	.4
Kisses, mild (Borden)	1 piece (6 grams)	18	.5
Kisses, tangy (Borden)	1 oz.	107	.3
Lagerkase, natural (Kraft)	1 oz.	107	.3
Leyden, natural (Kraft)	1 oz.	80	.7
Liederkranz (Borden)	1 oz.	86	.4
Limburger, natural (Kraft)	1 oz.	98	.6
Lite-Line (Borden)	¾-oz. slice	38	.8
MacLaren's, process, cold pack (Kraft)	1 oz.	109	.6
Monterey Jack:			
(Borden)	1 oz.	103	.6
(Frigo)	1 oz.	103	.4
(Kraft) natural	1 oz.	102	.4
Mozzarella:			
(Borden)	1 oz.	96	.8
(Frigo)	1 oz.	79	.3
Natural, low moisture, part skim (Kraft)	1 oz.	84	.3
Natural, low moisture, part skim, pizza (Kraft)	1 oz.	79	.3
Shredded (Kraft)	1 oz.	79	.3
Muenster:			
(Borden) natural	1 oz.	85	.7
(Kraft) natural	1 oz.	100	.3
(Kraft) process, slices	1 oz.	102	.6
Neufchâtel:			
Process (Borden)	1 oz.	73	6.5
Loaf (Kraft)	1 oz.	69	.7

(USDA): United States Department of Agriculture
(HEW/FAO): Health, Education and Welfare/Food and Agriculture Organization
* Prepared as Package Directs

Food and Description	Measure or Quantity	Calories	Carbohydrates (grams)
Natural (Kraft)			
Calorie-Wise	1 oz.	70	.7
Nuworld, natural (Kraft)	1 oz.	103	.7
Old English, process, loaf or			
slices (Kraft)	1 oz.	105	.5
Parmesan:			
Natural:			
(USDA)	1 oz.	111	.8
(Frigo)	1 oz.	107	.8
(Kraft)	1 oz.	107	.8
(Stella)	1 oz.	103	.9
Grated:			
(USDA) loosely packed	1 cup (3.7 oz.)	494	3.6
(USDA) loosely packed	1 T. (7 grams)	31	.2
(Borden)	1 oz.	143	8.8
(Buitoni)	1 oz.	118	.8
(Frigo)	1 T. (6 grams)	27	.2
(Kraft)	1 oz.	127	1.0
Shredded (Kraft)	1 oz.	114	.9
Parmesan & Romano,			
grated:			
(Borden)	1 oz.	135	2.2
(Kraft)	1 oz.	130	1.0
Pepato (Frigo)	1 oz.	110	.8
Pimiento American, process:			
(USDA)	1 oz.	105	.5
(Borden)	1 oz.	104	.5
Loaf or slices (Kraft)	1 oz.	103	.4
Pizza:			
(Borden)	1 oz.	85	.8
(Frigo)	1 oz.	73	.3
(Kraft)	1 oz.	73	.3
Port du Salut (Foremost			
Blue Moon)	1 oz.	100	Tr.
Port du Salut, natural			
(Kraft)	1 oz.	100	.3
Primost, natural (Kraft)	1 oz.	134	13.0
Provolone:			
(Borden)	1 oz.	93	1.0
(Frigo)	1 oz.	99	.5
(Kraft) natural	1 oz.	99	.5
Natural, sharp Casino	1 oz.	101	.6
Ricotta cheese (Sierra)	1 oz.	50	1.3

Food and Description	Measure or Quantity	Calories	Carbohydrates (grams)
Romano:			
Natural:			
(Borden) Italian pecorino	1 oz.	114	.8
(Frigo)	1 oz.	110	.8
(Stella)	1 oz.	106	.6
Grated:			
(Buitoni)	1 oz.	123	1.1
(Frigo)	1 T. (6 grams)	29	.2
(Kraft)	1 oz.	134	1.0
Shredded (Kraft)	1 oz.	121	.9
Romano & Parmesan, plain (Kraft)	1 oz.	133	1.0
Roquefort, natural:			
(Bordon) Napolean	1 oz.	107	.6
(Kraft)	1 oz.	105	.5
Sage, natural (Kraft)	1 oz.	113	.6
Sap Sago, natural (Kraft)	1 oz.	76	1.7
Sardo Romano, natural (Kraft)	1 oz.	109	.8
Scamorze			
(Frigo)	1 oz.	79	.3
(Kraft) natural	1 oz.	100	.3
Swiss, domestic:			
(Borden) process	¾-oz. slice	72	.8
(Fisher) natural	1 oz.	100	1.0
(Foremost Blue Moon) natural	1 oz.	105	1.0
(Kraft):			
Natural	1 oz.	105	.5
Process, loaf	1 oz.	92	.5
Process, slices	1 oz.	95	.6
Process, with muenster	1 oz.	98	.6
(Sealtest) natural	1 oz.	105	.5
Swiss, imported (Borden):			
Natural, Finland	1 oz.	104	.5
Natural, Switzerland	1 oz.	104	.5

(USDA): United States Department of Agriculture
(HEW/FAO): Health, Education and Welfare/Food and Agriculture Organization
* Prepared as Package Directs

Food and Description	Measure or Quantity	Calories	Carbo-hydrates (grams)
Washed curd, natural (Kraft)	1 oz.	107	.6
CHEESE CAKE and CHEESE CAKE MIX (See **CAKE** and **CAKE MIX**)			
CHEESE DIP (See **DIP**)			
CHEESE FONDUE:			
Home recipe (USDA)	4 oz.	301	11.3
(Borden)	6-oz. serving	354	15.3
CHEESE FOOD, process:			
American:			
(Borden)	1″ x 1″ x 1″ piece (.8 oz.)	71	2.5
(Borden) grated	1 oz.	129	8.4
(Fisher)	1 oz.	90	2.0
(Kraft) slices	1 oz.	94	2.4
(Pauly)	.8-oz. slice	74	1.6
Cheez 'n Bacon (Kraft)	¾-oz. slice	76	.8
Cheez 'n Crackers, process (Kraft)	1 piece (1.1 oz.)	127	9.3
Cheez-ola (Fisher) process	1 oz.	90	.5
Links (Kraft) *Handi-Snack:*			
Bacon	1 oz.	93	2.2
Jalapeño	1 oz.	92	2.2
Nippy	1 oz.	92	2.2
Smokelle	1 oz.	93	2.2
Swiss	1 oz.	90	1.4
Loaf, *Count-Down* (Fisher)	1 oz.	40	3.0
Mun-chee (Pauly) chunk	1 oz.	100	2.0
Munst-ett (Kraft)	1 oz.	100	1.7
Pimiento (Borden)	1 oz.	91	2.0
Pimiento (Pauly)	.8-oz. slice	73	.8
Pizzalone loaf (Kraft)	1 oz.	90	.5
Salami, slices (Kraft)	1 oz.	94	2.6
Sharp (Pauly)	1-oz. slice	100	.8
Super blend loaf (Kraft)	1 oz.	92	1.6
Swiss (Borden) cold pack	.7-oz. slice	62	1.1
Swiss, slices (Kraft)	1 oz.	92	2.3
Swiss (Pauly)	.8-oz. slice	74	1.6

Food and Description	Measure or Quantity	Calories	Carbo-hydrates (grams)
CHEESE PIE (Tastykake)	4-oz. pie	357	51.2
CHEESE PUFF, frozen (Durkee)	1 piece (.5 oz.)	59	3.0
CHEESE SOUFFLÉ:			
Home recipe (USDA)	¼ of 7″ soufflé (3.9 oz.)	240	6.8
Frozen (Stouffer's)	⅛ of 12-oz. pkg.	243	11.7
CHEESE SPREAD:			
American, process:			
(USDA)	1 T. (.5 oz.)	50	1.1
(Borden)	.7 oz.	57	1.5
(Fisher)	1 oz.	80	2.0
(Kraft)	1 oz.	78	1.9
(Nabisco) *Snack Mate*	1 tsp. (6 grams)	15	.3
Bacon (Borden) cheese & bacon	1 oz.	72	1.8
Bacon (Kraft) process	1 oz.	64	.5
Cheddar (Nabisco) *Snack Mate*	1 tsp. (6 grams)	15	.3
Cheese & bacon (Nabisco) *Snack Mate*	1 tsp. (6 grams)	15	.3
Cheez Whiz (Kraft) process	1 oz.	78	1.8
Chive & green onion (Nabisco) *Snack Mate*	1 tsp. (6 grams)	15	.3
Count Down (Fisher)	1 oz.	30	3.0
Garlic (Borden) process	1 oz.	72	1.8
Garlic (Kraft) process, *Swankyswig*	1 oz.	86	1.8
Imitation (Fisher) *Chef's Delight*	1 oz.	40	3.0
Imitation (Kraft) *Calorie-Wise*	1 oz.	48	3.6
Jalapeño (Kraft) *Cheez Whiz*	1 oz.	76	1.9
Limburger (Kraft)	1 oz.	69	.4

(USDA): United States Department of Agriculture
(HEW/FAO): Health, Education and Welfare/Food and Agriculture
         Organization
* Prepared as Package Directs

Food and Description	Measure or Quantity	Calories	Carbohydrates (grams)
Neufchâtel:			
(Borden) olive & pimiento	1 T. (.5 oz.)	36	1.8
(Borden) pineapple	1 T. (.5 oz.)	36	1.8
(Kraft) bacon & horseradish *Party Snacks*	1 oz.	74	.7
(Kraft) chipped beef, *Party Snacks*	1 oz.	67	1.2
(Kraft) chive, *Party Snacks*	1 oz.	69	.8
(Kraft) clam, *Party Snacks*	1 oz.	67	.8
(Kraft) Jalapeño peppers	1 oz.	68	2.2
(Kraft) olive & pimiento	1 oz.	68	1.9
(Kraft) onion, *Party Snacks*	1 oz.	66	1.6
(Kraft) pimiento	1 oz.	68	2.3
(Kraft) pineapple	1 oz.	70	3.0
(Kraft) relish	1 oz.	72	3.2
Old English (Kraft) sharp	1 oz.	85	.5
Pimiento:			
(Borden) *Country Store*	1 T. (.5 oz.)	36	1.7
(Kraft) *Cheez Whiz*	1 oz.	76	1.7
(Kraft) *Squeez-a-Snak*	1 oz.	86	.6
(Nabisco) *Snack Mate*	1 tsp. (.5 oz.)	15	.3
(Pauly)	¾-oz.	66	.9
Sharp (Kraft) *Squeez-a-Snak*	1 oz.	85	.6
Sharp (Pauly)	.8-oz.	77	.9
Sharpie (Kraft) process	1 oz.	90	.5
Smoke (Kraft) *Squeez-a-Snack*	1 oz.	83	4.8
Smokelle Swankyswig (Kraft) process	1 oz.	90	.5
Smokey cheese (Borden)	1 oz.	72	1.8
Swiss (Pauly) process	.8-oz.	76	1.2
Velva Kreme (Borden)	1 oz.	94	1.1
Velveeta (Kraft) process	1 oz.	85	2.5
CHEESE STRAW:			
(USDA)	5″ x ⅜″ x ⅜″ piece (6 grams)	27	2.1
(Durkee)	1 piece	29	1.0

Food and Description	Measure or Quantity	Calories	Carbohydrates (grams)
CHELOIS WINE (Great Western) 12% alcohol	3 fl. oz.	70	2.2
CHEESE & TOMATO PIE, frozen (Weight Watchers):			
1 pie	6-oz. pie	386	37.2
1 pie	7-oz. pie	450	43.4
CHENIN BLANC WINE:			
(Inglenook) Estate, 12% alcohol	3 fl. oz. (2.9 oz.)	60	1.3
(Louis M. Martini) dry, 12½% alcohol	3 fl. oz.	90	.2
CHERI SUISSE, Swiss liqueur (Leroux) 60 proof	1 fl. oz.	90	10.2
CHERRY:			
Sour:			
Fresh (USDA):			
Whole	1 lb. (weighed with stems)	213	52.5
Whole	1 lb. (weighed without stems)	242	59.7
Pitted	½ cup (2.7 oz.)	45	11.0
Canned, syrup pack, pitted (USDA):			
Light syrup	4 oz. (with liq.)	84	21.2
Heavy syrup	½ cup (with liq.)	116	29.5
Extra heavy syrup	4 oz. (with liq.)	127	32.4
Canned, water pack, pitted, solids & liq. (USDA)	½ cup (4.3 oz.)	52	13.1
Frozen, pitted (USDA):			
Sweetened	½ cup (4.6 oz.)	146	36.1
Unsweetened	4 oz.	62	15.2

(USDA): United States Department of Agriculture
(HEW/FAO): Health, Education and Welfare/Food and Agriculture
           Organization
* Prepared as Package Directs

Food and Description	Measure or Quantity	Calories	Carbohydrates (grams)
Sweet:			
Fresh (USDA):			
Whole	1 lb. (weighed with stems)	286	71.0
Whole, with stems	½ cup (2.3 oz.)	41	10.2
Pitted	½ cup (2.9 oz.)	57	14.3
Canned, syrup pack:			
Light syrup, pitted (USDA)	4 oz. (with liq.)	74	18.7
Heavy syrup, pitted (USDA)	½ cup (with liq., 4.2 oz.)	96	24.2
Extra heavy syrup, pitted (USDA)	4 oz. (with liq.)	113	29.0
(Del Monte) sweet, solids & liq.	½ cup (4.3 oz.)	106	25.2
(Del Monte) Royal Anne, solids & liq.	½ cup (4.3 oz.)	111	26.8
(Stokely-Van Camp) sweet, pitted, solids & liq.	½ cup (4.2 oz.)	50	11.0
Canned, dietetic or water pack:			
(Cellu) light, sweet, water pack, solids & liq.	½ cup	48	11.0
(Diet Delight) Royal Anne, solids & liq.	½ cup	73	16.9
CHERRY, BLACK, SYRUP, dietetic (No-Cal)	1 tsp.	0	0.
CHERRY BRANDY (DeKuyper) 70 proof	1 fl. oz. (1.1 oz.)	85	6.9
CHERRY, CANDIED (USDA)	1 oz.	96	24.6
CHERRY DRINK:			
(Ann Page)	1 cup (8.7 oz.)	124	30.9
(Hi-C)	6 fl. oz. (6.3 oz.)	93	23.0
*Mix (Wyler's)	6 fl. oz.	64	15.8

Food and Description	Measure or Quantity	Calories	Carbo-hydrates (grams)
CHERRY EXTRACT:			
(Ehlers) imitation	1 tsp.	16	
CHERRY HEERING, Danish liqueur, 49 proof	1 fl. oz.	80	10.0
CHERRY JELLY:			
Sweetened (Smucker's)	1 T. (.7 oz.)	53	13.5
Dietetic or low calorie:			
(Featherweight)	1 T.	18	4.0
(Slenderella)	1 T.	24	6.2
(Smucker's)	1 T.	5	1.2
CHERRY KARISE, liqueur (Leroux) 49 proof	1 fl. oz.	71	7.6
CHERRY KIJAFA, Danish wine, 17.5% alcohol	3 fl. oz.	148	15.3
CHERRY LIQUEUR:			
(Bols) 60 proof	1 fl. oz.	96	8.9
(DeKuyper) 50 proof	1 fl. oz.	75	8.5
(Hiram Walker) 60 proof	1 fl. oz.	82	8.2
(Leroux) 60 proof	1 fl. oz.	80	7.6
CHERRY, MARASCHINO			
(Liberty)	1 average cherry	8	1.9
CHERRY PIE:			
Home recipe, 2 crusts			
(USDA)	⅛ of 9″ pie		
	(5.6 oz.)	412	60.7
(Drake's)	2-oz. pie	203	26.3
(Hostess)	4½-oz. pie	435	58.8
(Tastykake) cherry-apple	4-oz. pie	373	56.8
Frozen:			
(Banquet)	⅛ of 20-oz. pie	228	33.8
(Morton)	⅙ of 24-oz. pie	300	42.0

(USDA): United States Department of Agriculture
(HEW/FAO): Health, Education and Welfare/Food and Agriculture
       Organization
* Prepared as Package Directs

Food and Description	Measure or Quantity	Calories	Carbohydrates (grams)
(Morton) mini pie	8-oz. pie	589	86.4
Tart (Pepperidge Farm)	3-oz. trat	277	34.3
CHERRY PIE FILLING:			
(Comstock)	1 cup (10¾-oz.)	334	84.6
(Lucky Leaf)	8 oz.	242	58.2
(Wilderness)	21-oz. can	720	168.3
CHERRY PRESERVE:			
Sweetened (Bama)	1 T. (.7 oz.)	54	13.5
Dietetic or low calorie:			
(Dia-Mel)	1 tsp.	2	0.
(Louis Sherry)	1 T. (.5 oz.)	2	0.
CHERRY TURNOVER, refrigerated (Pillsbury)	1 turnover	180	25.2
CHERRY WINE (Mogen David) 12% alcohol	3 fl. oz.	126	16.9
CHERVIL, raw (USDA)	1 oz.	16	3.3
CHESTNUT (USDA)			
Fresh, in shell	1 lb. (weighed in shell)	713	154.7
Fresh, shelled	4 oz.	220	47.7
Dried, in shell	1 lb. (weighed in shell)	1402	292.4
Dried, shelled	4 oz.	428	89.1
CHESTNUT FLOUR (See FLOUR, CHESTNUT)			
CHEWING GUM:			
Sweetened:			
(USDA)	1 piece (3 grams)	10	2.9
Bazooka, bubble, 1¢ size	1 piece	18	4.5
Bazooka, bubble, 5¢ size	1 piece	85	21.2
Beechies	1 tablet (2 grams)	6	1.6
Beech-Nut	1 stick (3 grams)	10	2.3
Beemans	1 stick	9	2.3
Big Red	1 stick	10	2.3
Black Jack	1 stick	9	2.3

Food and Description	Measure or Quantity	Calories	Carbo- hydrates (grams)
Chiclets	5¢ pkg.	65	
Chiclets, tiny size	1 piece	6	1.1
Cinnamint	1 stick	10	2.3
Clove	1 stick	9	2.3
Dentyne	1 piece	4	1.2
Doublemint	1 stick (3 grams)	10	2.3
Freedent	1 stick	10	2.3
Fruit Punch	1 stick	10	2.3
Juicy Fruit	1 stick (3 grams)	10	2.3
Orbit	1 stick	8	
Peppermint (Clark)	1 piece	10	2.3
Sour (Warner-Lambert)	1 stick	10	
Sour lemon (Clark)	1 stick	10	2.3
Spearmint (Wrigley's)	1 stick (3 grams)	10	2.3
Teaberry	1 stick	10	2.3
Unsweetened or dietetic:			
Bazooka, bubble, sugarless	1 piece	16	Tr.
*Care*Free* (Beech-Nut)	1 stick (3 grams)	7	Tr.
(Clark) all flavors	1 stick	7	1.7
(Estee) all flavors	1 section	4	.8
(Estee) bubble	1 piece (1 gram)	4	.9
(Harvey's)	1 stick	4	1.0
Peppermint (Amurol)	1 stick	5	1.8
Sug'r Like, all flavors	1 piece	4	.6

CHIANTI WINE:

(Antinori):			
Classico, 12½ % alcohol	3 fl. oz.	87	6.3
1955, 12½ % alcohol	3 fl. oz.	87	6.3
Vintage, 12½ % alcohol	3 fl. oz.	87	6.3
Brolio Classico, 13% alcohol	3 fl. oz.	66	.3
(Gancia) Classico, 12½ % al- cohol	3 fl. oz.	75	
(Italian Swiss Colony) 13% alcohol	3 fl. oz. (2.9 oz.)	83	2.9
(Louis M. Martini) 12½ % al- cohol	3 fl. oz.	90	.2

(USDA): United States Department of Agriculture
(HEW/FAO): Health, Education and Welfare/Food and Agriculture
     Organization
* Prepared as Package Directs

Food and Description	Measure or Quantity	Calories	Carbo-hydrates (grams)
CHICKEN (See also **CHICKEN, CANNED**): (USDA):			
Broiler, cooked, meat only	4 oz.	154	0.
Capon, raw, with bone	1 lb. (weighed ready-to-cook)	937	0.
Fryer:			
Raw:			
Ready-to-cook	1 lb. (weighed ready-to-cook)	382	0.
Breast	1 lb. (weighed with bone)	394	0.
Leg or drumstick	1 lb. (weighed with bone)	313	0.
Thigh	1 lb. (weighed with bone)	435	0.
Fried. A 2½-lb. chicken (Weighed before cooking with bone) will give you:			
Back	1 back (2.2 oz.)	139	2.7
Breast	½ breast (3⅛ oz.)	154	1.1
Leg or drumstick	1 leg (2 oz.)	87	.4
Neck	1 neck (2.1 oz.)	121	1.9
Rib	1 rib (.7 oz.)	42	.8
Thigh	1 thigh (2¼ oz.)	118	1.2
Wing	1 wing (1¾ oz.)	78	.8
Fried skin	1 oz.	119	2.6
Hen and cock:			
Raw	1 lb. (weighed ready-to-cook)	987	0.
Stewed:			
Meat only	4 oz.	236	0.
Chopped	½ cup (2.5 oz.)	150	0.
Diced	½ cup (2.4 oz.)	139	0.
Ground	½ cup (2 oz.)	116	0.
Roaster:			
Raw	1 lb. (weighed ready-to-cook)	791	0.
Roasted:			
Dark meat without skin	4 oz.	209	0.

Food and Description	Measure or Quantity	Calories	Carbo-hydrates (grams)
Light meat without skin	4 oz.	206	0.
CHICKEN A LA KING:			
Home recipe (USDA)	1 cup (8.6 oz.)	468	12.3
Canned:			
(College Inn)	5-oz. serving	150	4.0
(Richardson & Robbins)	1 cup (7.9 oz.)	272	14.4
(Swanson)	½ of 10½-oz. can	190	9.0
Frozen:			
(Banquet) cooking bag	5-oz. bag	138	10.4
(Green Giant) *Toast Topper*	5-oz. serving	170	8.0
CHICKEN BOUILLON/BROTH, cube or powder (See also **CHICKEN SOUP):**			
(Croyden House)	1 tsp. (5 grams)	12	2.5
(Herb-Ox)	1 cube (4 grams)	6	.6
(Herb-Ox)	1 packet (5 grams)	12	1.9
*(Knorr Swiss)	6 fl. oz.	13	
(Maggi)	1 cube	7	1.0
MBT	1 packet (.2 oz.)	12	2.0
(Steero)	1 cube (4 grams)	6	.4
(Wyler's)	1 cube	6	.7
(Wyler's) instant	1 envelope (4 grams)	8	.9
(Wyler's) no salt added	1 cube (4 grams)	11	1.6
CHICKEN CACCIATORE			
(Hormel)	1-lb. can	386	8.2
CHICKEN, CANNED:			
Boned:			
(USDA)	½ cup (3 oz.)	168	0.
(College Inn)	4 oz.	299	0.

(USDA): United States Department of Agriculture
(HEW/FAO): Health, Education and Welfare/Food and Agriculture Organization
* Prepared as Package Directs

Food and Description	Measure or Quantity	Calories	Carbo-hydrates (grams)
(Lynden Farms) solids & liq.	5-oz. jar	229	0.
(Swanson) chunk white	5-oz. can	220	0.
(Swanson) with broth	5-oz. can	220	0.
Whole (Lynden Farms)	52-oz. can	1170	0.
CHICKEN CROQUETTE DINNER, frozen (Morton)	10¼-oz. dinner	413	46.5
CHICKEN DINNER:			
Canned:			
(College Inn) & dumplings	5-oz. serving	170	12.0
(Lynden Farms) & noodle	12-oz. jar	413	31.8
(Lynden Farms) & noodle with vegetables	15-oz. can	434	38.2
(Swanson) & dumplings	7½-oz. can	230	18.0
Frozen:			
(Banquet):			
& dumplings, buffet	2-lb. bag	1209	128.2
& dumplings, dinner	12-oz. dinner	282	36.4
Fried	11-oz. dinner	530	48.4
Man Pleaser	17-oz. dinner	1026	89.2
& noodles	12-oz. dinner	374	50.7
(Morton):			
Boneless	10-oz. dinner	234	22.8
Country Table	15-oz. dinner	682	94.8
& dumplings	11-oz. dinner	272	31.2
Fried	11-oz. dinner	462	50.0
& noodles	10¼-oz. dinner	250	40.8
(Swanson):			
Boneless, *Hungry Man*	19-oz. dinner	730	74.0
Fried	11½-oz. dinner	570	28.0
Fried, barbecue-flavored	11¼-oz. dinner	530	47.0
Fried, *Hungry Man*	15¾-oz. dinner	910	78
Fried, barbecue-flavored, *Hungry Man*	16½-oz. dinner	766	72.0
Fried, crisp	10¾-oz. dinner	650	51.0
& noodle	10¼-oz. dinner	390	53.0
3-course	15-oz. dinner	630	64.0
(Weight Watchers):			
Creole style	13-oz. meal	256	11.8
Divan	9-oz. meal	251	7.9

Food and Description	Measure or Quantity	Calories	Carbohydrates (grams)
Chicken liver & onions	10½-oz. meal	210	11.0
Oriental style	15-oz. meal	346	32.0
With stuffing	16-oz. meal	411	36.8
White meat	9-oz. meal	291	13.0

CHICKEN & DUMPLINGS
(See **CHICKEN DINNER**)

CHICKEN ENTREE, frozen

(Green Giant) & biscuits, *Bake 'n Serve*	7-oz. entree	200	19.0
(Green Giant) & noodle, boil-in-bag	9-oz. bag	250	24.0
(Morton) fried, *Country Table*	12-oz. entree	583	27.3

CHICKEN FRICASSEE:

Home recipe (USDA)	1 cup (8.5 oz.)	386	7.7
Canned (Richardson & Robbins)	1 cup (7.9 oz.)	256	15.1

CHICKEN, FRIED, frozen:

(Banquet)	2-lb. pkg.	2591	117.3
(Swanson):			
Assorted pieces	3.2-oz. serving	260	10.0
Assorted pieces	16-oz. pkg.	1250	40.0
Assorted pieces	32-oz. pkg.	2600	100.0
Breast portion	3.2-oz. serving	250	8.0
Breast portion	32-oz. package	1719	55.0
Nibbler (wings)	3.2-oz. serving	290	12.0
Nibbler (wings)	28-oz. pkg.	2538	105.0
Thighs & drumsticks	3.2-oz. serving	260	7.0
Thighs & drumsticks	28-oz. pkg.	2275	55.7

CHICKEN GIZZARD (USDA):

Raw	2 oz.	64	.4
Simmered	2 oz.	84	.4

(USDA): United States Department of Agriculture
(HEW/FAO): Health, Education and Welfare/Food and Agriculture Organization
* Prepared as Package Directs

Food and Description	Measure or Quantity	Calories	Carbo-hydrates (grams)
CHICKEN LIVER (See LIVER)			
CHICKEN LIVER, CHOPPED (Mrs. Kornberg's)	6-oz. pkg.	260	
CHICKEN LIVER PUFF, frozen (Durkee)	1 piece	48	3.0
CHICKEN & NOODLES:			
Home recipe (USDA)	1 cup (8.5 oz.)	367	25.7
Canned (College Inn)	5-oz. serving	170	17.0
Frozen (Banquet) buffet	2-lb. pkg.	764	79.1
CHICKEN PARMIGIANA, frozen (Weight Watchers)	9-oz. meal	184	8.9
CHICKEN PIE:			
Home recipe, baked (USDA)	8-oz. pie (4¼" dia.)	533	41.5
Frozen:			
(Banquet)	8-oz. pie	427	39.0
(Morton)	8-oz. pie	384	31.9
(Swanson)	8-oz. pie	450	44.0
(Swanson) *Hungry Man*	16-oz. pie	780	66.0
CHICKEN PUFF, frozen (Durkee)	1 piece	49	3.0
CHICKEN RAVIOLI (Lynden Farms)	14½-oz. can	452	74.0
CHICKEN SALAD (Carnation)	1½-oz.	94	2.6
CHICKEN SOUP:			
Canned, regular pack: (USDA):			
Consommé, condensed	8 oz. (by wt.)	41	3.4
*Consommé, prepared with equal volume water	1 cup (8.5 oz.)	22	1.9

Food and Description	Measure or Quantity	Calories	Carbohydrates (grams)
Cream of, condensed	8 oz. (by wt.)	179	15.2
*Cream of, prepared with equal volume milk	1 cup (8.6 oz.)	179	14.5
*Cream of, prepared with equal volume water	1 cup (8.5 oz.)	94	7.9
Gumbo, condensed	8 oz. (by wt.)	104	13.8
*Gumbo, prepared with equal volume water	1 cup (8.5 oz.)	55	7.4
& noodle, condensed	8 oz. (by wt.)	120	15.0
*& noodle, prepared with equal volume water	1 cup (8.5 oz.)	65	8.2
& rice, condensed	8 oz. (by wt.)	89	10.7
*& rice, prepared with equal volume water	1 cup (8.5 oz.)	48	5.8
& vegetable, condensed	8 oz. (by wt.)	141	17.5
*& vegetable, prepared with equal volume water	1 cup (8.6 oz.)	76	9.6
(Ann Page):			
*Cream of	1 cup	104	9.3
*& noodle	1 cup	66	8.7
*& *Noodle-O's* style	1 cup	47	1.4
*& rice	1 cup	47	1.4
*& stars	1 cup	56	7.4
*& vegetable	1 cup	75	8.6
(Campbell):			
*Alphabet	8-oz. serving	88	12.0
*Broth	8-oz. serving	40	2.4
Chunky	10¾-oz. can	230	22.0
Cream of	8-oz. serving	102	8.0
*& dumplings	8-oz. serving	96	5.6
*Gumbo	8-oz serving	56	8.0
*& noodle	8-oz. serving	72	8.8
& noodle, *Soup For One*	7¾-oz. can	120	14.0
Noodle-O's	8-oz. serving	72	9.6

(USDA): United States Department of Agriculture
(HEW/FAO): Health, Education and Welfare/Food and Agriculture
Organization
* Prepared as Package Directs

Food and Description	Measure or Quantity	Calories	Carbo- hydrates (grams)
& rice, *Chunky*	19-oz. can	320	32.0
*with stars	8-oz. serving	64	7.2
*& vegetables	8-oz. serving	72	8.0
& vegetables, *Chunky*	10¾-oz. can	150	25.0
(College Inn) broth	1 cup	30	.1
(Lynden Farms) broth	1 cup (8 oz.)	14	0.
(Manischewitz):			
*Barley	8 oz. (by wt.)	83	12.3
*With kasha	1 cup	41	5.4
*& noodle	1 cup (8.1 oz.)	46	4.2
*& rice	8 oz. (by wt.)	47	5.3
*& vegetable	1 cup	55	7.8
(Progresso):			
With escarole	8-oz. serving	25	1.0
Chickarina	8-oz. serving	100	8.0
(Richardson & Robbins):			
Broth	1 cup (8.1 oz.)	32	1.6
Broth with rice	1 cup (8.1 oz.)	48	5.0
(Swanson) broth	½ of 13¾-oz. can	28	2.0
Canned, dietetic or low calorie:			
(Campbell) low sodium, *Chunky*	7¾-oz. can	170	13.0
(Claybourne) broth	8-oz. serving	9	0.
*(Dia-Mel) broth	8-oz. serving	18	1.0
*(Dia-Mel) & noodle	8-oz. serving	50	7.0
(Featherweight) & noodle, low sodium	8-oz. can	120	16.0
(Slim-ette) broth	8-oz. can	7	1.0
Mix:			
(Ann Page) & noodle	2-oz. pkg.	203	28.6
(Lipton):			
*Broth, *Cup-a-Broth*	6 fl. oz.	25	3.0
*Cream of, *Cup-a-Soup*	1 pkg.	80	10.0
Giggle Noodle	1 cup	80	12.0
Giggle Noodle, Cup-a-Soup	6 fl. oz.	40	8.0
*& noodle with broth	1 cup	60	8.0
*& noodle with meat	1 cup	70	9.0
& noodle with meat, Cup-a-Soup	6 fl. oz.	45	6.0
*& rice	1 cup	60	8.0
*& rice, *Cup-a-Soup*	6 fl. oz.	50	9.0

Food and Description	Measure or Quantity	Calories	Carbo-hydrates (grams)
*Ring-o-Noodle	1 cup	50	9.0
*Ring-o-Noodle, Cup-a-Soup	6 fl. oz.	50	9.0
*Ripple Noodle	1 cup	80	12.0
*& vegetable, Cup-a-Soup	6 fl. oz.	40	7.0
*(Nestlé) cream of, Souptime	6 fl. oz.	100	8.0
*(Nestlé) & noodle, Souptime	6 fl. oz.	30	4.0
(Wyler's) cream of	1 pkg. (.8 oz.)	93	14.7
*(Wyler's) & rice	6 fl. oz.	49	8.6
CHICKEN SPREAD:			
(Swanson)	5-oz. can	350	5.0
(Underwood)	1 oz.	63	1.1
CHICKEN STEW:			
Canned, regular pack:			
(B&M)	1 cup (7.9 oz.)	128	15.3
(Bounty)	7½-oz. can	175	17.5
(Libby's) with dumplings	⅓ of 24-oz. can	200	20.2
(Swanson)	½ of 15¼-oz. can	182	18.2
Canned, dietetic or low calorie:			
(Dia-Mel)	8-oz. can	150	19.0
(Featherweight)	7¼-oz. can	160	21.0
CHICKEN STOCK BASE			
(French's)	1 tsp. (3 grams)	8	1.0
CHICKEN TAMALE PIE, canned (Lynden Farms)	½ tamale pie with sauce (3.8 oz.)	143	12.0
CHICK PEAS or GARBANZOS, dry (USDA)	1 cup (7.1 oz.)	720	122.0

(USDA): United States Department of Agriculture
(HEW/FAO): Health, Education and Welfare/Food and Agriculture Organization
* Prepared as Package Directs

Food and Description	Measure or Quantity	Calories	Carbo-hydrates (grams)
CHICORY GREENS, raw (USDA):			
Untrimmed	½ lb. (weighed untrimmed)	37	7.0
Trimmed	4 oz.	23	4.3
CHICORY, WITLOOF, Belgian or French endive, raw, bleached head (USDA):			
Untrimmed	½ lb. (weighed untrimmed)	30	6.4
Trimmed, cut	½ cup (.9 oz.)	4	.8
CHILI or CHILI CON CARNE:			
Canned, beans only:			
(Gebhardt) spiced	1 cup	184	
(Van Camp) Mexican style	1 cup	250	43.0
Canned, with beans:			
(USDA)	1 cup (8.8 oz.)	339	31.1
(A&P)	½ of 15-oz. can	404	28.3
(Armour Star)	15½-oz. can	692	59.3
(Austex)	15½-oz. can	584	53.6
(Bounty)	7¾-oz. can	310	29.3
(Hormel)	7½-oz. can	320	23.6
(Libby's)	½ of 15-oz. can	379	10.7
(Morton House)	7½-oz. can	340	27.0
(Rosarita)	8-oz. can	376	27.2
(Swanson)	½ of 15½-oz. can	310	28.0
Canned, dietetic or low sodium:			
Dietetic (Dia-Mel)	8-oz. can	360	31.0
Low sodium (Campbell)	7¾-oz. can	310	30.0
Low sodium (Featherweight)	8-oz. can	300	26.0
Canned, without beans:			
(USDA)	1 cup (9 oz.)	510	14.8
(Armour Star)	15½-oz. can	835	25.5
(Austex)	15-oz. can	851	24.7
(Bunker Hill)	10¼-oz. can	657	
(Chef-Boy-Ar-Dee)	½ of 15¼-oz. can	328	14.0

Food and Description	Measure or Quantity	Calories	Carbo- hydrates (grams)
(Hormel)	½ of 15-oz can	340	7.6
(Libby's)	½ of 15-oz. can	276	32.2
(Morton House)	½ of 15-oz. can	340	14.0
(Nalley's)	8 oz.	311	12.9
(Rutherford)	8 oz.	447	
CHILI BEEF SOUP, canned:			
*(Campbell)	8-oz. serving	152	19.2
(Campbell) *Chunky*	11-oz. can	300	37.0
*CHILI CON CARNE MIX			
(Durkee)	1 cup	463	31.1
CHILI SAUCE:			
(USDA)	1 T. (.5 oz.)	16	3.7
(USDA) low sodium	1 T. (.5 oz.)	16	3.7
(Hunt's)	1 T. (.6 oz.)	19	4.9
Dietetic (Featherweight)	1 T. (.5 oz.)	8	1.5
CHILI SEASONING MIX:			
(Ann Page)	1¾-oz. pkg.	147	29.8
(Durkee)	1.7-oz. pkg.	148	33.0
*(Durkee)	1 cup	465	31.3
(French's) *Chili-O*	1¾-oz. pkg.	150	30.0
(Lawry's)	1.6-oz. pkg.	137	23.6
CHINESE DATE (See JUJUBE)			
CHINESE DINNER, frozen:			
Beef chop suey (Chun King)	11-oz. dinner	310	46.0
Chicken chow mein (Banquet)	12-oz. dinner	282	38.8
CHIPS (See POTATO CHIPS and CRACKERS, Corn Chips)			

(USDA): United States Department of Agriculture
(HEW/FAO): Health, Education and Welfare/Food and Agriculture
          Organization
* Prepared as Package Directs

Food and Description	Measure or Quantity	Calories	Carbo-hydrates (grams)
CHITTERLINGS, canned (Hormel)	1-lb., 2-oz. can	832	.5
CHIVES, raw (USDA)	½ lb.	64	13.2
CHOCO-DILES (Hostess)	1 piece (2.2 oz.)	259	37.5
CHOCOLATE, BAKING:			
Bitter or unsweetened:			
(Baker's)	1 oz. (1 sq.)	140	9.0
(Baker's) *Redi Blend*	1-oz. square	140	8.0
(Hershey's)	1 oz.	188	7.0
Sweetened:			
Chips, semisweet (Ghirardelli)	⅛ cup (2 oz.)	299	35.6
Chips, dark (Hershey's)	¼ cup (1.5 oz.)	226	26.6
Chips, milk (Hershey's)	¼ cup (1.5 oz.)	222	27.3
Chips, mini, semisweet (Hershey's)	¼ cup (1.5 oz.)	210	23.0
Choco-Bake (Nestlé)	1 oz.	170	12.0
German's (Baker's)	1 oz.	140	17.0
Morsels, semisweet (Nestlé)	1 oz.	150	18.0
Semisweet (Baker's)	1 oz.	130	17.0
CHOCOLATE CAKE (See CAKE, Chocolate)			
CHOCOLATE CAKE MIX (See CAKE MIX, Chocolate)			
CHOCOLATE CANDY (See Candy)			
CHOCOLATE DRINK, canned (Borden)	9½-fl.-oz. can	251	36.7
CHOCOLATE DRINK MIX:			
(USDA) hot	1 cup (4.9 oz.)	545	102.7
(USDA) hot	1 oz.	111	21.0
(Borden) Dutch, instant	2 heaping tsps.	87	18.9
(Ghirardelli) instant	1 T. (.4 oz.)	48	10.5

Food and Description	Measure or Quantity	Calories	Carbo-hydrates (grams)
Quik	2 heaping tsps.	56	14.4
*(Sealtest) dry	1 cup	180	24.0
CHOCOLATE EXTRACT, imitation (Ehlers)	1 tsp.	10	
CHOCOLATE, GROUND (Ghirardelli)	¼ cup	163	30.4
CHOCOLATE, HOT, home recipe (USDA)	1 cup (8.8 oz.)	238	26.0
CHOCOLATE ICE CREAM (See also individual brands):			
(Borden) 9.5% fat	¼ pt. (2.3 oz.)	126	16.9
(Dean) 11.7% fat	1 cup (5.6 oz.)	352	38.4
(Meadow Gold) 10% fat	¼ pt.	128	16.5
(Prestige) French	¼ pt. (2.6 oz.)	182	18.0
(Sealtest)	¼ pt. (2.3 oz.)	140	17.0
(Swift's) sweet cream	½ cup (2.3 oz.)	129	15.8
CHOCOLATE PIE:			
Home recipe (USDA) chiffon	⅙ of 9" pie (4.9 oz.)	459	61.2
Home recipe (USDA) meringue	⅙ of 9" pie (4.9 oz.)	533	46.9
(Tastykake) nut	4½-oz. pie	451	64.3
Frozen:			
(Banquet) cream	⅙ of 14-oz. pie	177	21.8
(Kraft) velvet nut	⅙ of 16¾-oz. pie	303	30.4
(Morton)	⅙ of 16-oz. pie	199	22.8
(Morton) mini pie	3½-oz. pie	266	28.8
Tart (Pepperidge Farm)	3-oz. pie tart	306	35.2
***CHOCOLATE PIE MIX,** cream (Pillsbury) *No Bake*	⅙ of pie	410	53.0

(USDA): United States Department of Agriculture

(HEW/FAO): Health, Education and Welfare/Food and Agriculture Organization

* Prepared as Package Directs

Food and Description	Measure or Quantity	Calories	Carbo-hydrates (grams)
CHOCOLATE PUDDING or PIE FILLING:			
Home recipe, sweetened (USDA) with starch base	½ cup (4.6 oz.)	192	33.4
Canned, regular pack:			
(Betty Crocker)	½ cup (5 oz.)	180	30.0
(Betty Crocker) fudge	½ cup (5 oz.)	180	30.0
(Del Monte)	5-oz. container	173	33.0
(Del Monte) fudge	5-oz. container	193	31.0
(Hunt's) *Snack Pack*	5-oz. can	180	24.0
(Hunt's) fudge, *Snack Pack*	5-oz. can	190	24.0
(Hunt's) mint, *Snack Pack*	5-oz. can	190	26.0
(Royal) *Dark 'n Sweet, Creamerino*	5-oz. container	250	39.0
(Royal) milk chocolate, *Creamerino*	5-oz. container	244	38.3
(Thank You)	½ cup	175	29.2
Chilled:			
(Breakstone) light	5-oz. container	256	35.5
(Breakstone) dark	5-oz. container	254	33.4
(Sanna) dark	4½-oz. container	191	28.6
(Sanna) light	4½-oz. container	198	30.4
Frozen (Rich's)	4½-oz. container	214	27.8
Mix:			
Sweetened, regular:			
(Ann Page)	¼ of 3⅝-oz. pkg.	102	23.7
*(Jell-O)	½ cup (5.2 oz.)	170	29.0
*(Jell-O) fudge	½ cup (5.2 oz.)	170	28.0
*(Jell-O) milk chocolate	½ cup (5.2 oz.)	170	29.0
*(My-T-Fine)	½ cup	133	28.0
*(My-T-Fine) almond	½ cup	169	27.0
*(My-T-Fine) fudge	½ cup (5 oz.)	151	27.0
*(Royal)	½ cup (5.1 oz.)	196	31.7
*(Royal) *Dark 'n Sweet*	½ cup (5.1 oz.)	195	30.7
Sweetened, instant:			
(Ann Page)	¼ of 4-oz. pkg.	110	25.6
*(Jell-O)	½ cup (5.4 oz.)	190	24.0
*(Jell-O) fudge	½ cup (5.4 oz.)	190	33.0
*(Royal)	½ cup (5.1 oz.)	194	31.8
*(Royal) *Dark 'n Sweet*	½ cup (5.1 oz.)	194	31.7

Food and Description	Measure or Quantity	Calories	Carbohydrates (grams)
*Dietetic or low calorie:			
(Dia-Mel)	4-oz. serving	60	8.2
(Estee)	½ cup	85	16.0
CHOCOLATE RENNET CUSTARD MIX (Junket):			
Powder:			
Dry	1 oz.	116	25.2
*With sugar	4 oz.	113	14.9
Tablet:			
Dry	1 tablet	1	.2
*With sugar	4 oz.	101	13.4
CHOCOLATE SYRUP:			
Sweetened:			
(USDA) fudge	1 T. (.7 oz.)	63	10.3
(USDA) thin type	1 T. (.7 oz.)	47	11.9
(Hershey's)	1 T. (.5 oz.)	37	8.3
(Smucker's)	1 T. (.6 oz.)	60	13.1
Dietetic or low calorie:			
(No-Cal)	1 tsp.	2	0.
(Slim-ette) Choco-top	1 T. (.5 oz.)	9	1.6
CHOP SUEY:			
Home recipe with meat			
(USDA)	1 cup (8.8 oz.)	300	12.8
Canned:			
(USDA) with meat	1 cup (8.8 oz.)	155	10.5
(Hung's) chicken	8 oz.	120	12.3
(Hung's) meatless	8 oz.	112	11.2
(Mow Sang) pork	20-oz. can	167	14.0
Frozen (Banquet):			
Beef, buffet	2-lb. pkg.	418	39.1
Beef, cooking bag	7-oz. bag	73	9.5
Beef, dinner	12-oz. dinner	282	38.8
Mix:			
(Durkee)	1⅝-oz. pkg.	128	19.0
*(Durkee)	1¾ cups	557	21.0

(USDA): United States Department of Agriculture
(HEW/FAO): Health, Education and Welfare/Food and Agriculture Organization
* Prepared as Package Directs

Food and Description	Measure or Quantity	Calories	Carbo-hydrates (grams)
CHOW CHOW:			
Sour (USDA)	1 oz.	8	1.2
Sweet (USDA)	1 oz.	33	7.7
(Crosse & Blackwell)	1 T. (.6 oz.)	6	1.0
CHOW MEIN:			
Home recipe (USDA)			
chicken, without noodles	8 oz.	231	9.1
Canned:			
(USDA) without noodles	8 oz.	86	16.2
(Chun King) beef	1 cup	150	11.0
(Chun King) chicken	1 cup	100	11.2
(Chun King) pork, *Divider-Pak*	7-oz. serving (¼ cup)	160	11.0
(Hung's) chicken	8 oz.	104	10.4
(Hung's) meatless	8 oz.	96	8.8
(La Choy) beef	1 cup	77	4.0
(La Choy) chicken	1 cup	74	5.0
(La Choy) chicken, bi-pack	1 cup	118	8.0
Frozen:			
(Banquet) chicken, buffet	2-lb. pkg.	345	36.4
(Banquet) chicken, cooking bag	7-oz. bag	89	9.7
(Banquet) chicken dinner	12-oz. dinner	282	38.8
(Green Giant) chicken, without noodle	9-oz. entree	130	15.0
(Temple) shrimp	1 cup	132	15.0
(Temple) vegetable	1 cup	68	12.0
CHOW MEIN NOODLES (See **NOODLES, CHOW MEIN**)			
CHUB, raw (USDA):			
Whole	1 lb. (weighed whole)	217	0.
Meat only	4 oz.	164	0.
CHUTNEY			
Major Grey's (Crosse & Blackwell)	1 T. (.8 oz.)	53	13.1

Food and Description	Measure or Quantity	Calories	Carbohydrates (grams)
CIDER (See **APPLE CIDER**)			
CINNAMON, GROUND:			
(USDA)	1 tsp. (2.3 grams)	6	1.8
(French's)	1 tsp. (1.7 grams)	6	1.4
CINNAMON STICKS, frozen			
(Aunt Jemima)	3 pieces (1¾ oz.)	145	21.3
CITRON, CANDIED			
(Liberty)	1 oz.	93	22.6
CITRUS COOLER:			
(Ann Page)	1 cup (8.7 oz.)	118	29.4
(Hi-C)	6 fl. oz. (6.3 oz.)	93	23.0
CITRUS SALAD, canned (See **GRAPEFRUIT & ORANGE SECTIONS**)			
CLAM:			
Raw, hard or round:			
(USDA) meat & liq.	1 lb. (weighed in shell)	71	6.1
(USDA) meat only	1 cup (8 oz.)	182	13.4
Raw, soft (USDA) meat & liq.	1 lb. (weighed in shell)	142	5.3
Raw, soft (USDA) meat only	1 cup (8 oz.)	186	3.0
Canned, all kinds (Doxsee):			
Chopped, solids & liq.	4 oz.	66	
Chopped & minced, solids & liq.	4 oz.	59	3.2
Chopped, meat only	4 oz.	111	2.1
Steamed, meat & broth	1 pt. (8 fl. oz.)	152	
Steamed, meat only	1 pt. (8 fl. oz.)	66	
Whole	4 oz.	62	

(USDA): United States Department of Agriculture
(HEW/FAO): Health, Education and Welfare/Food and Agriculture Organization
* Prepared as Package Directs

Food and Description	Measure or Quantity	Calories	Carbohydrates (grams)
Frozen (Mrs. Paul's):			
Deviled	3-oz. piece	180	14.0
Fried	½ of 5-oz. pkg.	266	20.2
CLAMATO COCKTAIL (Mott's)	6 fl. oz.	80	19.0
CLAM CAKE, frozen, thins (Mrs. Paul's)	2½-oz. cake	155	16.0
CLAM CHOWDER:			
Manhattan, canned:			
*(Campbell)	8-oz. serving	80	12.0
(Campbell) *Chunky*	19-oz. can	320	46.0
(Crosse & Blackwell)	6½-oz. serving	61	12.9
*(Doxsee)	1 cup (8.6 oz.)	112	17.7
(Progresso)	1 cup (8 oz. by wt.)	100	16.0
(Snow)	8-oz. serving	87	10.4
New England, canned:			
*(Campbell)	8-oz. serving	80	10.4
(Crosse & Blackwell)	6½-oz. serving	101	10.3
*(Doxsee)	1 cup (8.6 oz.)	214	27.0
(Snow)	½ of 15-oz. can	129	18.3
CLAM COCKTAIL (Sau-Sea)	4 oz.	80	19.1
CLAM FRITTERS, home recipe (USDA)	1.4-oz. fritter (2″ x 1¾″)	124	12.4
CLAM JUICE, canned:			
(USDA)	1 cup (8.3 oz.)	45	5.0
(Doxsee)	8 oz.	54	
(Snow)	½ cup (4 fl. oz.)	15	1.2
CLAM SOUP MIX (Wyler's)	.8-oz. pkg.	112	12.6
CLAM STEW, frozen (Snow)	8 oz.	198	12.9
CLAM STICKS, frozen (Mrs. Paul's)	½ of 8-oz. pkg.	249	29.2

Food and Description	Measure or Quantity	Calories	Carbo-hydrates (grams)
CLARET WINE:			
(Gold Seal) 12% alcohol	3 fl. oz.	82	.4
(Inglenook) Navalle, 12% alcohol	3 fl. oz.	60	.3
(Louis M. Martini) 12.5% alcohol	3 fl. oz.	90	.2
(Taylor) 12.5% alcohol	3 fl. oz.	72	2.4
CLARISTINE LIQUEUR			
(Leroux) 86 proof	1 fl. oz.	114	10.8
CLORETS:			
Chewing gum	1 piece	6	1.3
Mint	1 piece	6	1.6
CLOVE, GROUND:			
(USDA)	1 tsp. (2.1 grams)	7	1.3
(French)	1 tsp. (1.7 grams)	7	1.2
CLUB SODA (See SOFT DRINK)			
COCKTAIL HOST COCKTAIL, liquid mix			
(Holland House)	1½ fl. oz.	70	18.0
COCOA:			
Dry:			
Low fat (USDA)	1 T. (5 grams)	10	3.1
Medium-low fat (USDA)	1 T. (5 grams)	12	2.9
Medium-high fat (USDA)	1 T. (5 grams)	14	2.8
High fat (USDA)	1 T.	16	2.6
Unsweetened (Droste)	1 T. (7 grams)	21	2.9
Unsweetened (Hershey's)	⅓ cup (1 oz.)	116	13.0
Unsweetened (Sultana)	1 T. (7 grams)	30	3.5
Home recipe (USDA)	1 cup (8.8 oz.)	242	27.2

(USDA): United States Department of Agriculture
(HEW/FAO): Health, Education and Welfare/Food and Agriculture Organization
* Prepared as Package Directs

Food and Description	Measure or Quantity	Calories	Carbohydrates (grams)
Mix:			
(Carnation) instant, & marshmallow	1-oz. pkg.	112	22.0
(Carnation) instant, milk chocolate	1-oz. pkg.	112	22.0
(Carnation) instant, rich chocolate	1-oz. pkg.	112	22.0
(Hershey's) hot	1-oz. packet	115	21.0
(Hershey's) instant	3 T. (¾ oz.)	77	17.0
(Kraft)	1 oz.	105	21.3
*(Kraft)	1 cup	129	26.5
(Nestlé) hot	1-oz. packet	110	22.1
(Nestlé) instant, *Quik*	3 heaping tsps. (.7 oz.)	70	19.0
(Nestlé) instant, *Quik,* strawberry	3 heaping tsps. (.7 oz.)	80	21.0
Swiss Miss, instant	1 oz.	103	20.0
(Ovaltine) hot	1-oz. pkg.	119	22.0
Low calorie (Ovaltine) hot	.5-oz. pkg.	54	8.0
COCOA KRISPIES, cereal			
(Kellogg's)	1 cup (1 oz.)	110	26.0
COCOA PUFFS, cereal			
(General Mills)	1 cup (1 oz.)	110	25.0
COCONUT:			
Fresh (USDA):			
Whole	1 lb. (weighed in shell)	816	22.2
Meat only	4 oz.	392	10.7
Meat only	2″ x 2″ x ½″ piece (1.6 oz.)	156	4.2
Grated or shredded, loosely packed	½ cup (1.4 oz.)	225	6.1
Dried, canned or packaged: (Baker's):			
Angel Flake	¼ cup (.7 oz.)	95	7.9
Cookie	¼ cup (1 oz.)	137	12.2
Premium shred	¼ cup (.8 oz.)	101	9.1
(Durkee) shredded	¼ cup	69	2.0

Food and Description	*Measure or Quantity*	*Calories*	*Carbo-hydrates (grams)*
COCONUT PIE:			
Home recipe (USDA) custard	⅙ of 9" pie (5.4 oz.)	357	37.8
(Tastykake) cream	⅙ of 14-oz. pie	467	48.4
Frozen:			
Baked (USDA)	5 oz. serving	354	41.9
Unbaked (USDA)	5 oz. serving	291	38.5
(Banquet):			
Cream	⅙ of 14-oz. pie	174	19.1
Custard	⅙ of 20-oz. pie	203	28.3
(Morton):			
Cream	¼ of 16-oz. pie	197	22.0
Cream, mini pie	3½-oz. pie	266	28.8
Custard, mini pie	6½-oz. pie	369	53.6
Tart (Pepperidge Farm)	3-oz. pie tart	310	29.0
COCONUT PIE FILLING MIX (Also see **COCONUT PUDDING MIX**):			
Custard & pie, dry (USDA)	1 oz.	133	20.0
*Custard, prepared with egg yolk or milk (USDA)	5-oz. (including crust)	288	41.3
COCONUT PUDDNG MIX:			
(Ann Page) cream	3⅛-oz. pkg.	400	72.4
(Ann Page) toasted, instant	3¼-oz. pkg.	384	79.9
*(Jell-O) cream, instant	½ cup (5.3 oz.)	190	28.0
*(Royal) toasted, instant	½ cup (5.1 oz.)	184	27.3
COCO WHEATS, cereal	3 T. (1.3 oz.)	139	28.5
COD:			
Raw, whole (USDA)	1 lb. (weighed whole)	110	0.
Raw, meat only (USDA)	4 oz.	88	0.
Broiled (USDA)	4 oz.	193	0.

(USDA): United States Department of Agriculture
(HEW/FAO): Health, Education and Welfare/Food and Agriculture Organization
* Prepared as Package Directs

Food and Description	Measure or Quantity	Calories	Carbohydrates (grams)
Canned (USDA)	4 oz.	96	0.
Dehydrated, lightly salted (USDA)	4 oz.	425	0.
Dried, salted (USDA)	5½″ x 1½″ x ½″ (2.8 oz.)	104	0.
Frozen:			
(Groton)	⅓ of 1-lb. pkg.	117	0.
(Ship Ahoy)	⅓ of 1-lb. pkg.	112	0.
COFFEE:			
Ground:			
*Max-Pax	6 fl. oz.	2	0.
*(Maxwell House) regular	6 fl. oz.	2	0.
*Maxwell House Electra-Perk	6 fl. oz.	2	0.
*(Yuban) regular	6 fl. oz.	2	0.
*Yuban Electra Matic	6 fl. oz.	2	0.
Instant:			
(USDA) dry	1 rounded tsp. (2 grams)	1	.3
*(USDA)	1 cup (8.4 oz.)	3	.9
(Borden)	1 rounded tsp. (2 grams)	5	.9
(Borden) Kava	1 tsp. (1 gram)	3	.5
*(Chase & Sanborn)	5 fl. oz.	1	Tr.
*(Maxwell House)	6 fl. oz.	4	1.0
Nescafé	1 slightly rounded tsp. (2 grams)	4	1.0
*(Yuban)	6 fl. oz.	4	1.0
Freeze-dried:			
*Maxim	6 fl. oz.	4	1.0
Taster's Choice	1 slightly rounded tsp. (2 grams)	4	1.0
Decaffeinated:			
*Brim, regular, drip or electric perk	6 fl. oz.	2	0.
*Brim, freeze-dried	6 fl. oz.	4	1.0
Decaf	1 tsp. (2 grams)	4	1.0
Nescafé, freeze-dried	1 slightly rounded tsp.	4	1.0
*Sanka, regular, electric perk	6 fl. oz.	2	0.

Food and Description	Measure or Quantity	Calories	Carbohydrates (grams)
*Sanka, freeze-dried or instant	6 fl. oz.	4	1.0
Taster's Choice, freeze-dried	1 slightly rounded tsp. (2 grams)	4	1.0
COFFEE CAKE (See CAKE, coffee)			
COFFEE ICE CREAM (Breyer's)	¼ pt.	140	15.0
COFFEE SOUTHERN, liqueur	1 fl. oz.	79	8.8
COGNAC (See DISTILLED LIQUOR)			
COLA SOFT DRINK (See SOFT DRINK)			
COLA SYRUP, dietetic (No-Cal)	1 tsp. (5 grams)	0	Tr.
COLD DUCK WINE:			
(Great Western) pink, 12% alcohol	3 fl. oz.	92	7.7
(Taylor) 12.5% alcohol	3 fl. oz.	90	6.6
COLESLAW, not drained (USDA):			
Prepared with commercial French dressing	4 oz.	108	8.6
Prepared with homemade French dressing	4 oz.	146	5.8
Prepared with mayonnaise	4 oz.	163	5.4
Prepared with mayonnaise-type salad dressing	1 cup (4.2 oz.)	118	8.5

(USDA): United States Department of Agriculture
(HEW/FAO): Health, Education and Welfare/Food and Agriculture Organization
* Prepared as Package Directs

Food and Description	Measure or Quantity	Calories	Carbo-hydrates (grams)
COLLARDS:			
Raw (USDA):			
Leaves including stems	1 lb.	181	32.7
Leaves only	½ lb.	70	11.6
Boiled, drained (USDA):			
Leaves, cooked in large amount of water	½ cup (3.4 oz.)	29	4.6
Leaves & stems, cooked in small amount of water	½ cup (3.4 oz.)	31	4.8
Frozen:			
(USDA) not thawed	10-oz. pkg.	91	16.4
(USDA) boiled, chopped, drained	½ cup (3 oz.)	26	4.8
(Birds Eye) chopped	⅓ of 10-oz. pkg.	30	4.0
COLLINS MIX (Bar-Tender's)	1 serving (⅝ oz.)	70	17.4
COLLINS MIXER (See SOFT DRINK, Tom Collins)			
CONCENTRATE, cereal (Kellogg's)	⅓ cup (1 oz.)	110	15.0
CONCORD WINE:			
(Gold Seal) 13-14% alcohol	3 fl. oz.	125	9.8
(Mogen David) 12% alcohol	3 fl. oz.	120	16.0
Red (Pleasant Valley) 12.5% alcohol	3 fl. oz.	90	
CONSOMMÉ MADRILENE, canned, clear or red (Crosse & Blackwell)	6½-oz. serving	33	2.4
COOKIE (listed by type or brand name. See also **COOKIE, DIETETIC, COOKIE DOUGH, COOKIE, HOME RECIPE** and **COOKIE MIX**):			
Almond toast, *Mandel* (Stella D'oro)	1 piece (.5 oz.)	49	9.6

Food and Description	Measure or Quantity	Calories	Carbo-hydrates (grams)
Angelica Goodies (Stella D'oro)	1 piece (.8 oz.)	100	14.6
Anginetti (Stella D'oro)	1 piece (5 grams)	28	2.4
Animal cracker:			
(USDA)	1 oz.	122	22.7
(Nabisco) *Barnum's*	1 piece (3 grams)	12	1.9
(Sunshine) regular	1 piece (2 grams)	10	1.7
(Sunshine) iced	1 piece (5 grams)	26	3.7
Anisette sponge (Stella D'oro)	1 piece (.5 oz.)	39	10.0
Anisette toast (Stella D'oro)	1 piece (.4 oz.)	39	7.8
Applesauce (Sunshine)	1 piece (.6 oz.)	86	11.9
Arrowroot (Sunshine)	1 piece (4 grams)	16	3.0
Apple strudel (Nabisco)	1 piece (.4 oz.)	48	6.8
Assortments:			
(USDA)	1 oz.	136	20.1
(Stella D'oro) *Lady Stella Assortment*	1 piece (8 grams)	37	5.0
(Sunshine) *Lady Joan*	1 piece (9 grams)	42	5.8
(Sunshine) *Lady Joan*, iced	1 piece (.4 oz.)	47	6.1
Aunt Sally, iced (Sunshine)	1 piece (.8 oz.)	96	19.7
Bana-Bee (Nab)	1 pkg. (1¾ oz.)	253	31.4
Big Treat (Sunshine)	1 piece (1.3 oz.)	153	26.6
Bordeaux (Pepperidge Farm)	1 piece (8 grams)	36	5.1
Breakfast Treats (Stella D'oro)	1 piece (.8 oz.)	99	15.0
Brown edge wafers (Nabisco)	1 piece (6 grams)	28	4.2
Brownie:			
(USDA) frozen, with nuts & chocolate icing	1 oz.	119	17.2
(Drake's) junior	⅔-oz. cake	80	10.0
(Frito-Lay's) nut fudge	1.8-oz. piece	200	34.0
(Hostess)	1¼-oz. piece	157	24.1
(Hostess)	2-oz. piece	251	38.6
(Keebler) pecan fudge	1 pkg. (1.8 oz.)	230	27.9

(USDA): United States Department of Agriculture
(HEW/FAO): Health, Education and Welfare/Food and Agriculture
                Organization
* Prepared as Package Directs

Food and Description	Measure or Quantity	Calories	Carbo-hydrates (grams)
(Keebler) pecan fudge, bulk	.9-oz. square	115	13.9
(Pepperidge Farm) chocolate nut	1 piece (.4 oz.)	54	6.3
(Tastykake)	1 pkg. (2¼ oz.)	242	34.0
(Tastykake) peanut butter	1 pkg. (1¾ oz.)	239	32.0
Brussels (Pepperidge Farm)	1 piece (8 grams)	42	4.6
Butter:			
(Nabisco)	1 piece (5 grams)	23	3.3
(Sunshine)	1 piece (5 grams)	23	3.5
Buttercup (Keebler)	1 piece (5 grams)	24	3.6
Butterscotch Fudgies (Tastykake)	1 pkg. (1¾ oz.)	251	35.0
Capri (Pepperidge Farm)	1 piece (.6 oz.)	82	9.7
Caramel peanut logs (Nabisco) *Hey Days*	1 piece (.8 oz.)	122	13.4
Cardiff (Pepperidge Farm)	1 piece (4 grams)	18	4.5
Cherry Coolers (Sunshine)	1 piece (6 grams)	29	4.5
Chinese almond (Stella D'oro)	1 piece (1.2 oz.)	178	21.5
Chocolate & chocolate-covered:			
(USDA)	1 oz.	126	20.3
(Nabisco) *Pinwheels*	1 piece (1.1 oz.)	140	21.0
(Nabisco) wafers, *Famous*	1 piece (6 grams)	28	4.8
(Stella D'oro) *Como*	1 oz.	126	20.3
(Sunshine) snaps	1 piece (3 grams)	14	2.4
(Wise) chocolate creme	1 piece (7 grams)	32	4.9
Chocolate chip:			
(USDA)	1 oz.	134	19.8
(Drake's)	1 piece (.5 oz.)	74	9.9
(Keebler)	1 piece (.6 oz.)	80	11.0
(Nabisco) *Chips Ahoy!*	1 piece (.4 oz.)	53	7.3
(Pepperidge Farm)	1 piece (.4 oz.)	52	6.2
(Sunshine) *Chip-a-Roos*	1 piece (.4 oz.)	63	7.7
(Tastykake) *Choc-o-Chip*	1¾-oz. pkg.	283	34.8
Cinnamon crisp (Keebler)	1 piece (4 grams)	17	2.7
Cinnamon, spice, vanilla sandwich (Nab) *Crinkles*	1⅝-oz. pkg.	228	33.4
Cinnamon sugar (Pepperidge Farm)	1 piece (.4 oz.)	52	7.0
Cinnamon toast (Sunshine)	1 piece (3 grams)	13	2.3

Food and Description	Measure or Quantity	Calories	Carbo-hydrates (grams)
Coconut:			
(Keebler) chocolate drop	1 piece (.5 oz.)	75	8.5
(Nabisco) bars	1 piece (9 grams)	47	6.3
(Sunshine) bars	1 piece (.4 oz.)	47	6.2
(Sunshine) chocolate chip	1 piece (.6 oz.)	80	9.7
(Tastykake) *Coconut Kiss*	1¾-oz. pkg.	318	33.2
Commodore (Keebler)	1 piece (.5 oz.)	65	10.1
Cream Lunch (Sunshine)	1 piece (.4 oz.)	45	7.3
Cream wafer stick (Dutch Twin)	1 piece (7 grams)	36	5.9
Creme wafer stick (Nabisco)	1 piece (9 grams)	50	6.0
Cup Custard (Sunshine):			
Chocolate	1 piece (.5 oz.)	70	9.3
Vanilla	1 piece (.5 oz.)	71	9.3
Devil's food cake (Sunshine)	1 piece (.5 oz.)	55	10.9
Dixie Vanilla (Sunshine)	1 piece (.5 oz.)	60	13.1
Dresden (Pepperidge Farm)	1 piece (.6 oz.)	83	10.0
Egg Jumbo (Stella D'oro)	1 piece (.4 oz.)	40	7.6
Fig bar:			
(USDA)	1 oz.	101	21.4
(Keebler)	1 piece (.7 oz.)	71	14.4
(Nabisco) *Fig Newton*	1 piece	55	11.5
(Sunshine)	1 piece	45	9.2
Fortune (Chun King)	1 piece	31	4.6
Fudge:			
(Keebler) *Fudge Stripes*	1 piece (.4 oz.)	57	7.5
(Pepperidge Farm) chip	1 piece (.4 oz.)	51	6.7
(Planters) creme	1 oz.	140	20.0
(Sunshine)	1 piece (.5 oz.)	72	9.4
Gingersnaps:			
(USDA)	1 oz.	119	22.6
(USDA) crumbs	1 cup (4.1 oz.)	483	91.8
(Keebler)	1 piece (6 grams)	24	4.3
(Nabisco) old fashioned	1 piece (7 grams)	30	5.5
(Sunshine)	1 piece (6 grams)	24	4.4
Golden Bars (Stella D'oro)	1 piece (oz.)	123	16.0
Golden Fruit (Sunshine)	1 piece (.7 oz.)	61	14.4

(USDA): United States Department of Agriculture
(HEW/FAO): Health, Education and Welfare/Food and Agriculture Organization
* Prepared as Package Directs

Food and Description	Measure or Quantity	Calories	Carbo- hydrates (grams)
Graham cracker (See **CRACKER**, Graham)			
Hermit bar, frosted (Tastykake)	1 pkg. (2 oz.)	321	60.8
Home Plate (Keebler)	1 piece (.5 oz.)	58	9.9
Hostess With The Mostest (Stella D'oro)	1 piece (8 grams)	39	5.2
Hydrox (Sunshine):			
Regular or mint	1 piece (.4 oz.)	48	7.1
Vanilla	1 piece (.4 oz.)	50	7.1
Jan Hagel (Keebler)	1 piece (10 grams)	44	6.7
Keebies (Keebler)	1 piece (.4 oz.)	51	7.1
Ladyfingers (USDA)	.4-oz. ladyfinger (3¼″ x 1⅜″ x 1⅛″)	40	7.1
Lemon:			
(Pepperidge Farm) nut crunch	1 piece (.4 oz.)	57	6.4
(Planters) creme	1 oz.	140	20.0
(Sunshine)	1 piece (.5 oz.)	76	9.8
(Sunshine) *Lemon Coolers*	1 piece (6 grams)	29	4.5
Lido (Pepperidge Farm)	1 piece (.6 oz.)	91	10.0
Lisbon (Pepperidge Farm)	1 piece (5 grams)	28	3.3
Macaroon:			
(USDA)	1 oz.	135	18.7
(Hostess) fudge	1 piece (1.3 oz.)	213	32.7
(Nabisco) *Bake Shop,* coconut	1 piece (.7 oz.)	87	12.1
(Tastykake) almond	2-oz. pkg. (2 pieces)	336	35.1
(Van de Kamp's) coconut	1 piece (.7 oz.)	89	
Margherite (Stella D'oro):			
Chocolate	1 piece (.6 oz.)	73	10.6
Vanilla	1 piece (.6 oz.)	73	10.5
Marquisitte (Pepperidge Farm)	1 piece (8 grams)	45	5.0
Marshmallow:			
(USDA)	1 oz.	116	20.5
(Nabisco) *Mallomars*	1 piece (.5 oz.)	55	9.0
(Nabisco) puffs, chocolate coated	1 piece (.7 oz.)	85	13.0
(Nabisco) sandwich	1 piece (8 grams)	33	6.0
(Planters) banana pie	1 oz.	127	22.0

Food and Description	Measure or Quantity	Calories	Carbohydrates (grams)
(Planters) chocolate pie	1 oz.	127	22.0
(Sunshine) *Mallo Puff*	1 piece (.6 oz.)	63	12.2
Milano (Pepperidge Farm)	1 piece (.4 oz.)	62	7.2
Milano, mint (Pepperidge Farm)	1 piece (.5 oz.)	76	8.4
Mint sandwich (Nabisco) *Mystic*	1 piece (.6 oz.)	88	10.6
Molasses (USDA)	1 oz.	120	21.5
Molasses & spice (Sunshine)	1 piece (.6 oz.)	67	11.9
Naples (Pepperidge Farm)	1 piece (6 grams)	33	3.7
Nassau (Pepperidge Farm)	1 piece (.6 oz.)	83	9.2
Oatmeal:			
(USDA) raisin	1 oz.	128	20.8
(Drake's)	1 piece (.5 oz.)	69	10.1
(Drake's) whole wheat	1 piece (.5 oz.)	75	11.4
(Keebler) old-fashioned	1 piece (.6 oz.)	79	11.7
(Nabisco)	1 piece (.6 oz.)	75	11.5
(Nabisco) raisin, *Bake Shop*	1 piece (.6 oz.)	77	11.5
(Pepperidge Farm) Irish	1 piece (.5 oz.)	50	7.1
(Pepperidge Farm) raisin	1 piece (.4 oz.)	55	7.5
(Sunshine)	1 piece (.4 oz.)	58	8.9
(Sunshine) iced	1 piece (.5 oz.)	69	11.6
(Sunshine) peanut butter	1 piece (.6 oz.)	79	10.5
(Tastykake) raisin bar	1 pkg. (2¼ oz.)	298	47.6
(Van de Kamp's)	1 piece (.6 oz.)	59	
Old Country Treats (Stella D'oro)	1 piece (.5 oz.)	64	7.1
Orleans (Pepperidge Farm)	1 piece (6 grams)	30	3.5
Peach-apricot pastry (Stella D'oro)	1 piece (.8 oz.)	99	15.0
Peanut & peanut butter:			
(USDA)	1 oz.	134	19.0
(Nabisco) *Cheda-Nut*	1 piece (7 grams)	38	4.5
(Nabisco) creme patties	1 piece (7 grams)	35	4.0
(Nabisco) sandwich, *Nutter Butter*	1 piece (.5 oz.)	70	9.5
(Sunshine) patties	1 piece (7 grams)	33	4.2

(USDA): United States Department of Agriculture
(HEW/FAO): Health, Education and Welfare/Food and Agriculture Organization
* Prepared as Package Directs

Food and Description	Measure or Quantity	Calories	Carbo-hydrates (grams)
Pecan Sandies (Keebler)	1 piece (.6 oz.)	85	9.2
Penguins (Keebler)	1 piece (.8 oz.)	111	14.0
Pfefferneuse, spice drop (Stella D'oro)	1 piece	40	
Pirouette (Pepperidge Farm):			
Chocolate laced	1 piece (7 grams)	38	4.5
Lemon or original	1 piece (7 grams)	37	4.4
Pitter Patter (Keebler)	1 piece (.6 oz.)	84	10.9
Pizzelle, Carolines (Stella D'oro)	1 piece (.4 oz.)	49	6.7
Raisin:			
(USDA)	1 oz.	108	22.9
(Nabisco) fruit biscuit	1 piece (.5 oz.)	55	12.0
Rich 'n Chips (Keebler)	1 piece (.5 oz.)	73	8.9
Rochelle (Pepperidge Farm)	1 piece (.6 oz.)	81	9.6
Sandwich, creme:			
(USDA)	1 oz.	140	19.6
(Keebler):			
Chocolate fudge	1 piece (.7 oz.)	99	13.0
Vanilla	1 piece (.6 oz.)	82	11.1
(Nabisco):			
Cameo	1 piece (.5 oz.)	70	10.5
Assorted, *Cookie Break*	1 piece (.4 oz.)	50	7.3
Vanilla, *Cookie Break*	1 piece (.4 oz.)	50	7.3
Oreo	1 piece (.4 oz.)	51	7.3
Oreo, Double Stuf	1 piece (.5 oz.)	70	9.0
Mystic Mint	1 piece (.6 oz.)	85	10.5
Social Tea	1 piece (.4 oz.)	20	3.5
Swiss	1 piece (.4 oz.)	82	11.1
(Sunshine):			
Orbit	1 piece (.4 oz.)	51	7.0
Vienna Finger	1 piece (.5 oz.)	71	10.5
Sesame, *Regina* (Stella D'oro)	1 piece (.4 oz.)	51	6.9
Shortbread or shortcake:			
(USDA)	1 oz.	141	18.5
(USDA)	1¾" sq. (8 grams)	40	5.2
(Nabisco) *Lorna Doone*	1 piece (8 grams)	40	4.8
(Nabisco) pecan	1 piece (.5 oz.)	80	8.5
(Pepperidge Farm)	1 piece (.5 oz.)	72	8.3
(Sunshine) *Scotties*	1 piece (8 grams)	39	5.0

Food and Description	Measure or Quantity	Calories	Carbo- hydrates (grams)
(Tastykake) vanilla	6 pieces (2¼-oz. pkg.)	352	43.8
Social Tea Biscuit (Nabisco)	1 piece (5 grams)	21	3.5
Spiced wafers (Nabisco)	1 piece (10 grams)	33	5.8
Sprinkles (Sunshine)	1 piece (.6 oz.)	57	11.4
Sugar cookie:			
(Keebler) old-fashioned	1 piece (.6 oz.)	78	12.4
(Nabisco) rings	1 piece (.5 oz.)	70	10.5
(Pepperidge Farm)	1 piece (.4 oz.)	51	7.0
(Pepperidge Farm) brown	1 piece (.4 oz.)	48	6.9
(Sunshine)	1 piece (.6 oz.)	86	11.9
(Van de Kamp's)	1 piece (.6 oz.)	79	
Sugar wafer:			
(USDA)	1 oz.	137	20.8
(Dutch Twin)	1 piece (7 grams)	34	4.7
(Keebler) *Krisp Kreem*	1 piece (6 grams)	31	3.7
(Nabisco) *Biscos*	1 piece (4 grams)	19	2.5
(Sunshine)	1 piece (9 grams)	43	6.6
(Sunshine) lemon	1 piece (9 grams)	44	6.5
Swedish Kreme (Keebler)	1 piece (5.7 oz.)	98	12.2
Tahiti (Pepperidge Farm)	1 piece (.5 oz.)	84	8.6
Toy (Sunshine)	1 piece (3 grams)	13	2.1
Vanilla creme (Planters)	1 oz.	116	20.0
Vanilla creme (Wise)	1 piece (7 grams)	33	5.0
Vanilla wafer:			
(USDA)	1 oz.	131	21.1
(Keebler)	1 piece (4 grams)	19	2.6
(Nabisco) *Nilla*	1 piece (4 grams)	19	3.0
(Sunshine) small	1 piece (3 grams)	15	2.2
Venice (Pepperidge Farm)	1 piece (9 grams)	48	6.2
Waffle creme (Dutch Twin)	1 piece (9 grams)	48	6.2
Waffle creme (Nabisco) *Biscos*	1 piece (8 grams)	43	6.0
Yum Yums (Sunshine)	1 piece (.5 oz.)	83	10.4
COOKIE, DIETETIC:			
Angel Puffs (Stella D'oro)	1 piece (3 grams)	17	1.5
Apple pastry (Stella D'oro)	1 piece (.8 oz.)	94	13.6

(USDA): United States Department of Agriculture
(HEW/FAO): Health, Education and Welfare/Food and Agriculture Organization
* Prepared as Package Directs

Food and Description	Measure or Quantity	Calories	Carbo-hydrates (grams)
Assorted (Estee)	1 piece (5 grams)	26	3.0
Bittersweet chocolate wafer (Estee)	1 piece (.7 oz.)	115	10.0
Chocolate chip (Estee)	1 piece (7 grams)	30	4.0
Chocolate chip, *Sug'r Like*	1 piece	41	4.0
Chocolate-flavored bar, *Sug'r Like*	1 piece	45	3.0
Chocolate crescent, *Sug'r Like*	1 piece	41	4.0
Chocolate wafer (Estee)	1 piece (5 grams)	27	2.4
Chocolate wafer, *Sug'r Like*	1 piece	34	4.0
Fig pastry (Stella D'oro)	1 piece (.9 oz.)	100	15.5
Fruit wafer (Estee)	1 piece (5 grams)	27	2.7
Have-a-Heart (Stella D'oro)	1 piece (.7 oz.)	97	11.3
Kichel (Stella D'oro)	1 piece (1 gram)	8	.7
Lemon, *Sug'r Like*	1 piece	41	4.0
Lemon thin (Estee)	1 piece (6 grams)	25	4.0
Milk chocolate wafer (Estee)	1 piece (.7 oz.)	110	10.0
Oatmeal raisin (Estee)	1 piece (7 grams)	30	4.0
Peach-apricot pastry (Stella D'oro)	1 piece (.8 oz.)	104	15.2
Prune pastry (Stella D'oro)	1 piece (.8 oz.)	92	14.3
Rich crisp bar, *Sug'r Like*	1 piece	45	3.5
Royal Nuggets (Stella D'oro)	1 piece	2	.1
Sandwich (Estee)	1 piece (.4 oz.)	50	8.0
Vanilla, *Sug'r Like*	1 piece	41	4.0
Vanilla thin (Estee)	1 piece (6 grams)	25	4.0
Wafer, assorted (Estee)	1 piece (5 grams)	30	3.0
COOKIE DOUGH:			
Refrigerated:			
Unbaked (USDA) plain	1 oz.	127	16.7
Baked (USDA) plain	1 oz.	141	18.4
(Pillsbury):			
Butterscotch nut	1 cookie	53	6.7
Chocolate chip	1 cookie	50	7.3
Oatmeal & chocolate chip	1 piece	57	7.3
Oatmeal raisin	1 cookie	60	8.7
Peanut butter	1 cookie	53	6.3

Food and Description	Measure or Quantity	Calories	Carbohydrates (grams)
COOKIE, HOME RECIPE			
(USDA):			
Brownie with nuts	1¾" x 1¾" x ⅞"	97	10.2
Chocolate chip	1 oz.	146	17.0
Sugar, soft, thick	1 oz.	126	19.3
COOKIE MIX:			
Brownie:			
(Betty Crocker):			
Chocolate chip butterscotch	⅟₁₆ pkg.	130	20.0
Fudge	⅟₁₆ pkg.	120	21.0
Fudge, supreme	⅟₂₄ pkg.	120	20.0
German chocolate	⅟₁₆ pkg.	150	26.0
Walnut	⅟₁₆ pkg.	140	22.0
(Pillsbury):			
*Fudge	1½" sq.	60	9.5
*Fudge, family style	1½" sq.	65	10.0
*Walnut	1½" sq.	65	10.0
*Walnut, family style	1½" sq.	65	10.0
*Chocolate chip (Betty Crocker) *Big Batch*	1 cookie	75	9.0
Date bar (Betty Crocker)	⅟₃₂ pkg.	60	9.0
*Macaroon, coconut (Betty Crocker)	⅟₂₄ pkg.	80	10.0
Lemon (Nestlé's)	1 oz.	132	20.1
*Oatmeal (Betty Crocker) *Big Batch*	1 cookie	70	9.0
*Peanut butter (Betty Crocker) *Big Batch*	1 cookie	70	8.0
*Sugar (Betty Crocker) *Big Batch*	1 cookie	65	9.0
Sugar (Nestlé's)	1 oz.	132	20.1
Toll House with morsels (Nestlé's)	1 piece (.4 oz.)	52	7.2
Toll House without morsels (Nestlé's)	1 piece (8 grams)	42	5.7

(USDA): United States Department of Agriculture
(HEW/FAO): Health, Education and Welfare/Food and Agriculture Organization
* Prepared as Package Directs

Food and Description	Measure or Quantity	Calories	Carbo-hydrates (grams)
Vienna Dream Bar (Betty Crocker)	½₄ pkg.	90	10.0
COOKING FATS (See **FATS**)			
COOKING SPRAY *Mazola No Stick*	2-second spray	7	0.
CORDIAL (See individual kinds of liqueur by flavor or brand name)			
CORDON D' ALSACE, Alsatian wine, 12% alcohol (Wilm)	3 fl. oz.	66	3.6
CORDON DE BORDEAUX, French Bordeaux, red or white (Chanson) 11¼ % alcohol	3 fl. oz.	60	6.3
CORDON DE BOURGOGNE, French white Burgundy, (Chanson) 11½ % alcohol	3 fl. oz.	81	6.3
CORDON DU RHONE, French red Rhone wine, (Chanson) 12% alcohol	3 fl. oz.	84	6.3
CORIANDER SEED (French's)	1 tsp. (1.4 grams)	6	.8
CORN: Fresh, white or yellow (USDA):			
Raw, untrimmed, on cob	1 lb. (weighed in husk)	157	36.1
Raw, trimmed, on cob	1 lb. (husk removed)	240	55.1
Boiled, kernels, cut from cob, drained	1 cup (5.8 oz.)	138	31.2
Boiled, whole	4.9-oz. ear (5″ x 1¾″)	70	16.2

Food and Description	Measure or Quantity	Calories	Carbo-hydrates (grams)
Canned, regular pack:			
(USDA) golden or yellow, whole kernel, solids & liq., vacuum pack	½ cup (3.7 oz.)	88	21.7
(USDA):			
Golden or yellow, whole kernel, wet pack	½ cup (4.5 oz.)	84	20.1
Golden or yellow, whole kernel, drained solids, wet pack	½ cup (3 oz.)	72	17.0
White kernel, solids & liq.	½ cup (4.5 oz.)	84	20.1
White kernel, solids & drained solids	½ cup (2.8 oz.)	67	15.8
White whole kernel, drained liq., wet pack	4 oz.	29	7.8
Cream style	½ cup (4.4 oz.)	102	25.0
(Butter Kernel):			
Cream style	½ cup (4.1 oz.)	92	22.5
Golden or yellow, whole kernel, drained solids	½ cup (4.1 oz.)	75	18.0
(Del Monte):			
Cream style	½ cup (4.4 oz.)	102	22.2
Cream style, white, wet pack	½ cup (4.3 oz.)	97	21.3
Golden, whole kernel, solids & liq.	½ cup (4 oz.)	78	16.6
Golden, whole kernel, drained solids	½ cup	100	21.3
Golden or yellow, vacuum pack	½ cup	101	21.6
White, whole kernel, solids & liq.	½ cup	78	16.6
White, whole kernel, drained solids	½ cup	102	21.4

(USDA): United States Department of Agriculture
(HEW/FAO): Health, Education and Welfare/Food and Agriculture Organization
* Prepared as Package Directs

Food and Description	Measure or Quantity	Calories	Carbo-hydrates (grams)
(Green Giant):			
Cream style, golden kernel	½ cup	105	22.5
Golden or yellow kernel, solids & liq.	½ cup	80	16.5
Golden or yellow kernel, vacuum pack, Niblets	½ cup	75	15.0
Golden, whole kernel, solids & liq.			
Mexicorn with peppers	½ cup	75	15.0
(Kounty Kist; Lindy):			
Cream style, golden kernel	½ cup	115	25.0
Golden, whole kernel, solids & liq.	½ cup	90	19.0
Golden, whole kernel, vacuum pack	½ cup	80	17.5
(Le Sueur) golden, whole kernel, solids & liq.	½ cup	85	17.5
(Libby's):			
Cream style	½ cup	85	21.0
Whole kernel, solids & liq.	½ cup	80	18.5
(Stokely-Van Camp):			
Cream style, white or golden	½ cup	105	23.5
Golden or yellow, whole kernel, solids & liq.	½ cup (4.5 oz.)	90	19.5
Golden, vacuum pack	½ cup	120	26.5
White, solids & liq.	½ cup	95	20.5
Canned, dietetic or low calorie:			
(USDA):			
Cream style	4 oz.	93	21.0
White or yellow, whole kernel, solids & liq.	4 oz.	65	15.4
White or yellow, whole kernel, drained solids	4 oz.	86	20.4
(Blue Boy):			
Cream style	4 oz.	105	20.6
Whole kernel, solids & liq.	4 oz.	78	16.0

Food and Description	Measure or Quantity	Calories	Carbo-hydrates (grams)
(Cellu) whole kernel, solids & liq., low sodium	½ cup	65	15.0
(Diet Delight) whole kernel, solids & liq.	½ cup (4.4 oz.)	71	14.6
(Featherweight):			
Cream style	½ cup	80	18.0
Whole kernel, solids & liq.	½ cup	70	16.0
(S and W Nutradiet):			
Cream style	4 oz.	95	20.1
Whole kernel, solids & liq.	4 oz.	59	12.2
(Tillie Lewis)	½ cup	83	15.4
Frozen:			
(USDA) boiled, drained	4 oz.	107	24.5
(Birds Eye):			
On the cob	1 ear (4.9 oz.)	130	28.0
On the cob, *Little Ears*	1 ear	70	16.0
Kernel	⅓ pkg.	70	18.0
(Green Giant):			
On the cob	5½″ ear	160	33.0
On the cob, *Nibblers*	3″ ear	90	18.0
Cream style	½ cup	90	20.0
Mexicorn	½ cup	95	15.0
Niblets	½ cup	95	15.0
White kernel, in butter sauce	½ cup	95	15.0
CORNBREAD, home recipe (USDA):			
Corn pone, prepared with white, whole-ground cornmeal	4 oz.	231	41.1
Johnnycake, prepared with yellow, degermed cornmeal	4 oz.	303	51.6

(USDA): United States Department of Agriculture
(HEW/FAO): Health, Education and Welfare/Food and Agriculture Organization
* Prepared as Package Directs

Food and Description	Measure or Quantity	Calories	Carbohydrates (grams)
Southern-style, prepared with degermed cornmeal	2½″ x 2½″ x 1⅝″ piece	254	39.9
Southern-style, prepared with whole-ground cornmeal	4 oz.	234	33.0
Spoon bread, prepared with white, whole-ground cornmeal	4 oz.	221	19.2
CORNBREAD MIX:			
Dry (USDA)	1 oz.	122	20.1
*Prepared with egg & milk (USDA)	2⅜″ muffin (1.4 oz.)	93	13.2
(Albers)	1 oz.	109	19.6
*(Aunt Jemima)	⅙ pkg. (2.4 oz.)	228	34.9
*(Dromedary)	2″ x 2″ piece	130	19.0
*(Pillsbury) *Ballard*	1⁄16 of recipe	160	26.0
CORN CHEX, cereal	1 cup (1 oz.)	110	25.0
CORN CHIPS (See **CRACKERS**)			
CORN CHOWDER (Snow) New England	8 oz.	159	19.6
CORNED BEEF:			
Uncooked (USDA) boneless, medium fat	1 lb.	1329	0.
Cooked (USDA) boneless, medium fat	4 oz.	422	0.
Canned:			
(Armour Star)	4 oz.	322	0.
(Austex)	15-oz. can	769	45.5
(Bounty)	7½-oz. can	372	22.2
(Hormel) *Mary Kitchen*	7½-oz.	400	21.0
(Libby's)	4 oz.	192	14.3
(Libby's) home style	4 oz.	226	13.2
(Nally's)	4 oz.	179	9.1
(Wilson)	15½-oz. can	792	31.6
CORNED BEEF HASH DINNER, frozen (Banquet)	10-oz. dinner	372	42.6

Food and Description	Measure or Quantity	Calories	Carbo-hydrates (grams)
CORNED BEEF SPREAD			
(Underwood)	1-oz.	55	Tr.
CORN FLAKE CRUMBS			
(Kellogg's)	¼ cup	110	25.0
CORN FLAKES, cereal:			
(USDA)	1 cup (1 oz.)	112	24.7
(USDA) crushed	1 cup (2.5 oz.)	270	59.7
(USDA) frosted	1 cup (1.4 oz.)	154	36.5
(General Mills) *Country*	1 cup (1 oz.)	110	24.0
(Kellogg's)	1 cup (1 oz.)	110	25.0
(Post) *Post Toasties*	1½ cups (1 oz.)	110	24.0
(Ralston Purina)	1 cup (1 oz.)	110	24.0
(Van Brode) regular	1¼ cups (1 oz.)	107	24.4
(Van Brode) sugar toasted	¾ cup (1 oz.)	107	25.6
Low sodium (Cellu)	1 oz.	110	25.0
Low sodium (Van Brode)	1 oz.	110	25.1
CORN FRITTER:			
Home recipe (USDA)	4 oz.	428	45.0
Frozen (Mrs. Paul's)	½ of 8-oz. pkg.	243	31.7
CORN GRITS (See HOMINY)			
CORNMEAL, WHITE or YELLOW:			
Dry:			
Bolted (USDA)	1 cup (4.3 oz.)	442	90.9
Bolted (Aunt Jemima/Quaker)	1 cup (4 oz.)	408	84.8
Degermed:			
(USDA)	1 cup (4.9 oz.)	502	108.2
(Aunt Jemima/Quaker)	1 cup (4 oz.)	404	88.8
Self-rising degermed:			
(USDA)	1 cup (5 oz.)	491	105.9
(Aunt Jemima)	1 cup (6 oz.)	582	126.0

(USDA): United States Department of Agriculture
(HEW/FAO): Health, Education and Welfare/Food and Agriculture Organization
* Prepared as Package Directs

Food and Description	Measure or Quantity	Calories	Carbo-hydrates (grams)
Self-rising whole ground (USDA)	1 cup (5 oz.)	489	101.4
Self-rising (Aunt Jemima)	1 cup (6 oz.)	594	122.4
Whole-ground, unbolted (USDA)	1 cup (4.3 oz.)	433	90.0
Cooked:			
(USDA)	1 cup (8.5 oz.)	120	25.7
Degermed (Albers)	1 cup	119	25.5
Mix:			
Bolted (Aunt Jemima/Quaker)	1 cup (4 oz.)	392	80.4
Degermed (Aunt Jemima/Quaker)	1 cup (4 oz.)	392	84.0
CORN PUDDING, home recipe (USDA)	1 cup (8.6 oz.)	255	31.9
CORN SALAD, raw (USDA):			
Untrimmed	1 lb. (weighed untrimmed)	91	15.7
Trimmed	4 oz.	24	4.1
CORNSTARCH:			
(USDA)	1 cup (4.5 oz.)	463	112.1
(Argo)	1 T. (8 grams)	34	8.3
(Kingsford's)	1 T. (8 grams)	34	8.3
(Duryea's)	1 T. (8 grams)	34	8.3
CORN STICK (See CORNBREAD)			
CORN SYRUP, light & dark blend (USDA)	1 T. (.7 oz.)	61	15.8
CORN TOTAL, cereal	1 cup (1 oz.)	110	24.0
CORNY-SNAPS, cereal (Kellogg's)	1 cup (1 oz.)	120	24.0
COTTAGE PUDDING, home recipe (USDA):			
Without sauce	2 oz.	195	30.8

Food and Description	Measure or Quantity	Calories	Carbo-hydrates (grams)
With chocolate sauce	2 oz.	180	32.1
With strawberry sauce	2 oz.	166	27.4
COUGH DROP:			
(Beech-Nut)	1 drop (2 grams)	10	2.4
(H-B)	1 drop	8	1.9
(Luden's):			
Honey lemon	1 drop	8	
Honey licorice	1 drop	8	
Menthol	1 drop	9	2.1
Wild cherry	1 drop	9	
(Pine Bros.)	1 drop (3 grams)	8	2.0
(Smith Brothers)	1 drop	7	2.1
COUNT CHOCULA, cereal (General Mills)	1 cup (1 oz.)	110	24.0
COUNTRY MORNING, cereal (Kellogg's):			
Regular	⅓ cup (1 oz.)	130	18.0
With raisins & dates	⅓ cup (1 oz.)	130	19.0
COUNTRY-STYLE SAUSAGE, smoked links (USDA)	1 oz.	98	0.
COWPEA (USDA):			
Immature seeds:			
Raw, whole	1 lb. (weighed in pods)	317	54.4
Raw, shelled	½ cup (2.5 oz.)	91	15.7
Boiled, drained solids	½ cup (2.9 oz.)	88	14.8
Canned, solids & liq.	4 oz.	79	14.1
Frozen (See **BLACK-EYED PEAS,** frozen)			

(USDA): United States Department of Agriculture
(HEW/FAO): Health, Education and Welfare/Food and Agriculture
Organization
* Prepared as Package Directs

Food and Description	Measure or Quantity	Calories	Carbo-hydrates (grams)
Young pods with seeds:			
Raw, whole	1 lb. (weighed untrimmed)	182	39.3
Boiled, drained solids	4 oz.	39	7.9
Mature seeds, dry:			
Raw	1 lb.	1556	279.9
Raw	½ cup (3 oz.)	288	51.8
Boiled	½ cup (4.4 oz.)	94	17.1
CRAB, all species:			
Fresh (USDA):			
Steamed, whole	1 lb. (weighed in shell)	202	1.1
Steamed, meat only	4 oz.	105	.6
Canned:			
(USDA) drained solids	4 oz.	115	1.2
(Icy Point) Alaska King, drained solids	7½-oz. can	215	2.3
(Pillar Rock) Alaska King, drained solids	7½-oz. can	215	2.3
Frozen:			
(Wakefield's) Alaska King, thawed & drained	4 oz.	96	.6
(Ship Ahoy) King crab	8-oz. pkg.	211	.5
CRAB APPLE, fresh (USDA):			
Whole	1 lb. (weighed whole)	284	74.3
Flesh only	4 oz.	77	20.2
CRAB CAKE, frozen (Mrs. Paul's), thins	½ of 10-oz. pkg.	325	30.8
CRAB COCKTAIL, King crab (Sau-Sea)	4-oz. jar	80	18.4
CRAB, DEVILED:			
Home recipe (USDA)	1 cup (8.5 oz.)	451	31.9
Frozen (Mrs. Paul's)	½ of 6-oz. pkg.	165	17.0
Frozen (Mrs. Paul's) miniatures	½ of 7-oz. pkg.	221	25.9

Food and Description	Measure or Quantity	Calories	Carbo-hydrates (grams)
CRAB IMPERIAL, home recipe (USDA)	1 cup (7.8 oz.)	323	8.6
CRAB SOUP (Crosse & Blackwell)	½ of 13-oz. can	59	8.3
CRACKER, PUFFS and CHIPS:			
American Harvest (Nabisco)	1 piece (3 grams)	16	2.0
Arrowroot biscuit (Nabisco)	1 piece (5 grams)	22	3.5
Bacon-flavored thins (Nabisco)	1 piece (2 grams)	11	1.3
Bacon Nips	1 oz.	147	15.6
Bacon Rinds (Wonder)	1 oz.	146	0.
Bacon toast (Keebler)	1 piece (3 grams)	15	2.0
Bakon-Snacks	1 oz.	150	14.3
Bakon Tasters (Old London)	½-oz. bag	62	8.8
Bugles (General Mills)	15 pieces (1 oz.)	150	17.0
Butter (USDA)	1 oz.	130	19.1
Butter thins (Nabisco)	1 piece (3 grams)	14	2.2
Cheese-flavored (See also individual brand names in this grouping):			
(USDA)	1 oz.	136	17.1
Cheddar Bitz (Frito-Lay's)	1 oz.	129	18.9
Cheese Balls (Planters)	1 oz.	160	4.3
Cheese'n Cracker (Kraft)	4 crackers & ¾ oz. cheese	138	.7
Cheese Curls (Planters)	1 oz.	160	4.3
Cheese Nips (Nabisco)	1 piece (1 gram)	6	.7
Cheese Pixies (Wise)	1-oz. bag	155	15.7
Chee*Tos, cheese-flavored puffs	1 oz.	156	15.4
Cheez Doodles (Old London)	1-oz. bag	155	15.7
Cheez-Its (Sunshine)	1 piece (1 gram)	6	.6
Cheez Waffles (Austin's)	1 piece	26	

(USDA): United States Department of Agriculture
(HEW/FAO): Health, Education and Welfare/Food and Agriculture Organization

* Prepared as Package Directs

Food and Description	Measure or Quantity	Calories	Carbo- hydrates (grams)
Cheez Waffles (Old London)	1 piece (2 grams)	11	1.3
Che-zo (Keebler)	1 piece	5	.6
Combo Cheez (Austin's)	1 piece	26	
Parmesan swirl (Nabisco)	1 piece (2.2 grams)	11	1.2
Sandwich (Planters)	1 piece	29	3.0
Swiss cheese (Nabisco)	1 piece (1.9 oz.)	10	1.1
Thins (Pepperidge Farm)	1 piece (3 grams)	12	1.8
Thins, dietetic (Estee)	1 piece (1 gram)	5	.8
Tid-Bit (Nabisco)	1 piece (<1 gram)	5	.5
Toast (Keebler)	1 piece (3 grams)	16	1.9
Twists (Bachman)	1 oz.	150	17.0
Twists (Nalley)	1 oz.	155	14.2
Twists (Wonder)	1 oz.	154	14.7
Cheese & peanut butter sandwich:			
(USDA)	1 oz.	139	15.9
(Austin's)	1⅛-oz. pkg.	194	19.0
Chicken in a Biskit (Nabisco)	1 piece (2 grams)	10	1.1
Chipos (General Mills)	1 oz.	150	17.0
Chipsters (Nabisco)	1 piece	2	.3
Clam-flavored crisps (Snow)	1 oz.	147	14.9
Club (Keebler)	1 piece	15	2.0
Corn Capers (Wonder)	1 oz.	158	15.4
Corn cheese (Tom Houston)	10 pieces (5 grams)	29	1.9
Corn chips:			
Cornetts	1 oz.	153	16.3
Dipsy Doodles (Old London)	1 oz.	162	15.5
Fritos	1 oz.	156	15.5
Fritos, barbecue-flavored	1 oz.	150	15.5
Korkers (Nabisco)	1 piece (2 grams)	8	.8
(Old London) barbecue	1-oz. bag	155	16.7
(Planters)	1 oz.	159	4.0
(Wise) barbecue	1¾-oz. bag	274	27.5
(Wise) rippled	1-oz. bag	162	15.6
(Wonder)	1 oz.	162	14.8
Crown Pilot (Nabisco)	1 piece (.6 oz.)	73	12.4
Diggers (Nabisco)	1 piece	4	.5
Doo Dads (Nabisco)	1 piece	2	.3
Escort (Nabisco)	1 piece	21	2.7

Food and Description	Measure or Quantity	Calories	Carbo-hydrates (grams)
Flings, cheese-flavored curls (Nabisco)	1 piece (2 grams)	10	.8
Goldfish (Pepperidge Farm):			
Cheddar cheese	10 pieces (6 grams)	28	3.3
Lightly salted	10 pieces (6 grams)	28	3.6
Parmesan cheese	10 pieces (6 grams)	28	3.4
Pizza	10 pieces (6 grams)	29	5.0
Pretzel	10 pieces (7 grams)	29	5.0
Onion	10 pieces (6 grams)	28	3.6
Sesame garlic	10 pieces (6 grams)	29	3.5
Graham:			
(USDA)	2½" sq. (7 grams)	27	5.1
(Nabisco)	1 piece (7 grams)	30	5.3
(Nabisco) *Cinnamon Treats*	1 piece (.2 oz.)	28	5.0
Chocolate- or cocoa-covered:			
(USDA)	1 oz.	135	19.2
(Keebler) deluxe	1 piece (9 grams)	42	5.6
(Nabisco)	1 piece	57	7.0
(Nabisco) *Fancy Dip*	1 piece (.5 oz.)	65	8.5
Sugar-honey coated (USDA)	1 oz.	117	21.7
Sugar-honey coated (Nabisco) *Honey Maid*	1 piece (7 grams)	30	5.5
Hi-Ho (Sunshine)	1 piece (4 grams)	18	2.1
Hot Potatas (Old London)	⅝-oz. bag	82	12.0
Matzo (see **MATZO**)			
Melba toast (see **MELBA TOAST**)			
Milk lunch (Nabisco) *Royal Lunch*	1 piece (.4 oz.)	55	7.9
Munchos	1 oz.	159	14.5
Onion-flavored			
(Frito-Lay) *Funyuns*	1 oz.	137	18.9
(General Mills) *Onyums*	30 pieces (.5 oz.)	79	7.7
(Keebler) toast	1 piece (3 grams)	18	2.1

(USDA): United States Department of Agriculture
(HEW/FAO): Health, Education and Welfare/Food and Agriculture Organization
* Prepared as Package Directs

Food and Description	Measure or Quantity	Calories	Carbo- hydrates (grams)
(Nabisco) French	1 piece (2 grams)	12	1.5
(Old London) rings	½-oz. bag	68	10.4
(Pepperidge Farm) thins	1 piece (3 grams)	12	2.0
(Snow) crisps	1 oz.	157	15.9
(Wise) rings	½-oz. bag	65	11.1
(Wonder) rings	1 oz.	133	19.5
Oyster:			
(USDA)	10 pieces (.4 oz.)	44	7.1
(USDA)	1 cup (1 oz.)	124	20.0
(Nabisco) *Dandy*	1 piece	3	.6
(Nabisco) *Oysterettes*	1 piece	3	.6
(Sunshine) mini	1 piece	3	.6
Peanut butter 'n cheez crackers (Kraft)	4 crackers & ¾ oz. peanut butter	191	13.4
Peanut butter sandwich:			
(Planters) cheese crackers	1 piece (7 grams)	29	3.0
(Wise) cheese crackers	1 piece (6 grams)	30	3.4
(Wise) toasted crackers	1 piece (6 grams)	30	3.7
Pizza Wheels (Wise)	¾-oz. bag	90	16.1
Ritz (Nabisco)	1 piece (3 grams)	17	2.0
Roman Meal Wafers	1 piece (4 grams)	15	2.4
Rye, *Wasa Crisp:*			
Golden	1 piece	37	8.0
Lite	1 piece	30	6.0
Seasoned	1 piece	34	7.0
Rye thins (Pepperidge Farm)	1 piece (3 grams)	10	2.0
Rye toast (Keebler)	1 piece (4 grams)	17	2.2
Rye wafers (Nabisco)	1 piece (4 grams)	23	4.5
Saltine:			
Flavor-Kist, any kind	1 piece	12	2.2
(Keebler) *Zesta*	1 section (3 grams)	12	2.0
(Nabisco) *Premium*	1 piece (3 grams)	12	2.0
(Sunshine) *Krispy,* salted tops	1 piece (3 grams)	11	2.0
(Sunshine) Krispy, unsalted tops	1 piece (3 grams)	12	2.1
Sea toast (Keebler)	1 piece (.5 oz.)	62	11.1
Sesame:			
(Keebler) wafer	1 piece (3 grams)	16	2.0
(Nabisco) butter-flavored	1 piece (3 grams)	17	1.9

Food and Description	Measure or Quantity	Calories	Carbo-hydrates (grams)
(Nabisco) *Teeko*, glazed crisp	1 piece (.2 oz.)	22	3.0
(Sunshine) *La Lanne*	1 piece (3 grams)	15	1.8
Wasa Crisp	1 piece (.4 grams)	60	9.0
Sesa Wheat (Austin's)	1 piece	34	3.7
Sociables (Nabisco)	1 piece (2 grams)	10	1.3
Soda:			
(USDA)	1 oz.	124	20.0
(USDA)	2½″ sq. (6 grams)	24	3.9
(Sunshine)	1 piece	20	3.3
Star Lites (Wise)	1 cup (.5 oz.)	63	9.9
Tortilla chip (Wonder) taco	1 oz.	144	15.9
Tortilla chip, taco, *Doritos*	1 oz.	142	17.9
Tater Puffs (Nabisco)	1 piece (1.3 grams)	7	.8
Town House	1 piece (3 grams)	18	2.0
Triscuit (Nabisco)	1 piece (4 grams)	21	3.0
Uneeda Biscuit (Nabisco) unsalted tops	1 piece (5 grams)	22	3.7
Unsalted (Cellu)	1 piece	150	2.5
Wafer-ets (Hol-Grain):			
Rice, salted	1 piece (3 grams)	12	2.5
Rice, unsalted	1 piece (3 grams)	12	2.5
Wheat, salted	1 piece (2 grams)	7	1.4
Wheat, unsalted	1 piece (2 grams)	7	1.4
Waldorf, low salt (Keebler)	1 piece (3 grams)	14	2.4
Waverly wafer (Nabisco)	1 piece (4 grams)	18	2.6
Wheat Thins (Nabisco)	1 piece (2 grams)	9	1.2
Whistles (General Mills)	17 pieces (.5 oz.)	71	8.0
Whole Wheat (USDA)	1 oz.	114	19.3
CRACKER CRUMBS, GRAHAM:			
(USDA)	1 cup (3 oz.)	330	63.0
(Keebler)	3 oz.	368	64.1
(Nabisco)	⅛ of 9″ pie shell (.5 oz.)	70	12.0

(USDA): United States Department of Agriculture
(HEW/FAO): Health, Education and Welfare/Food and Agriculture Organization
* Prepared as Package Directs

Food and Description	Measure or Quantity	Calories	Carbo-hydrates (grams)
CRACKER JACK (See POPCORN)			
CRACKER MEAL:			
(USDA)	1 T. (.4 oz.)	44	7.1
(Keebler):			
Fine, medium or coarse	3 oz.	316	68.5
Zesty	3 oz.	363	61.5
CRACKER PIE CRUST MIX (See PIECRUST MIX)			
CRANAPPLE (Ocean Spray):			
Regular	6 fl. oz.	146	36.3
Low calorie	6 fl. oz.	32	7.8
CRANBERRY:			
Fresh:			
(USDA) untrimmed	1 lb. (weighed with stems)	200	47.0
(USDA) trimmed, stems removed	1 cup (4 oz.)	52	12.2
(Ocean Spray)	1 cup (2 oz.)	26	6.1
Dehydrated (USDA)	1 oz.	104	23.9
CRANBERRY-APPLE JUICE DRINK, canned (Ann Page)	½ cup	91	22.6
CRANBERRY JUICE COCKTAIL:			
(Ann Page)	½ cup	79	19.8
(Ocean Spray) regular	6 fl. oz.	108	22.0
(Ocean Spray) low calorie	6 fl. oz.	39	9.3
*Frozen (Ocean Spray)	6 fl. oz.	113	28.3
CRANBERRY-ORANGE RELISH:			
Uncooked (USDA)	4 oz.	202	51.5
(Ocean Spray)	1 T. (.6 oz.)	33	8.2
CRANBERRY PIE (Tastykake)	4-oz. pie	376	57.7

Food and Description	Measure or Quantity	Calories	Carbohydrates (grams)
CRANBERRY SAUCE:			
Home recipe (USDA) sweetened, unstrained	4 oz.	202	51.6
Canned:			
(USDA) sweetened, strained	½ cup (4.8 oz.)	199	51.0
(Ocean Spray) jellied	2 oz.	89	21.8
(Ocean Spray) whole berry	2 oz.	89	22.0
CRANBREAKER MIX (Bar-Tender's)	⅝-oz. serving	70	17.4
CRANGRAPE, drink (Ocean Spray)	6 fl. oz.	101	24.6
CRANICOT, drink (Ocean Spray)	6 fl. oz.	134	32.8
CRANPRUNE JUICE DRINK (Ocean Spray)	6 fl. oz.	133	32.8
CRAPPIE, white, raw, meat only (USDA)	4 oz.	90	0.
CRAYFISH, freshwater (USDA):			
Raw, in shell	1 lb. (weighed in shell)	39	.7
Raw, meat only	4 oz.	82	1.4
CRAZY COW, cereal (General Mills):			
Chocolate	1 cup (1 oz.)	110	24.0
Strawberry	1 cup (1 oz.)	110	25.0
CREAM (See also **CREAM SUBSTITUTE**):			
Half & half:			
(Dean)	1 T. (.5 oz.)	22	.7

(USDA): United States Department of Agriculture
(HEW/FAO): Health, Education and Welfare/Food and Agriculture
Organization
* Prepared as Package Directs

Food and Description	Measure or Quantity	Calories	Carbohydrates (grams)
(Meadow Gold)	1 T.	30	.6
(Sealtest) 10.5% fat	1 T.	18	1.0
Light, table or coffee:			
(USDA)	1 T. (.5 oz.)	32	.6
(Sealtest) 16% fat	1 T. (.5 oz.)	26	.6
(Sealtest) 18% fat	1 T. (.5 oz.)	28	.6
Light whipping:			
(USDA)	1 cup (8.4 oz.)	717	8.6
(USDA)	1 T. (.5 oz.)	45	.5
(Sealtest) 30% fat	1 T. (.5 oz.)	45	1.0
Whipped topping, pressurized:			
(USDA)	1 cup (2.1 oz.)	155	.6
(USDA)	1 T. (3 grams)	10	.1
Heavy whipping:			
Unwhipped (USDA)	1 cup (8.4 oz.)	838	7.4
(Dean)	1 T. (.5 oz.)	51	.5
(Sealtest) 36% fat	1 T. (.5 oz.)	52	.5
(Sealtest) 40% fat	1 T.	60	.5
Sour:			
(USDA)	1 cup (8.1 oz.)	485	9.9
(Axelrod's)	8-oz. container	433	8.8
(Breakstone)	1 T. (.5 oz.)	29	.6
(Dean)	1 T. (.5 oz.)	28	.6
(Sealtest)	1 T. (.5 oz.)	28	.5
Imitation:			
(Borden) Zesta, 13.5% vegetable fat	1 T.	24	.9
(Dean) Sour Slim	1 T. (1.1 oz.)	30	3.3
(Pet)	1 T. (.5 oz.)	25	1.0
Sour dressing, cultured (Breakstone)	1 T.	27	.7
*CREAM OF RICE, cereal	4 oz.	82	17.9
CREAMSICLE (Popsicle Industries)	2½ fl. oz.	78	12.8
CREAM SUBSTITUTE:			
(USDA) liquid, frozen	1 T. (.5 oz.)	20	2.0
(USDA) powdered	1 tsp. (2 grams)	10	1.0
(Borden) Cremora	1 tsp.	11	1.1
(Carnation) Coffee-mate	1 tsp. (1.9 grams)	11	1.1

Food and Description	Measure or Quantity	Calories	Carbo-hydrates (grams)
Coffee Rich, frozen, liquid	½ oz.	22	2.1
(Meadow Gold) half & half	1 T.	27	1.2
N-Rich	1 tsp. (3 grams)	10	1.7
Perx	1 tsp. (5.3 grams)	8	.6
(Pet) non-dairy	1 tsp. (2 grams)	10	1.0
Poly Perx	1 oz.	40	4.1
Poly Rich, frozen, liquid	½ oz.	22	2.1
Pream	1 tsp. (2.2 grams)	11	1.1
(Sanna)	1 plastic cup	24	2.0
(Sealtest) *Coffee Twin*	½ fl. oz.	18	1.0
CREAM OF WHEAT, cereal:			
Instant, dry	2½ T. (1 oz.)	100	21.0
Mix 'n Eat:			
Regular	1 packet (1 oz.)	100	21.0
Baked apple & cinnamon	1¼-oz. packet	130	29.0
Banana & spice	1½-oz. packet	130	29.0
Maple & brown sugar	1½-oz. packet	130	29.0
Quick, dry	2½ T. (1 oz.)	100	21.0
Regular	2½ T. (1 oz.)	100	22.0
CREME DE CACAO			
LIQUEUR, brown or white:			
(Bols) 54 proof	1 fl. oz.	101	11.8
(Garnier) 54 proof	1 fl. oz.	97	13.1
(Hiram Walker) 54 proof	1 fl. oz.	104	15.0
(Leroux) brown, 54 proof	1 fl. oz.	101	14.3
(Leroux) white, 54 proof	1 fl. oz.	98	13.3
CREME DE CAFE			
LIQUEUR (Leroux) 60 proof	1 fl. oz.	104	13.6
CREME DE CASSIS			
LIQUEUR:			
(Garnier) 36 proof	1 fl. oz.	83	13.5
(Leroux) 35 proof	1 fl. oz.	88	14.9

(USDA): United States Department of Agriculture
(HEW/FAO): Health, Education and Welfare/Food and Agriculture Organization
* Prepared as Package Directs

Food and Description	Measure or Quantity	Calories	Carbohydrates (grams)
CREME DE MENTHE LIQUEUR, green or white:			
(Bols) 60 proof	1 fl. oz.	122	13.0
(Garnier) 60 proof	1 fl. oz.	110	15.3
(Hiram Walker) 60 proof	1 fl. oz.	94	11.2
(Leroux) green, 60 proof	1 fl. oz.	110	15.2
(Leroux) white, 60 proof	1 fl. oz.	101	12.8
CREPE, frozen (Mrs. Paul's):			
Crab	5½-oz. pkg.	297	13.8
Shrimp	5½-oz. pkg.	264	24.7
CRISP RICE, cereal (Van Brode)	1 cup (1 oz.)	113	23.0
CRISPY CRITTERS, cereal	1 cup (1 oz.)	113	23.0
CRISPY RICE, cereal (Ralston Purina)	1 cup (1 oz.)	110	25.0
CROAKER (USDA):			
Atlantic:			
Raw, whole	1 lb. (weighed whole)	148	0.
Raw, meat only	4 oz.	109	0.
Baked	4 oz.	151	0.
White, raw, meat only	4 oz.	95	0.
Yellowfin, raw, meat only	4 oz.	101	0.
CROQUETTES, frozen (Mrs. Paul's) seafood	½ of 6-oz. pkg.	181	23.9
CROUTON:			
(Arnold):			
American style	½ oz.	66	8.7
Bavarian rye	½ oz.	65	9.5
Danish style	½ oz.	67	8.8
English style	½ oz.	66	9.5
French style	½ oz.	66	9.2
Italian or Mexican style	½ oz.	66	9.1
(Kellogg's) *Croutettes*	.7 oz.	70	15.0

CRULLER (See DOUGHNUT)

Food and Description	Measure or Quantity	Calories	Carbo-hydrates (grams)
CRUMB CAKE (Hostess)	1¼-oz. cake	131	21.7
CUCUMBER, fresh (USDA):			
Eaten with skin	½ lb. (weighed whole)	31	7.4
Eaten without skin	½ lb. (weighed with skin)	23	5.3
Unpared, 10-oz. cucumber	7½″ x 2″ pared cucumber (7.3 oz.)	29	6.6
Pared	6 slices (2″ x ⅛″)	7	1.6
Pared & diced	½ cup (2.5 oz.)	10	2.3
CUMIN SEED (French's)	1 tsp. (1.6 oz.)	7	.7
CUPCAKE:			
Home recipe (USDA):			
Without icing	1.4-oz. cupcake	146	22.4
With chocolate icing	1.8-oz. cupcake	184	29.7
With boiled white icing	1.8-oz. cupcake	176	30.9
With uncooked white icing	1.8-oz. cupcake	184	31.6
Commercial:			
Chocolate:			
(Drake's) creme filled	1½-oz. cupcake	187	25.6
(Hostess)	1¾-oz. cupcake	166	29.9
(Tastykake):			
Chocolate	1 cupcake (1 oz.)	191	33.0
Creme filled	1¼-oz. cupcake	128	23.2
Coconut (Tastykake)	1-oz. cupcake	92	16.7
Lemon, creme filled (Tastykake)	⅞-oz. cupcake	124	17.1
Orange (Hostess)	1½-oz. cupcake	149	26.8
Vanilla, creme filled (Tastykake)	1⅞-oz. cupcake	123	16.4
*CUPCAKE MIX (Flako)	1/12 of pkg.	140	21.9
CURACAO LIQUEUR:			
Blue (Bols) 64 proof	1 fl. oz.	105	10.3

(USDA): United States Department of Agriculture
(HEW/FAO): Health, Education and Welfare/Food and Agriculture
          Organization
* Prepared as Package Directs

Food and Description	Measure or Quantity	Calories	Carbo-hydrates (grams)
Orange (Bols) 64 proof	1 fl. oz.	100	8.8
(Garnier) 60 proof	1 fl. oz.	100	12.7
(Hiram Walker) 60 proof	1 fl. oz.	84	9.5
(Leroux) 60 proof	1 fl. oz.	84	9.5
CURRANT:			
Fresh (USDA):			
Black European:			
Whole	1 lb. (weighed with stems)	240	58.2
Stems removed	4 oz.	61	14.9
Red & white:			
Whole	1 lb. (weighed with stems)	220	53.2
Stems removed	1 cup (3.9 oz.)	55	13.3
Dried, Zante (Del Monte)	½ cup (2.4 oz.)	205	47.8
CURRANT JELLY			
(Smucker's)	1 T. (.7 oz.)	50	12.9
CURRY POWDER (Crosse & Blackwell)	1 T. (6 grams)	21	3.9
CUSTARD:			
Home recipe (USDA) baked	½ cup (4.7 oz.)	152	14.7
Chilled (Sealtest)	4 oz.	149	24.3
CUSTARD APPLE, bullock's-heart, raw, (USDA):			
Whole	1 lb. (weighed with skin & seeds)	266	66.3
Flesh only	4 oz.	115	28.6
CUSTARD PIE:			
Home recipe (USDA)	⅛ of 9″ pie	331	35.6
Frozen (Banquet)	5 oz.	274	41.2
CUSTARD PUDDING MIX:			
(Ann Page) egg	2¾-oz. pkg.	292	61.6
(Lynden Farms) real egg	4-oz. pkg.	441	69.2
*(Royal) regular	½ cup	132	18.5

Food and Description	Measure or Quantity	Calories	Carbohydrates (grams)
C.W. POST, cereal:			
Family style	¼ cup (1 oz.)	140	19.0
Family style with raisins	¼ cup (1 oz.)	130	19.0

D

DAIQUIRI COCKTAIL:			
(Hiram Walker) 52.5 proof	3 fl. oz.	177	12.0
(National Distillers) *Duet*, 12% alcohol	8-fl.-oz. can	280	24.0
(Party Tyme) canned, banana, 12.5% alcohol	2 fl. oz.	66	5.7
Dry mix (Bar-Tender's)	1 serving (⅝ oz.)	70	17.2
Dry mix (Holland House)	.6-oz. pkg.	69	7.0
Dry mix, banana (Holland House)	.6-oz. pkg.	66	16.0
DAMSON PLUM (See PLUM)			
DANDELION GREENS, raw (USDA):			
Trimmed	1 lb.	204	41.7
Boiled, drained	½ cup (3.2 oz.)	30	5.8
DANISH PASTRY (See CAKE, coffee)			
DATE, dry:			
Domestic:			
(USDA):			
With pits	1 lb. (weighed with pits)	1081	287.7
Without pits	4 oz.	311	82.7
Without pits, chopped	1 cup (6.1 oz.)	477	126.8

(USDA): United States Department of Agriculture
(HEW/FAO): Health, Education and Welfare/Food and Agriculture Organization
* Prepared as Package Directs

Food and Description	Measure or Quantity	Calories	Carbo-hydrates (grams)
(Cal-Date):			
Whole	1 date (.8 oz.)	62	16.4
Diced	2 oz.	161	42.8
(Dromedary):			
Chopped	1 cup (5. oz.)	493	114.2
Pitted	1 cup (5 oz.)	470	112.3
Imported (Bordo) Iraq:			
Diced	½ cup (2 oz.)	159	39.8
Whole	4 average dates (.9 oz.)	73	18.2
DEVIL DOGS (Drake's):			
Family size	1 piece (1.6 oz.)	178	24.9
Senior size	1 piece (2.3 oz.)	244	33.4
DEVIL'S FOOD CAKE (See **CAKE**, Devil's Food)			
DEVIL'S FOOD CAKE MIX (See **CAKE MIX**, Devil's Food)			
DEWBERRY, fresh (See **BLACKBERRY,** fresh)			
DILL SEED (French's)	1 tsp. (2.1 grams)	9	1.2
DING DONG (Hostess)	1 cake (1.3 oz.)	170	21.1
DIP (See also **DIP MIX**):			
Bacon & horseradish:			
(Borden)	1 oz.	58	1.7
(Breakstone)	1 T. (.6 oz.)	31	.7
(Kraft) *Teez*	1 oz.	57	1.6
Barbecue (Borden)	1 oz.	58	1.7
Blue cheese (Breakstone)	1 oz.	58	1.3
Blue cheese (Dean) Tang	1 oz.	61	2.3
Blue cheese (Sealtest) *Dip'n Dressing*	1 oz.	49	1.5
Blue cheese, Neufchâtel cheese (Kraft) *Ready Dip*	1 oz.	69	1.6
Casino (Sealtest) *Dip'n Dressing*	1 oz.	44	2.1

Food and Description	Measure or Quantity	Calories	Carbohydrates (grams)
Clam (Borden) & lobster	1 oz.	58	1.7
Clam (Kraft) *Teez*	1 oz.	45	1.5
Cucumber & onion (Breakstone)	1 oz.	50	1.6
Dill pickle & Neufchâtel cheese (Kraft) *Ready Dip*	1 oz.	67	2.4
Enchilada, *Fritos*	1 oz.	37	3.9
Garden spice (Borden)	1 oz.	66	2.1
Garlic (Dean)	1 oz.	58	2.0
Garlic (Kraft) *Teez*	1 oz.	47	1.5
Green goddess (Kraft) *Teez*	1 oz.	46	1.5
Jalapeño bean:			
(Amigos)	3½-oz. can	128	16.2
Fritos	1 oz.	34	3.7
(Gebhardt)	1 oz.	30	4.0
Onion:			
(Borden) French	1 oz.	58	1.7
(Kraft) Neufchâtel cheese, *Ready Dip*	1 oz.	68	2.0
(Kraft) French onion, *Teez*	1 oz.	43	1.5
(Sealtest) French onion, *Dip'n Dressing*	1 oz.	46	2.2
Pizza (Borden)	1 oz.	58	1.7
Shrimp Dip (Dean)	1 oz.	27	2.4
Tasty Tartar (Borden)	1 oz.	48	1.8
Western Bar-Q (Borden)	1 oz.	48	1.8
DIP MIX (Lawry's):			
Green onion	1 pkg. (.6 oz.)	50	10.6
Guacamole	1 pkg. (.6 oz.)	50	5.5
Toasted onion	1 pkg. (.6 oz.)	48	9.8

DISTILLED LIQUOR. The values below would apply to unflavored bourbon whiskey, brandy, Canadian whiskey, gin, Irish whiskey, rum, rye

(USDA): United States Department of Agriculture
(HEW/FAO): Health, Education and Welfare/Food and Agriculture Organization
* Prepared as Package Directs

Food and Description	Measure or Quantity	Calories	Carbo- hydrates (grams)
whiskey, Scotch whisky, tequila and vodka. The caloric content of distilled liquors depends on the percentage of alcohol. The proof is twice the alcohol percent and the following values apply to all brands (USDA):			
80 proof	1 fl. oz.	65	Tr.
86 proof	1 fl. oz.	70	Tr.
90 proof	1 fl. oz.	74	Tr.
94 proof	1 fl. oz.	77	Tr.
100 proof	1 fl. oz.	83	Tr.
DOCK, including **SHEEP SORREL** (USDA):			
Raw, whole	1 lb. (weighed untrimmed)	89	17.8
Boiled, drained	4 oz.	22	4.4
DOLLY VARDEN, raw, meat & skin (USDA)	4 oz.	163	0.
DOUGHNUT:			
(USDA) cake type	1 piece (1.1 oz.)	125	16.4
(USDA) yeast-leavened	1 piece (.6 oz.)	82	8.6
(Hostess):			
Cinnamon	1 piece (1 oz.)	111	14.5
Crunch	1 piece (1 oz.)	105	16.5
Plain	1 piece (1 oz.)	120	12.8
Powdered	1 piece (1 oz.)	117	15.1
Frozen (Morton):			
Bavarian creme	1 piece (2 oz.)	180	22.1
Boston creme	1 piece (2.3 oz.)	208	28.5
Chocolate iced	1 piece (1.5 oz.)	148	19.6
Glazed	1 piece (1.5 oz.)	150	19.2
Jelly	1 piece (1.8 oz.)	175	22.9
Mini	1 piece (1.1 oz.)	122	16.0
DOZY OATS (Drake's):			
1 piece	1.1 oz.	134	22.4
1 piece	2 oz.	236	38.6
1 piece	2¼ oz.	269	44.2

Food and Description	Measure or Quantity	Calories	Carbo-hydrates (grams)
DRAMBUIE LIQUEUR, 80 proof (Hiram Walker)	1 fl. oz.	110	11.0
DREAMSICLE (Popsicle Industries)	2½ fl. oz.	70	13.1
DRUM, raw (USDA): Freshwater:			
Whole	1 lb. (weighed whole)	143	0.
Meat only	4 oz.	137	0.
Red:			
Whole	1 lb. (weighed whole)	149	0.
Meat only	4 oz.	91	0.
DUCK, raw (USDA): Domesticated:			
Ready-to-cook	1 lb. (weighed with bones)	1213	0.
Meat only	4 oz.	187	0.
Wild:			
Dressed	1 lb. (weighed dressed)	613	0.
Meat only	4 oz.	156	0.
DUMPLINGS, canned, dietetic (Dia-Mel) stuffed, with chicken	8-oz. can	200	28.0
ECLAIR: Home recipe (USDA) with custard filling & chocolate icing	4 oz.	271	26.3
Frozen (Rich's) chocolate	1 piece (2.6 oz.)	234	30.0

(USDA): United States Department of Agriculture
(HEW/FAO): Health, Education and Welfare/Food and Agriculture Organization
* Prepared as Package Directs

Food and Description	Measure or Quantity	Calories	Carbo- hydrates (grams)
EEL (USDA):			
Raw, meat only	4 oz.	264	0.
Smoked, meat only	4 oz.	374	0.
EGG BEATERS (Fleischmann)	¼ cup (2.1 oz.)	101	1.8
EGG, CHICKEN (USDA):			
Raw:			
White only	1 large egg (1.2 oz.)	17	.3
White only	1 cup (9 oz.)	130	2.0
Yolk only	1 large egg (.6 oz.)	59	.1
Yolk only	1 cup (8.5 oz.)	835	1.4
Whole, small	1 egg (1.3 oz.)	60	.3
Whole, medium	1 egg (1.5 oz.)	71	.4
Whole, large	1 egg (1.8 oz.)	81	.4
Whole	1 cup (8.8 oz.)	409	2.3
Whole, extra large	1 egg (2 oz.)	94	.5
Whole, jumbo	1 egg (2.3 oz.)	105	.6
Cooked:			
Boiled	1 large egg (1.8 oz.)	81	.4
Fried in butter	1 large egg	99	.1
Omelet, mixed with milk & cooked in fat	1 large egg	107	1.5
Poached	1 large egg	78	.4
Scrambled, mixed with milk & cooked in fat	1 large egg	111	1.5
Scrambled, mixed with milk & cooked in fat	1 cup (7.8 oz.)	381	5.3
Dried:			
Whole	1 cup (3.8 oz.)	639	4.4
White, powder	1 oz.	105	1.6
Yolk	1 cup (3.4 oz.)	637	2.4
EGG, DUCK, raw (USDA)	1 egg (2.8 oz.)	153	.6
EGG, GOOSE, raw (USDA)	1 egg (5.8 oz.)	303	2.1
EGG, TURKEY, raw (USDA)	1 egg (3.1 oz.)	150	1.5

Food and Description	Measure or Quantity	Calories	Carbo-hydrates (grams)
EGG FOO YOUNG, frozen (Chun King)	6 oz. (½ pkg.)	120	10.9
EGG McMUFFIN (See McDONALD'S)			
EGG MIX (Durkee):			
Omelet:			
With bacon	1.3-oz. pkg.	128	18.0
*With bacon	½ pkg.	210	10.0
With cheese	1.3-oz. pkg.	125	12.0
*With cheese	½ of pkg.	309	24.0
Puffy	1.3-oz. pkg.	113	19.0
*Puffy	½ of pkg.	302	10.5
Western	1.1-oz. pkg.	110	20.0
*Western	½ of pkg.	302	11.0
Scrambled:			
With bacon	1.3-oz. pkg.	181	6.0
Plain	.8-oz. pkg.	124	4.0
EGG NOG, dairy:			
(Borden):			
4.69% fat	½ cup (4.2 oz.)	132	16.3
6.0% fat	½ cup (4.4 oz.)	154	16.6
8.0% fat	½ cup (4.4 oz.)	175	16.0
(Meadow Gold)	½ cup	164	25.5
(Sealtest):			
6% fat	½ cup (4.6 oz.)	174	18.0
8% fat	½ cup (4.6 oz.)	192	17.3
EGG NOG ICE CREAM (Breyer's)	¼ pt.	150	16.0
EGGPLANT:			
Raw (USDA) whole	1 lb. (weighed untrimmed	92	20.6
Boiled (USDA) drained, diced	1 cup (7.1 oz.)	38	8.2

(USDA): United States Department of Agriculture
(HEW/FAO): Health, Education and Welfare/Food and Agriculture
           Organization
* Prepared as Package Directs

Food and Description	Measure or Quantity	Calories	Carbo-hydrates (grams)
Frozen:			
(Buitoni) parmesan	4 oz.	189	16.2
(Mrs. Paul's):			
Parmigiana	½ of 11-oz. pkg.	259	23.4
Slices, breaded & fried	⅓ of 9-oz. pkg.	199	21.3
Sticks, breaded & fried	½ of 7-oz. pkg.	264	28.0
(Weight Watchers) parmigiana	13-oz. meal	251	25.1
EGG ROLL, frozen:			
(Chun King) chicken	½-oz. egg roll	28	3.2
(Chun King) meat & shrimp	½-oz. egg roll	29	3.7
(Chun King) shrimp	½-oz. egg roll	24	3.8
(Hung's)	1 piece	131	15.7
(Mow Sang) chicken & mushroom	1 egg roll	69	7.0
(Mow Sang) pork, barbecue	1 egg roll	74	6.0
(Mow Sang) shrimp	1 egg roll	64	6.0
(Mow Sang) vegetable	1 egg roll	66	7.0
(Temple) shrimp	1 roll	376	47.0
EGG, SCRAMBLED, frozen (Swanson) & sausage with coffee cake	6¼-oz. breakfast	460	22.0
***EGGSTRA** (Tillie Lewis)	½ of 7-oz. dry pkg. (1 large egg substitute)	54	4.0
ELDERBERRY, fresh (USDA):			
Whole	1 lb. (weighed with stems)	307	69.9
Stems removed	4 oz.	82	18.6
ELDERBERRY JELLY (Smucker's)	1 T. (.7 oz.)	52	13.3
ENCHILADA, frozen:			
Beef:			
(Banquet) with sauce, cooking bag	2 enchilada with sauce	207	28.9

Food and Description	Measure or Quantity	Calories	Carbo-hydrates (grams)
(Banquet) with cheese & chili gravy, buffet	2-lb. pkg.	1118	118.2
(Patio) with chili gravy	1 piece (4 oz.)	371	23.7
Cheese (Patio)	1 piece (4 oz.)	130	18.9
ENCHILADA DINNER, frozen:			
Beef:			
(Banquet)	12-oz. dinner	479	63.6
(Patio) 3-compartment	13-oz. dinner	320	34.0
(Swanson)	15-oz. dinner	570	72.0
Cheese:			
(Banquet)	12-oz. dinner	459	58.8
(Patio) 3-compartment	12-oz. dinner	330	40.0
ENCHILADA MIX (Lawry's)	1.6-oz. pkg.	144	27.3
ENDIVE, BELGIAN or FRENCH (See CHICORY WITLOOF)			
ENDIVE, CURLY, raw (USDA):			
Untrimmed	1 lb. (weighed untrimmed)	80	16.4
Trimmed	½ lb.	45	9.3
Cut up or shredded	1 cup (2.5 oz.)	14	2.9
ESCAROLE, raw (USDA):			
Untrimmed	1 lb. (weighed untrimmed)	80	16.4
Trimmed	½ lb.	46	9.2
Cut up or shredded	1 cup (2.5 oz.)	14	2.9
ESCAROLE SOUP, canned (Progresso) in chicken broth	1 cup (8 oz. by wt.)	25	1.0
EULACHON or SMELT, raw, meat only (USDA)	4 oz.	134	0.

(USDA): United States Department of Agriculture
(HEW/FAO): Health, Education and Welfare/Food and Agriculture Organization
* Prepared as Package Directs

Food and Description	Measure or Quantity	Calories	Carbo-hydrates (grams)
EXTRACT (See individual listings)			

F

Food and Description	Measure or Quantity	Calories	Carbo-hydrates (grams)
FARINA (See also **CREAM OF WHEAT**):			
Regular:			
Dry:			
(USDA)	1 cup (6 oz.)	627	130.1
(H-O) cream, enriched	1 cup (6.1 oz.)	625	133.8
(H-O) cream, enriched	1 T.	41	8.8
Malt-O-Meal	1 oz.	96	21.1
Cooked:			
*(USDA)	1 cup (8.4 oz.)	100	20.7
*(USDA)	4 oz.	48	9.9
*(Pillsbury) made with milk & salt	⅔ cup	200	26.0
*(Pillsbury) made with water & salt	⅔ cup	80	2.0
Quick-cooking:			
Dry (USDA)	1 oz.	103	21.2
Dry, *Malt-O-Meal*	1 oz.	100	22.0
Cooked (USDA)	1 cup (8.6 oz.)	105	21.8
Instant-cooking (USDA):			
Dry	1 oz.	103	21.2
Cooked	4 oz.	62	12.9
FAT, COOKING, vegetable:			
(USDA)	1 cup (7.1 oz.)	1768	0.
(USDA)	1 T. (.4 oz.)	106	0.
Crisco	1 T. (.4 oz.)	110	0.
Fluffo	1 T. (.4 oz.)	110	0.
Spry	1 T. (.4 oz.)	95	0.
FENNEL LEAVES, raw (USDA):			
Untrimmed	1 lb. (weighed untrimmed)	118	21.5
Trimmed	4 oz.	32	5.8

FIG [177]

Food and Description	Measure or Quantity	Calories	Carbohydrates (grams)
FENNEL SEED (French's)	1 tsp. (2.1 grams)	8	1.3
FESTIVAL MAIN MEAL MEAT, canned (Wilson-Sinclair):			
Beef roast	3 oz.	100	0.
Corned beef brisket	3 oz.	135	0.
Ham	3 oz.	129	.8
Picnic	3 oz.	137	.8
Pork loin, smoked	3 oz.	114	.8
Pork roast	3 oz.	133	0.
Turkey & dressing	3 oz.	159	8.5
Turkey roast	3 oz.	87	0.
FIG:			
Fresh:			
(USDA)	1 lb.	363	92.1
(USDA) small	1.3-oz. fig (1½" dia.)	30	7.7
Candied (Bama)	1 T. (.7 oz.)	37	9.6
Canned, regular pack, solids & liq. (USDA):			
Light syrup	4 oz.	74	19.1
Heavy syrup	3 figs & 2 T. syrup (4 oz.)	96	24.9
Heavy syrup	½ cup (4.4 oz.)	106	27.5
Extra heavy syrup	4 oz.	117	30.3
(Del Monte)	½ cup (4.3 oz.)	114	28.1
Canned, unsweetened or dietetic pack:			
(USDA) water pack, solids & liq.	4 oz.	54	14.1
(Diet delight) Kadota, solids & liq.	½ cup (4.4 oz.)	76	18.2
(Featherweight) Kadota, water pack, solids & liq.	½ cup	60	18.0

(USDA): United States Department of Agriculture
(HEW/FAO): Health, Education and Welfare/Food and Agriculture Organization
* Prepared as Package Directs

Food and Description	Measure or Quantity	Calories	Carbohydrates (grams)
(S and W) *Nutradiet*, whole, unsweetened	6 figs (3.5 oz.)	52	12.7
Dried (USDA):			
Chopped	1 cup (6 oz.)	469	118.2
Whole	.7-oz. fig (2″ x 1″)	58	14.5
FIG JUICE			
Real Fig	½ cup (4.5 oz.)	61	15.8
FIGURINES (Pillsbury), all flavors	1 bar	138	10.5
FILBERT or HAZELNUT (USDA):			
Whole	4 oz. (weighed in shell)	331	8.7
Shelled	1 oz.	180	4.7
FISH (See individual listings)			
FISH CAKE:			
Home recipe (USDA) fried	2 oz.	98	5.3
Frozen:			
(Commodore)	2 oz.	102	9.8
(Mrs. Paul's) breaded & fried	½ of 8-oz. pkg.	208	20.5
(Mrs. Paul's) thins, breaded & fried	⅛ of 10-oz. pkg.	326	35.3
FISH & CHIPS, frozen:			
(Gorton)	½ of 1-lb. pkg.	395	39.0
(Mrs. Paul's) batter fried	½ of 12-oz. pkg.	364	7.2
(Swanson)	10¼-oz. dinner	450	40.0
(Swanson)	5-oz. entree	290	25.0
(Swanson) *Hungry Man*	15¾-oz. dinner	760	68.0
FISH CHOWDER, New England (Snow)	½ cup	78	8.6
FISH DINNER, frozen:			
(Banquet)	8¾-oz. dinner	382	43.6
(Morton)	9-oz. dinner	253	20.5

Food and Description	Measure or Quantity	Calories	Carbo- hydrates (grams)
FISH FILLET, frozen (Mrs. Paul's):			
Batter fried	½ of 9-oz. pkg.	307	34.6
Breaded & fried	½ of 8-oz. pkg.	205	17.4
Buttered	2½-oz. piece	154	.7
Miniature, light batter fried	⅓ of 9-oz. pkg.	154	15.3
FISH FLAKES, canned (USDA)	4 oz.	126	0.
FISH LOAF, home recipe (USDA)	4 oz.	141	8.3
FISH PARMESAN, frozen (Mrs. Paul's)	½ of 10-oz. pkg.	226	20.2
FISH PUFF, frozen (Gordon)	½ of 8-oz. pkg.	265	9.0
FISH STICK, frozen:			
(USDA) cooked, commercial, 3¾″ x 1″ x ½″ sticks	10 sticks (8-oz. pkg.)	400	14.8
(Commodore)	4 oz.	200	7.6
(Gorton)	½ of 8-oz. pkg.	200	8.0
(Mrs. Paul's) batter fried	1 stick (.9 oz.)	58	6.4
(Mrs. Paul's) breaded & fried	⅓ of 9-oz. pkg.	156	16.0
FLAN PUDDING:			
Chilled (Breakstone)	5-oz. container	185	37.5
*Mix, regular (Royal)	½ cup (4.9 oz.)	141	20.9
FLORIDA PUNCH, canned (HI-C)	6 fl. oz.	95	24.0
FLOUNDER: Raw:			
(USDA) whole	1 lb. (weighed whole)	118	0.

(USDA): United States Department of Agriculture
(HEW/FAO): Health, Education and Welfare/Food and Agriculture
                    Organization
* Prepared as Package Directs

Food and Description	Measure or Quantity	Calories	Carbo-hydrates (grams)
(USDA) meat only	4 oz.	90	0.
Baked (USDA)	4 oz.	229	0.
Frozen:			
(Gorton)	1 lg. pkg.	360	0.
(Mrs. Paul's) fillets, breaded & fried	½ of 8-oz. pkg.	276	23.2
(Ship Ahoy)	1-lb. pkg.	316	0.
(Weight Watchers) 2-compartment	8½-oz. meal	169	13.0
(Weight Watchers) 3-compartment	16-oz. meal	261	14.1
FLOUR:			
(USDA):			
Buckwheat, dark, sifted	1 cup (3.5 oz.)	326	70.6
Buckwheat, light, sifted	1 cup (3.5 oz.)	340	77.9
Carob or St. John's-bread	1 oz.	51	22.9
Chestnut	1 oz.	103	21.6
Corn	1 cup (3.9 oz.)	405	84.5
Cottonseed	1 oz.	101	9.4
Fish, from whole fish	1 oz.	95	0.
Lima bean	1 oz.	97	17.9
Potato	1 oz.	100	22.7
Rice, stirred, spooned	1 cup (5.6 oz.)	574	125.6
Rye:			
Light:			
Unsifted, spooned	1 cup (3.6 oz.)	361	78.7
Sifted, spooned	1 cup (3.1 oz.)	314	68.6
Medium:	1 oz.	99	21.2
Dark:			
Unstirred	1 cup (4.5 oz.)	419	87.2
Stirred	1 cup (4.5 oz.)	415	86.5
Soybean, defatted, stirred	1 cup (3.6 oz.)	329	38.5
Soybean, high fat	1 oz.	108	9.4
Sunflower seed, partially defatted	1 oz.	96	10.7
Wheat:			
All-purpose:			
Unsifted, dipped	1 cup (5 oz.)	521	108.8
Unsifted, spooned	1 cup (4.4 oz.)	459	95.9
Sifted, spooned	1 cup (4.1 oz.)	422	88.3
Bread:			
Unsifted, dipped	1 cup (4.8 oz.)	496	101.6

Food and Description	Measure or Quantity	Calories	Carbo-hydrates (grams)
Unsifted, spooned	1 cup (4.3 oz.)	449	91.9
Sifted, spooned	1 cup (4.1 oz.)	427	87.4
Cake:			
Unsifted, dipped	1 cup (4.2 oz.)	433	94.5
Unsifted, spooned	1 cup (3.9 oz.)	404	88.1
Sifted, spooned	1 cup (3.5 oz.)	360	78.6
Gluten:			
Unsifted, dipped	1 cup (5 oz.)	537	67.0
Unsifted, spooned	1 cup (4.8 oz.)	510	63.7
Sifted, spooned	1 cup (4.8 oz.)	514	64.2
Self-rising:			
Unsifted, dipped	1 cup (4.6 oz.)	458	96.5
Unsifted, spooned	1 cup (4.5 oz.)	447	94.2
Sifted, spooned	1 cup (3.7 oz.)	373	78.7
Whole wheat	1 oz.	94	20.1
(Aunt Jemima) self-rising	¼ cup (1 oz.)	109	23.6
Ballard, all-purpose	1 cup	400	87.0
Ballard, self-rising	1 cup	380	84.0
Bisquick (Betty Crocker)	½ cup	240	38.0
Gold Medal (Betty Crocker) all-purpose	1 cup	483	100.7
Gold Medal (Betty Crocker) self-rising	1 cup	476	100.5
Masa Trigo (Quaker)	⅛ cup	149	24.7
(Pillsbury):			
All-purpose	1 cup	400	87.0
Instant blending	1 cup	50	11.0
Medium rye	1 cup	420	89
Self-rising	1 cup	380	84.0
Unbleached	1 cup	400	86.0
Whole wheat	1 cup	400	86.0
Presto, self-rising	1 cup (3.9 oz.)	399	87.8
Robin Hood, all-purpose	1 cup (4 oz.)	400	85.0
Robin Hood, self-rising	1 cup (4 oz.)	380	81.0
(Swans Down) cake	¼ cup	100	22.0
(Swans Down) cake, self-rising	¼ cup	90	20.0

(USDA): United States Department of Agriculture
(HEW/FAO): Health, Education and Welfare/Food and Agriculture Organization
＊ Prepared as Package Directs

Food and Description	Measure or Quantity	Calories	Carbo- hydrates (grams)
FOLLE BLANCHE WINE (Louis M. Martini) 12.5% alcohol	3 fl. oz.	90	.2
FOOD STICKS (Pillsbury), all flavors	1 stick	45	6.8
FOUR FRUIT PRESERVE (Smucker's)	1 T.	53	13.7
FOURNIER NATURE (Gold Seal) 12% alcohol	3 fl. oz.	82	.4
FRANKEN*BERRY, cereal (General Mills)	1 cup	110	24.0
FRANKFURTER, raw or cooked: (USDA):			
Raw, all kinds	1 frankfurter (10 per lb.)	140	.8
Raw, all meat	1 frankfurter (10 per lb.)	134	1.1
Raw, with cereal	1 frankfurter (10 per lb.)	112	<.1
Cooked, all kinds	1 frankfurter (10 per lb.)	136	.7
(Armour Star) all meat	1 frankfurter (10 per lb.)	155	0.
(Hormel): All beef	1 frankfurter (1.6 oz.)	140	.6
All meat	1 frankfurter (1.6 oz.)	140	.8
Wrangler	1 frankfurter (2 oz.)	175	1.6
(Hygrade): Beef	1 frankfurter (1.6 oz.)	146	1.4
Beef, *Ball Park*	1 frankfurter (2 oz.)	169	<.1
Meat	1 frankfurter (1.6 oz.)	147	1.5

Food and Description	Measure or Quantity	Calories	Carbo-hydrates (grams)
Meat, *Ball Park*	1 frankfurter (2 oz.)	175	<.1
(Oscar Mayer):			
beef	1 frankfurter (1.6 oz.)	141	1.4
Beef	1 frankfurter (2 oz.)	180	1.8
Machiach Brand	1 frankfurter (2 oz.)	179	1.8
Little wiener	1 weiner (.3 oz.)	31	.3
Wiener	1 frankfurter (1.6 oz.)	145	1.3
Wiener	1 frankfurter (2 oz.)	184	1.6
(Swift)	1 frankfurter (1.6 oz.)	150	1.2
(Vienna) beef	1 frankfurter	132	1.0
(Wilson):			
All beef	1 frankfurter (1.6 oz.)	136	.8
Skinless	1 frankfurter (1.6 oz.)	140	.8
Canned (USDA)	2 oz.	125	.1
Canned (Hormel)	12-oz. can	966	2.4

FRANKS AND BEANS (See **BEANS & FRANKS**)

FRANKS-N-BLANKETS, frozen (Durkee)	1 piece	45	1.0

FRENCH TOAST, frozen:			
(Aunt Jemima)	1 slice (1.5 oz.)	85	13.2
(Aunt Jemima) cinnamon swirl	1 slice (1.5 oz.)	97	13.7
(Eggo)	1 slice (1.5 oz.)	80	12.0
(Swanson) with sausage	4½-oz. breakfast	300	22.0

(USDA): United States Department of Agriculture
(HEW/FAO): Health, Education and Welfare/Food and Agriculture
Organization
* Prepared as Package Directs

Food and Description	Measure or Quantity	Calories	Carbo-hydrates (grams)
FROG LEGS, raw (USDA):			
Bone in	1 lb. (weighed with bone)	215	0.
Meat only	4 oz.	83	0.
FROOT LOOPS, cereal (Kellogg's)	1 cup (1 oz.)	110	25.0
FROSTED RICE, cereal (Kellogg's)	1 cup (1 oz.)	110	26.0
FROSTED SHAKE, any flavor (Borden)	9¼-oz. can	320	43.0
FROSTED TREAT (Weight Watchers)	1 serving (4.8 oz.)	140	23.5
FROSTING (See **CAKE ICING**)			
FROSTY O's, cereal (General Mills)	1 cup (1 oz.)	110	24.0
FROZEN CUSTARD (See **ICE CREAM**)			
FRUIT BRUTE, cereal (General Mills)	1 cup (1 oz.)	110	24.0
FRUIT CAKE (See **CAKE,** fruit)			
FRUIT COCKTAIL:			
Canned, regular pack, solids & liq.:			
(USDA) light syrup	4 oz.	68	17.8
(USDA) heavy syrup	½ cup (4.5 oz.)	97	25.2
(USDA) extra heavy syrup	4 oz.	104	26.9
(Del Monte) heavy syrup	½ cup (4.3 oz.)	95	23.1
(Hunt's) heavy syrup	½ cup (4.5 oz.)	89	23.9
(Libby's) heavy syrup	½ cup (4.5 oz.)	94	24.7

Food and Description	Measure or Quantity	Calories	Carbohydrates (grams)
(Stokely-Van Camp)	½ cup (4.5 oz.)	95	23.0
Canned, unsweetened or dietetic pack, solids & liq.:			
(USDA) water pack	4 oz.	42	11.0
(Cellu) water pack	½ cup	40	10.0
(Diet Delight) unsweetened	½ cup	60	14.3
(Diet Delight) water pack	½ cup	40	10.0
(Featherweight) juice pack	½ cup	50	14.0
(Libby's) water pack	½ cup (4.3 oz.)	40	10.4
(S and W) *Nutradiet,* low calorie	4 oz.	41	9.7
(Tillie Lewis)	½ cup (4.3 oz.)	49	12.2
FRUIT CUP (Del Monte):			
Mixed, solids & liq.	5-oz. container	110	26.7
Peaches, cling, diced, solids & liq.	5-oz. container	116	27.8
FRUIT DOODLE (Drake's)			
Apple	1 piece (1⅝ oz.)	178	22.7
Cherry	1 piece (1⅝ oz.)	173	21.7
FRUIT, MIXED, frozen, quick thaw (Birds Eye)	½ cup (5 oz.)	130	34.0
FRUIT PUNCH:			
Canned (Alegre) red tropical	6 fl. oz.	98	24.2
Canned (Ann Page) tropical	1 cup (8.7 oz.)	122	30.4
*Mix (Wyler's)	6 fl. oz.	64	15.8
FRUIT SALAD:			
Bottled (Kraft) chilled	4 oz.	57	13.3
Canned, regular pack, solids & liq.:			
(USDA) light syrup	4 oz.	67	17.6
(USDA) heavy syrup	½ cup (4.3 oz.)	85	22.0

(USDA): United States Department of Agriculture
(HEW/FAO): Health, Education and Welfare/Food and Agriculture
                Organization

* Prepared as Package Directs

Food and Description	Measure or Quantity	Calories	Carbohydrates (grams)
(USDA) extra heavy syrup	4 oz.	102	26.5
(Del Monte) fruit for salad	½ cup (4.3 oz.)	94	23.0
(Del Monte) tropical	½ cup (4.4 oz.)	107	26.0
(Libby's) heavy syrup	½ cup (4.4 oz.)	89	24.0
(Stokely-Van Camp)	½ cup (4.5 oz.)	95	22.0
Canned, unsweetened or dietetic pack, solids & liq.:			
(USDA) water pack	4 oz.	40	10.3
(Cellu) water pack	½ cup	30	8.0
(Diet Delight) unsweetened	½ cup (4.4 oz.)	69	16.5
(Featherweight)	½ cup	45	13.0
(S and W) *Nutradiet,* unsweetened	4 oz.	43	10.3
FRUIT-SICLE (Popsicle Industries)	2½ fl. oz.	59	
FUDGE CAKE MIX (See CAKE MIX, Fudge)			
FUDGE ICE BAR (Sealtest)	2½ fl. oz.	90	19.0
FUDGE PUDDING (Thank You)	½ cup (4.5 oz.)	202	34.3
FUDGSICLE (Popsicle Industries):			
Banana	2½ fl. oz.	102	23.5
Chocolate	2½ fl. oz.	153	20.0
FUNNY BONES (Drake's)	1¼-oz. cake	153	20.0
*FUNNY FACE (Pillsbury), all flavors	8 fl. oz.	80	20.0

G

GARBANZO, dry (See CHICK PEAS)

Food and Description	Measure or Quantity	Calories	Carbo-hydrates (grams)
GARLIC, raw (USDA):			
Whole	2 oz. (weighed with skin)	68	15.4
Peeled	1 oz.	39	8.7
GARLIC FLAKES (Gilroy)	1 tsp. (1.5 grams)	5	1.1
GARLIC POWDER (Gilroy)	1 tsp.	9	1.8
GARLIC SPREAD (Lawry's)	1 T. (.5 oz.)	79	1.2
GAZPACHO SOUP, canned (Crosse & Blackwell)	½ can (6½ fl. oz.)	61	6.8
GELFILTE FISH, canned (Manischewitz):			
4-portion can	1 piece (3.7 oz.)	100	3.9
2-lb. jar	1 piece (2.4 oz.)	64	2.5
Fish balls	1 piece (1.5 oz.)	40	1.6
Fishlet	1 piece (7 grams)	70	.3
2-lb. jar	1 piece (1.7 oz.)	40	1.5
GELATIN, unflavored, dry:			
(USDA)	1 envelope (7 grams)	23	0.
(Ann Page)	¼-oz. envelope	24	0.
GELATIN DESSERT:			
Powder:			
Regular:			
(USDA)	3-oz. pkg.	315	74.8
*(USDA)	½ cup (4.2 oz.)	71	16.9
*(USDA) with fruit added	½ cup (4.2 oz.)	81	19.8
(Ann Page)	¼ of 3-oz. pkg.	83	19.0
*(Jell-O) all fruit flavors	½ cup (4.9 oz.)	80	19.0
*(Jells Best) all flavors	½ cup	80	18.7
*(Royal) all flavors	½ cup (4.2 oz.)	82	18.9

(USDA): United States Department of Agriculture
(HEW/FAO): Health, Education and Welfare/Food and Agriculture
            Organization
* Prepared as Package Directs

Food and Description	Measure or Quantity	Calories	Carbo-hydrates (grams)
Dietetic or low calorie:			
*(D-Zerta) all flavors	½ cup (4.3 oz.)	8	0.
*(Dia-Mel) *Gel-a-Thin*, all flavors	4-oz. serving	10	1.0
(Estee) all flavors	½ cup	40	9.0
*(Louis Sherry) *Shimmer*, all flavors	½ cup (4.4 oz.)	10	1.0
Canned:			
Dietetic (Dia-Mel) *Gel-a-Thin*, all flavors	4-oz. container	1	.2
GELATIN DRINK (Knox)			
orange	1 envelope	70	10.0
GERMAN DINNER, frozen (Swanson)	11-oz. dinner	430	40.0
GIN, unflavored (See **DISTILLED LIQUOR**)			
GIN, SLOE:			
(Bols) 66 proof	1 fl. oz.	85	4.7
(DeKuyper) 60 proof	1 fl. oz.	70	5.2
(Garnier) 60 proof	1 fl. oz.	82	8.5
(Hiram Walker) 60 proof	1 fl. oz.	68	4.8
GINGERBREAD			
Home recipe (USDA)	1.9-oz. piece (2″ x 2″ x 2″)	174	28.6
Mix:			
(USDA) dry	4 oz.	482	88.7
*(USDA)	⅑ of 8″ sq. (2.2 oz.)	174	32.2
*(Betty Crocker)	⅑ of cake	210	36.0
*(Dromedary)	2″ x 2″ sq.	100	19.0
*Pillsbury)	3″ sq.	190	36.0
GINGER, CANDIED (USDA)			
GINGER ROOT, fresh (USDA):			
With skin	1 oz.	13	2.5
Without skin	1 oz.	14	2.7
	1 oz.	96	24.7

Food and Description	Measure or Quantity	Calories	Carbo-hydrates (grams)
GIN SOUR COCKTAIL			
(Calvert) 60 proof	3 fl. oz.	195	10.4
GOLD-O-MINT LIQUEUR			
(Leroux) 25 proof	1 fl. oz.	110	15.2
GOOD HUMOR:			
Chocolate eclair	3-oz. piece	220	25.0
Sandwich	2.5-oz. piece	200	34.0
Strawberry shortcake	3-oz. piece	200	21.0
Toasted almond bar	3-oz. piece	170	25.0
Vanilla, chocolate coated bar	3-oz. piece	170	12.0
Whammy:			
Assorted	1.6-oz. piece	100	9.0
Crisp crunch	1.6-oz. piece	110	10.0
Vanilla	1.4-oz. piece	137	11.2
Ice	1.5-oz. piece	50	13.0
GOOSE, domesticated (USDA):			
Raw	1 lb. (weighed ready-to-cook)	1172	0.
Roasted, meat & skin	4 oz.	500	0.
Roasted, meat only	4 oz.	264	0.
GOOSEBERRY (USDA):			
Fresh	1 lb.	177	44.0
Fresh	1 cup (5.3 oz.)	58	14.6
Canned, water pack, solids & liq.	4 oz.	29	7.5
GOOSE, GIZZARD, raw (USDA)	4 oz.	158	0.
GRAHAM CRACKER (See CRACKER)			

(USDA): United States Department of Agriculture
(HEW/FAO): Health, Education and Welfare/Food and Agriculture Organization
* Prepared as Package Directs

Food and Description	Measure or Quantity	Calories	Carbo-hydrates (grams)
GRANOLA:			
Heartland:			
Coconut	¼ cup (1 oz.)	130	18.0
Plain or raisin	¼ cup (1 oz.)	120	18.0
Puffs, regular or cinnamon spice	½ cup (1 oz.)	120	20.0
Nature Valley:			
Cinnamon & raisin	⅓ cup (1 oz.)	130	19.0
Coconut & honey	⅓ cup (1 oz.)	130	18.0
Fruit & nut	⅓ cup (1 oz.)	130	20.0
Oats & honey	⅓ cup (1 oz.)	130	19.0
Sun Country:			
Almonds	½ cup (2 oz.)	250	34.0
Raisin	½ cup (2 oz.)	250	37.0
Vita-Crunch:			
Date	½ cup	284	47.0
Raisin	½ cup	289	46.4
GRANOLA BARS			
Nature Valley:			
Cinnamon and honey 'n oats	1 bar (.8 oz.)	110	16.0
Coconut & peanut	1 bar (.8 oz.)	120	15.0
GRAPE:			
Fresh:			
American type (slip skin), Concord, Delaware, Niagara, Catawba & Scuppernong:			
(USDA)	½ lb. (weighed with stem, skin & seeds)	98	22.4
(USDA)	½ cup (2.7 oz.)	52	11.9
(USDA)	3½″ x 3″ bunch (3.5 oz.)	43	9.9
European type (adherent skin), Malaga, Muscat, Thompson seedless, Emperor & Flame Tokay:			
(USDA)	½ lb. (weighed with stem & seeds)	135	34.9

Food and Description	Measure or Quantity	Calories	Carbo-hydrates (grams)
(USDA) whole	20 grapes (¾″ dia.)	54	13.8
(USDA) whole	½ cup (.3 oz.)	58	15.1
(USDA) halves	½ cup (.3 oz.)	58	14.9
Canned, solids & liq.:			
(USDA) Thompson, seedless, heavy syrup	4 oz.	87	22.7
(USDA) Thompson, seedless, water pack	4 oz.	58	15.4
(Featherweight) water pack, seedless	½ cup	50	12.0
GRAPEADE, chilled			
(Sealtest)	6 fl. oz.	96	24.2
GRAPE DRINK:			
(Ann Page)	1 cup (8.7 oz.)	125	31.1
(Hi-C)	6 fl. oz.	89	22.0
(Wagner's)	8 fl. oz.	129	32.4
GRAPE JELLY:			
Sweetened (Smucker's)	1 T.	53	13.3
Dietetic or low calorie:			
(Dia-Mel)	1 tsp.	2	0.
(Diet Delight)	1 T. (.6 oz.)	11	2.7
(Featherweight)	1 T.	16	4.0
(Kraft)	1 oz.	34	8.4
(Louis Sherry) pure	1 tsp.	16	4.0
(Slenderella)	1 T. (.6 oz.)	23	5.8
(Tillie Lewis)	1 T.	12	3.0
GRAPE JUICE:			
Canned:			
(USDA)	½ cup (4.4 oz.)	83	20.9
(Seneca) unsweetened	½ cup (4.4 oz.)	84	20.9
(Seneca) sweetened	½ cup (4.4 oz.)	115	29.0
(S and W) *Nutradiet,* unsweetened	4 oz. (by wt.)	68	17.5

(USDA): United States Department of Agriculture
(HEW/FAO): Health, Education and Welfare/Food and Agriculture Organization
* Prepared as Package Directs

Food and Description	Measure or Quantity	Calories	Carbo-hydrates (grams)
Frozen, concentrate, sweetened:			
(USDA)	6-fl.-oz. can	395	100.0
*(USDA) diluted	½ cup (4.4 oz.)	66	16.6
*(Minute Maid)	6 fl. oz.	99	25.0
*(Seneca)	½ cup (4.4 oz.)	66	17.2
GRAPE JUICE DRINK, canned, approx. 30% grape juice (USDA)	1 cup (8.8 oz.)	135	34.5
GRAPE NUTS, cereal (Post)	¼ cup (1 oz.)	110	22.0
GRAPE NUTS FLAKES, cereal (Post)	¼ cup (1 oz.)	100	23.0
GRAPE PIE (Tastykake)	4-oz. pie	369	51.8
GRAPEFRUIT:			
Fresh:			
White (USDA):			
Seeded type	1 lb. (weighed with seeds & skin)	84	22.0
Seedless type	1 lb. (weighed with skin)	87	22.4
Seeded type	½ med. grapefruit (3¾" dia., 8.5 oz.)	44	11.7
Sections, seedless (Sunkist)	1 cup (7 oz.)	78	20.2
	½ grapefruit (8.5 oz.)	44	11.0
Pink and red (USDA):			
Seeded type	1 lb. (weighed with seeds & skin)	87	22.6
Seedless type	1 lb. (weighed with skin)	93	24.1
Seeded type	½ med. grapefruit (3¾" dia., 8.5 oz.)	46	12.0
Canned, syrup pack, solids & liq. (Del Monte)	½ cup	74	17.5
Canned, unsweetened or dietetic pack, solids & liq.:			
(USDA) water pack	½ cup (4.2 oz.)	36	9.1
(Del Monte) sections	½ cup	46	10.5

Food and Description	Measure or Quantity	Calories	Carbo-hydrates (grams)
(Diet Delight) sections	½ cup (4.3 oz.)	47	11.1
(Featherweight) sections	½ cup	40	9.0
(Tillie Lewis)	½ cup (4.4 oz.)	45	11.2
GRAPEFRUIT DRINK:			
Natural (Ann Page)	6 fl. oz. (6.5 oz.)	83	20.7
Sweetened (Wagner)	6 fl. oz.	86	21.8
GRAPEFRUIT JUICE:			
Fresh, pink, red or white, all varieties (USDA)	½ cup (4.3 oz.)	48	11.3
Bottled (Kraft) chilled, unsweetened	½ cup (4.3 oz.)	48	11.1
Bottled (Kraft) chilled, sweetened	½ cup (4.3 oz.)	60	14.0
Canned:			
Sweetened:			
(USDA)	½ cup (4.4 oz.)	66	16.0
(Del Monte)	6 fl. oz.	89	20.8
Sweetened:			
(USDA)	½ cup (4.4 oz.)	51	12.2
Del Monte	6 fl. oz.	72	16.6
(Featherweight)	½ cup	43	9.0
(Ocean Spray)	6 fl. oz. (6.5 oz.)	71	16.3
Frozen, concentrate:			
Sweetened			
(USDA)	6-fl.-oz. can	348	84.8
*(USDA) diluted with 3 parts water	½ cup (4.4 oz.)	58	14.1
Unsweetened			
(USDA)	6-fl.-oz. can	300	71.6
*(USDA) diluted with 3 parts water	½ cup (4.4 oz.)	51	12.2
*(Minute Maid)	6 fl. oz.	75	18.3
Dehydrated, crystals:			
(USDA)	4-oz. can	429	102.4
*(USDA) reconstituted	½ cup (4.4 oz.)	50	11.9

(USDA): United States Department of Agriculture
(HEW/FAO): Health, Education and Welfare/Food and Agriculture Organization
* Prepared as Package Directs

Food and Description	Measure or Quantity	Calories	Carbohydrates (grams)
GRAPEFRUIT PEEL, CANDIED (Liberty)	1 oz.	93	22.6
GRAVES WINE (See also individual regional, vineyard or brand names):			
(Barton & Guestier) 12.5% alcohol	3 fl. oz.	65	.6
(Cruse) 11.5% alcohol	3 fl. oz.	69	
GRAVY, canned:			
Beef (Ann Page)	10½-oz. can	118	18.3
Beef (Franco-American)	10¼-oz. can	154	15.4
Brown:			
(Dawn Fresh) with mushroom broth	2 oz. serving	20	4.0
(Franco-American) with onion	10½-oz. can	131	21.0
Ready Gravy	¼ cup serving	44	7.4
Chicken (Franco-American)	10½-oz. can	263	15.8
Chicken giblet (Franco-American)	10½-oz. can	184	15.8
Mushroom (Franco-American)	10½-oz. can	184	21.0
GRAVY MASTER	1 fl. oz. (1.3 oz.)	66	13.9
GRAVY with MEAT or TURKEY:			
Canned:			
(Bunker Hill):			
Beef chunks	15-oz. can	788	16.0
Chopped beef	10½-oz. can	516	10.0
Sliced beef	15-oz. can	716	16.0
Sliced beef liver	15-oz. can	398	30.0
(Morton House):			
Sliced beef	½ of 12½-oz. can	190	8.0
Sliced pork	½ of 12½-oz. can	190	9.0
Sliced turkey	½ of 12½-oz. can	140	7.0
Frozen:			
(Banquet):			
Giblet gravy and sliced turkey	5-oz. cooking bag	98	5.3

Food and Description	Measure or Quantity	Calories	Carbo-hydrates (grams)
Giblet gravy and sliced turkey	2-lb. pkg.	564	28.2
Sliced beef	5-oz. cooking bag	116	4.8
Sliced beef	2-lb. pkg.	782	34.5
(Green giant) *Toast Topper*:			
Sliced beef	5-oz. serving	130	7.0
Sliced turkey	5-oz. can	100	7.0
Mix:			
Au jus:			
(Ann Page)	¾-oz. pkg.	52	10.9
(Durkee)	1-oz. pkg.	62	13.0
(Durkee) *Roastin' Bag*	1-oz. pkg.	64	14.0
(French's) *Gravy Makins*	¾-oz. pkg.	63	12.0
Brown:			
(Ann Page)	¾-oz. pkg.	78	12.0
(Durkee)	.8-oz. pkg.	59	10.0
(Durkee) with mushrooms	.7-oz. pkg.	59	11.0
(Durkee) with onions	.8-oz. pkg.	66	13.0
*(Ehler's)	¼-cup serving	22	3.5
(French's) *Gravy Makins*	¾-oz. pkg.	78	13.7
*(Kraft)	2 oz. serving	21	2.8
(Lawry's)	1½-oz. pkg.	136	16.3
(McCormick)	⅞-oz. pkg.	100	10.0
*(McCormick)	2-oz. serving	25	2.5
*(Pillsbury)	¼ cup serving	15	3.0
*(Spatini)	1-oz. serving	10	3.0
Chicken:			
(Ann Page)	1-oz. pkg.	107	16.7
(Durkee)	1-oz. pkg.	87	14.0
(Durkee) creamy	1.2-oz. pkg.	156	14.0
(Durkee) *Roastin Bag*	1.5-oz. pkg.	122	24.0
(Durkee) *Roastin Bag,* creamy	2-oz. pkg.	242	22.0

(USDA): United States Department of Agriculture
(HEW/FAO): Health, Education and Welfare/Food and Agriculture
Organization

* Prepared as Package Directs

Food and Description	Measure or Quantity	Calories	Carbo-hydrates (grams)
(Durkee) Roastin Bag, Italian style	1.5-oz. pkg.	144	31.0
*(Ehler's)	¼ cup serving	21	4.0
(French's) Gravy Makins	.9-oz. pkg.	94	14.8
(Lawry's)	1-oz. pkg.	110	13.6
*(McCormick)	2-oz. serving	20	3.0
*(Pillsbury)	¼ cup serving	15	3.0
(Swiss)	1¼-oz. pkg.	107	22.7
*(Wyler's)	2-oz. serving	25	3.7
*Herb (McCormick)	2-oz. serving	22	2.5
Homestyle (Durkee)	.8-oz. pkg.	70	11.0
Homestyle (French's) Gravy Makins	.9-oz. pkg.	89	14.5
*Homestyle (Pillsbury)	¼ cup serving	15	3.0
Meatloaf (Durkee) Roastin' Bag	1.5-oz. pkg.	129	18.0
Mushroom:			
(Ann Page)	¾-oz. pkg.	76	12.1
(Durkee)	.8-oz. pkg.	60	11.0
(French's) Gravy Makins	¾-oz. pkg.	70	13.7
(Lawry's)	1.3-oz. pkg.	145	15.6
*(McCormick)	2-oz. serving	17	2.5
*(Wyler's)	2-oz. serving	15	1.8
Onion:			
(Ann Page)	1-oz. pkg.	106	17.7
(Durkee)	1-oz. pkg.	84	15.0
(French's) Gravy Makins	1-oz. pkg.	84	17.3
*(Kraft)	2-oz. serving	22	3.7
*(McCormick)	2-oz. serving	29	3.5
*(Wyler's)	2-oz. serving	17	2.7
Pork:			
(Durkee)	1-oz. pkg.	70	14.0
(Durkee) Roastin' Bag	1.5-oz. pkg.	130	26.0
(French's) Gravy Makins	.7-oz. pkg.	77	13.4
Pot roast (Durkee) Roastin' Bag	1.5-oz. pkg.	125	25.0
Pot roast (Durkee) Roastin' Bag, & onion	1.5-oz. pkg.	125	24.0
Swiss steak (Durkee)	1-oz. pkg.	68	16.0

Food and Description	Measure or Quantity	Calories	Carbo-hydrates (grams)
Swiss steak (Durkee) *Roastin' Bag*	1.5-oz. pkg.	115	28.0
Turkey (Durkee)	1-oz. pkg.	93	14.0
Turkey (French's) *Gravy Makins*	.9-oz. pkg.	89	14.0
GREEN PEA (See PEA)			
GRENADINE SYRUP:			
(Garnier) nonalcoholic	1 fl. oz.	103	26.0
(Giroux) nonalcoholic	1 fl. oz.	100	25.0
(Leroux) 25 proof	1 fl. oz.	81	15.2
GRITS (See HOMINY GRITS)			
GROUND-CHERRY, Poha or Cape Gooseberry:			
Whole (USDA)	1 lb. (weighed with husks & stems)	221	46.7
Flesh only (USDA)	4 oz.	60	12.7
GROUPER, raw (USDA):			
Whole	1 lb. (weighed whole)	170	0.
Meat only	4 oz.	99	0.
GUAVA, COMMON, fresh (USDA):			
Whole	1 lb. (weighed untrimmed)	273	66.0
Whole	1 guava (2.8 oz.)	48	11.7
Flesh only	4 oz.	70	17.0
GUAVA, STRAWBERRY, fresh (USDA)			
Whole	1 lb. (weighed untrimmed)	289	70.2
Fresh only	4 oz.	74	17.9

(USDA): United States Department of Agriculture
(HEW/FAO): Health, Education and Welfare/Food and Agriculture Organization
* Prepared as Package Directs

Food and Description	Measure or Quantity	Calories	Carbo-hydrates (grams)
GUINEA HEN, raw (USDA):			
Ready-to-cook	1 lb. (weighed ready-to-cook)	594	0.
Meat & skin	4 oz.	179	0.

H

HADDOCK:			
Raw:			
Whole (USDA)	1 lb. (weighed whole)	172	0.
Meat only	4 oz.	90	0.
Fried, breaded (USDA)	4" x 3" x ½" fillet (3.5 oz.)	165	5.8
Frozen:			
(Banquet) Dinner	8¾-oz. dinner	419	45.4
(Gorgon)	⅓ of 1-lb. pkg.	120	0.
(Mrs. Paul's) breaded & fried	½ of 8-oz. pkg.	236	23.6
(Mrs. Paul's) buttered fillets	½ of 10-oz. pkg.	200	1.2
(Weight Watchers) 2-compartment meal	8¾-oz. meal	169	13.9
(Weight Watchers) 3-compartment meal	16-oz. meal	261	13.2
Smoked, canned or not (USDA)	4 oz.	117	0.
HAKE, raw (USDA):			
Whole	1 lb. (weighed whole)	144	0.
Meat only	4 oz.	84	0.
HALF & HALF (milk & cream) (See **CREAM**)			
HALF & HALF WINE:			
(Gallo) 20% alcohol	3 fl. oz.	100	5.7
(Lejon) 18.5% alcohol	3 fl. oz.	116	6.7

Food and Description	Measure or Quantity	Calories	Carbo-hydrates (grams)
HALIBUT (USDA):			
Atlantic & Pacific:			
Raw:			
Whole	1 lb. (weighed whole)	268	0.
Meat only	4 oz.	113	0.
Broiled	4 oz.	194	0.
Broiled, steak	4" x 3" x ½" steak (4.4 oz.)	254	0.
Smoked	4 oz.	254	0.
California, raw, meat only	4 oz.	110	0.
Greenland (See **TURBOT**)			
HAM (See also **PORK**):			
Cooked:			
(Hormel)	1 oz.	35	0.
(Hormel) chopped, sliced	1 oz.	70	<1.0
Canned:			
(Armour Golden Star)	1 oz.	36	0.
(Armour Star)	1 oz.	53	0.
(Hormel) *Tender Chunk*	1 oz.	47	0.
(Oscar Mayer) *Jubilee*, extra lean, cooked	½₁₂ of 3-lb. ham (4 oz.)	132	.5
(Swift) *Hostess*	¼" slice (3.5 oz.)	141	.8
(Swift) *Premium*	1¾-oz. slice (5" x 2" x ¼")	111	.3
(Wilson)	1 oz.	48	.3
(Wilson) *Tender Made*	1 oz.	44	.3
Chopped or minced, canned:			
(Armour Star)	1 oz.	84	.4
(Hormel)	1 oz. (8-lb. can)	90	<1.0
Deviled, canned:			
(USDA)	1 T. (.5 oz.)	46	0.
(Armour Star)	1 oz.	79	0.
(Libby's)	1 oz.	85	.3
(Underwood)	1 oz.	97	Tr.

(USDA): United States Department of Agriculture
(HEW/FAO): Health, Education and Welfare/Food and Agriculture Organization
* Prepared as Package Directs

Food and Description	*Measure or Quantity*	*Calories*	*Carbo-hydrates (grams)*
Packaged (Oscar Mayer):			
Chopped	1 oz.	62	.3
Sliced, *Jubilee*	2-oz. slice	69	.5
Steak, *Jubilee*	8-oz. steak	257	0.
Spiced or unspiced, canned (Hormel)	1 oz. (5-lb. can)	78	.4
HAMBURGER (See **BEEF,** Ground; **McDONALD'S; BURGER KING**)			
HAMBURGER MIX:			
(Ann Page):			
Beef noodle	⅕ of 7-oz. pkg.	146	48.2
Cheeseburger macaroni	⅕ of 8-oz. pkg.	175	29.1
Chili tomato	⅕ of 8-oz. pkg.	156	32.5
Hash	⅕ of 6-oz. pkg.	121	27.7
Potato stroganoff	⅕ of 7-oz. pkg.	141	28.2
**Hamburger Helper* (General Mills):			
Beef noodle	⅕ of pkg.	320	26.0
Cheeseburger macaroni	⅕ of pkg.	360	28.0
Chili tomato	⅕ of pkg.	330	29.0
Hash dinner	⅕ of pkg.	300	24.0
Lasagne	⅕ of pkg.	330	32.0
Pizza dish	⅕ of pkg.	340	33.0
Potato stroganoff	⅕ of pkg.	330	29.0
Rice oriental	⅕ of 8-oz. pkg.	340	35.0
Spaghetti	⅕ of pkg.	330	31.0
Stew, hamburger	⅕ of pkg.	290	23.0
Make-a-Better-Burger (Lipton) mildly seasoned or onion	⅛ of pkg.	30	3.0
HAMBURGER SEASONING MIX:			
(Durkee)	1-oz. pkg.	110	15.0
*(Durkee)	1 cup	663	7.5
(French's)	1-oz. pkg.	100	20.0
HAM SALAD, canned (Carnation)	1½ oz.	78	3.4

Food and Description	Measure or Quantity	Calories	Carbo-hydrates (grams)
HAM & CHEESE LOAF			
(Oscar Mayer)	1-oz. slice	75	.3
HAM DINNER, frozen:			
(Banquet)	10-oz. dinner	369	47.7
(Morton)	10-oz. dinner	449	56.9
(Swanson)	10¼-oz. dinner	380	47.0
HAWAIIAN PUNCH:			
Canned:			
Cherry	6 fl. oz.	87	22.8
Grape	6 fl. oz.	93	23.4
Orange	6 fl. oz.	97	24.4
Red	6 fl. oz.	84	21.3
Very Berry	6 fl. oz.	87	21.6
*Mix, red punch	8 fl. oz.	100	25.0
HAWS, SCARLET, raw			
(USDA):			
Whole	1 lb. (weighed with core)	316	75.5
Flesh & skin	4 oz.	99	23.6
HAZELNUT (See **FILBERT**)			
HEADCHEESE (USDA)	1 oz.	76	.3
HERRING (USDA):			
Raw:			
Atlantic, whole	1 lb. (weighed whole)	407	0.
Atlantic, meat only	4 oz.	200	0.
Pacific, meat only	4 oz.	111	0.
Canned:			
Plain, solids & liq.	4 oz.	236	0.
Bismarck, drained (Vita)	5-oz. jar	273	6.9
Cocktail, drained (Vita)	8-oz. jar	342	24.8

(USDA): United States Department of Agriculture
(HEW/FAO): Health, Education and Welfare/Food and Agriculture
Organization
* Prepared as Package Directs
(USDA): United States Department of Agriculture

Food and Description	Measure or Quantity	Calories	Carbohydrates (grams)
In cream sauce (Vita)	8-oz. jar	397	18.1
In tomato sauce, solids & liq.	4 oz.	200	4.2
In wine sauce, drained (Vita)	8-oz. jar	401	16.6
Lunch, drained (Vita)	8-oz. jar	483	13.1
Matjes, drained (Vita)	8-oz. jar	304	26.2
Party Snacks, drained (Vita)	8-oz. jar	401	16.6
Tastee Bits, drained (Vita)	8-oz. jar	361	24.7
Pickled, Bismarck type	4 oz.	253	0.
Salted or brined	4 oz.	247	0.
Smoked:			
Bloaters	4 oz.	222	0.
Hard	4 oz.	340	0.
Kippered	4 oz.	239	0.
HICKORY NUT (USDA):			
Whole	1 lb. (weighed in shell)	1068	20.3
Shelled	4 oz.	763	14.5
HOB-NOB, any flavor (Drake's)	1 cake	68	9.1
HO-HO (Hostess)	1 cake (1 oz.)	124	16.5
HOMINY GRITS:			
Dry:			
(USDA):			
Degermed	1 oz.	103	22.1
Degermed	½ cup (2.8 oz.)	282	60.9
(Albers) quick, degermed	1½ oz.	150	33.0
(Aunt Jemima/Quaker)	1 T. (1 oz.)	101	22.4
(Pocono) creamy	1 oz.	101	23.6
(Quaker):			
Instant	.8-oz. packet	79	17.7
Instant, with imitation bacon bits	1-oz. packet	101	21.6
Instant, with imitation ham	1-oz. packet	99	21.3
Cooked (USDA) Degermed	⅔ cup (5.6 oz.)	84	18.0

Food and Description	Measure or Quantity	Calories	Carbo-hydrates (grams)
HONEY, strained:			
(USDA)	½ cup (5.7 oz.)	496	134.1
(USDA)	1 T. (.7 oz.)	61	16.5
HONEYCOMB, cereal (Post)	1⅓ cup (1 oz.)	110	25.0
HONEYDEW, fresh (USDA):			
Whole	1 lb. (weighed whole)	94	22.0
Wedge	2" x 7" wedge (5.3 oz.)	31	7.2
Flesh only	4 oz.	37	8.7
Flesh only, diced	1 cup (5.9 oz.)	55	12.9
HOPPING JOHN, frozen (Green Giant)	½ cup	150	21.0
HORSERADISH:			
Raw (USDA):			
Whole	1 lb. (weighed unpared)	288	65.2
Pared	1 oz.	25	5.6
Prepared:			
(USDA)	1 oz.	11	2.7
(Kraft)	1 oz.	3	.4
(Kraft) cream style	1 oz.	9	.7
(Kraft) oil style	1 oz.	20	.5
***HOT DOG BEAN SOUP** (Campbell)	8-oz. serving	168	20.0
HYACINTH BEAN (USDA):			
Young pod, raw:			
Whole	1 lb. (weighed untrimmed)	140	29.1
Trimmed	4 oz.	40	8.3
Dry seeds	4 oz.	383	69.2

(HEW/FAO): Health, Education and Welfare/Food and Agriculture
(USDA): United States Department of Agriculture
                Organization

* Prepared as Package Directs

Food and Description	Measure or Quantity	Calories	Carbo-hydrates (grams)

ICE CREAM and FROZEN CUSTARD (See also listing by flavor or brand name, e.g., **CHOCOLATE ICE CREAM** or **DREAMSICLE** or **GOOD HUMOR**):
Sweetened:
 (USDA):

10% fat	1 cup (4.7 oz.)	257	27.7
12% fat	1 cup (5 oz.)	294	29.3
12% fat, brick-type	2½-oz. slice	147	14.6
12% fat	small container (3½ fl. oz.)	128	12.8
16% fat	1 cup (5.2 oz.)	329	26.6
(Dean) fruit, 10.4% fat	1 cup (5.6 oz.)	336	41.1

Dietetic (See **FROZEN DESSERT**)

ICE CREAM BAR,
 chocolate-coated (Sealtest)   1 bar (2½ fl. oz.)   150   12.0

ICE CREAM CONE, cone only:

(Comet) any color	1 piece (4 grams)	19	3.9
(Comet) rolled sugar, any color	1 piece (.4 oz.)	49	10.2

ICE CREAM CUP, cup only:

(Comet) any color	1 piece (5 grams)	20	4.1
(Comet) *Pilot*	1 piece (4 grams)	19	3.9

ICE CREAM SANDWICH
 (Sealtest)   1 sandwich (3 fl. oz.)   170   26.0

ICE MILK:
 (USDA):

Hardened	1 cup (4.6 oz.)	199	29.3
Soft-serve	1 cup (6.2 oz.)	266	39.2

Food and Description	Measure or Quantity	Calories	Carbo-hydrates (grams)
(Borden):			
2.5% fat	1 cup (4.6 oz.)	186	35.2
3.25% fat	1 cup (4.7 oz.)	194	36.2
Lite Line, any flavor	1 cup	198	32.0
(Dean):			
Count Calorie, 2.1% fat	1 cup (4.8 oz.)	155	17.1
5% fat	1 cup (4.9 oz.)	227	35.0
Light'n Easy:			
Chocolate	½ cup (2¼ oz.)	108	17.7
Strawberry	½ cup (2¼ oz.)	104	17.7
Vanilla	½ cup (2¼ oz.)	105	17.2
(Meadow Gold) Vanilla, 4% fat	¼ pt.	95	16.5
(Sealtest) *Light 'n Lively*:			
Banana	1 cup (4.8 oz.)	206	39.4
Banana strawberry twirl	1 cup (5 oz.)	220	40.0
Buttered almond	1 cup (4.8 oz.)	240	36.0
Caramel nut	1 cup (4.8 oz.)	240	37.4
Cherry pineapple	1 cup (4.8 oz.)	200	36.0
Chocolate	1 cup (4.8 oz.)	220	40.0
Coffee	1 cup (4.8 oz.)	200	36.0
Lemon chiffon	1 cup (4.8 oz.)	236	48.6
Orange-pineapple	1 cup	200	36.0
Peach	1 cup (4.8 oz.)	200	36.0
Raspberry	1 cup (4.8 oz.)	198	35.6
Strawberry	1 cup (4.8 oz.)	200	36.0
Strawberry royale	1 cup (5 oz.)	224	43.2
Toffee	1 cup (4.8 oz.)	220	38.2
Toffee crunch	1 cup (4.8 oz.)	238	40.4
Vanilla	1 cup (4.8 oz.)	200	36.0
Vanilla with chocolate & strawberry	1 cup	200	36.0
Vanilla fudge royale	1 cup (5 oz.)	220	42.0
ICE MILK BAR, chocolate-coated (Sealtest)	1 bar (2½ fl. oz.)	130	14.0

(USDA): United States Department of Agriculture
(HEW/FAO): Health, Education and Welfare/Food and Agriculture Organization
* Prepared as Package Directs

Food and Description	Measure or Quantity	Calories	Carbo-hydrates (grams)
ICE STICK, twin pop (Sealtest)	3 fl. oz.	70	18.0
ICES (See individual fruit ice flavors)			
ICING (See CAKE ICING)			
INSTANT BREAKFAST (See individual brand name or company listings)			
IRISH WHISKEY (See DISTILLED LIQUORS)			
ITALIAN DINNER, frozen:			
(Banquet)	11-oz. dinner	446	44.6
(Swanson)	13-oz. dinner	420	55.0

J

JACKFRUIT, fresh (USDA):			
Whole	1 lb. (weighed with seeds & skin)	124	32.3
Flesh only	4 oz.	111	28.8
JACK MACKEREL, raw, meat only (USDA)	4 oz.	162	0.
JACK ROSE MIX (Bar-Tender's)	1 serving (⅝ oz.)	70	17.2
JAM, sweetened (See also individual listings by flavor):			
(USDA)	1 oz.	77	19.8
(USDA)	1 T. (.7 oz.)	54	14.0
(Ann Page) all flavors	1 tsp. (6.8 grams)	19	4.8
JELLY, sweetened (See also individual listings by flavor):			
(USDA)	1 T. (.6 oz.)	49	12.7

Food and Description	Measure or Quantity	Calories	Carbo-hydrates (grams)
(Ann Page) all flavors	1 tsp.	19	4.6
(Bama)	1 T. (.7 oz.)	51	12.7
(Crosse & Blackwell)	1 T. (.7 oz.)	51	12.8
(Kraft)	1 oz.	74	18.4
(Ma Brown)	1 oz.	73	17.0
(Polaner)	1 T.	54	13.5
(Smucker's)	1 T. (.7 oz.)	49	12.4
JERUSALEM ARTICHOKE:			
(USDA):			
Unpared	1 lb. (weighed with skin)	207	52.3
Pared	4 oz.	75	18.9
JOHANNISBERGER RIESLING WINE:			
(Deinhard) 11% alcohol	3 fl. oz.	72	4.5
(Inglenook) Estate, 12% alcohol	3 fl. oz.	61	.9
(Louis M. Martini) 12.5% alcohol	3 fl. oz.	90	.2
JORDAN ALMOND (See CANDY)			
JUICE (See individual flavors)			
JUJUBE or CHINESE DATE			
(USDA):			
Fresh, whole	1 lb. (weighed with seeds)	443	116.4
Fresh, flesh only	4 oz.	119	31.3
Dried, whole	1 lb. (weighed with seeds)	1159	297.1
Dried, flesh only	4 oz.	325	83.5
JUNIOR FOOD (See BABY FOOD)			

(USDA): United States Department of Agriculture
(HEW/FAO): Health, Education and Welfare/Food and Agriculture Organization
* Prepared as Package Directs

Food and Description	Measure or Quantity	Calories	Carbo-hydrates (grams)
JUNIORS (Tastykake):			
Chocolate	1 pkg. (2¾ oz.)	397	70.8
Chocolate devil food	1 pkg. (2¾ oz.)	284	45.2
Coconut	1 pkg. (2¾ oz.)	415	83.5
Coconut devil food	1 pkg. (2¾ oz.)	318	60.4
Jelly square	1 pkg. (3¼ oz.)	429	91.7
Koffee Kake	1 pkg. (2½ oz.)	395	59.7
Lemon	1 pkg. (2¾ oz.)	422	84.8
JUNKET (See individual flavors)			

K

KABOOM, cereal (General Mills)	1 cup (1 oz.)	110	24.0
KAFE VIN (Lejon) 19.7% alcohol	3 fl. oz.	183	22.8
KALE:			
Raw (USDA) leaves only	1 lb. (weighed untrimmed)	154	26.1
Boiled (USDA) leaves including stems	½ cup (1.9 oz.)	15	2.2
Frozen (Birds Eye) chopped	⅓ of pkg.	30	5.0
KARO, syrup:			
Dark corn	1 T. (.7 oz.)	60	15.0
Imitation maple	1 T. (.1 oz.)	59	14.6
Light corn	1 T. (.7 oz.)	60	14.9
Pancake & waffle	1 T. (.7 oz.)	60	14.9
KEFIR (Alta-Dena Dairy):			
Plain	1 cup (8.6 oz.)	180	13.0
Flavored	1 cup (7.3 oz.)	190	24.0
KETCHUP (See **CATSUP**)			
KIDNEY (USDA):			
Beef, raw	4 oz.	147	1.0

Food and Description	Measure or Quantity	Calories	Carbo- hydrates (grams)
Beef, braised	4 oz.	286	.9
Calf, raw	4 oz.	128	.1
Hog, raw	4 oz.	120	1.2
Lamb, raw	4 oz.	119	1.0
KIELBASA (Vienna)	2½-oz. serving	206	1.1
KINGFISH, raw (USDA):			
Whole	1 lb. (weighed whole)	210	0.
Meat only	4 oz.	119	0.
KING VITAMAN, cereal (Quaker)	¾ cup (1 oz.)	120	23.3
KIPPERS (See **HERRING**)			
KIRSCH LIQUEUR (Garnier) 96 proof	1 fl. oz.	83	8.8
KIRSCHWASSER (Leroux) 96 proof	1 fl. oz.	80	0.
KIX, cereal	1½ cups (1 oz.)	110	24.0
KNOCKWURST (USDA)	1 oz.	79	.6
KOHLRABI (USDA):			
Raw, whole	1 lb. (weighed with skin, without leaves)	96	21.9
Raw, diced	1 cup (4.8 oz.)	40	9.1
Boiled, drained	4 oz.	27	6.0
Boiled, drained	1 cup (5.5 oz.)	37	8.2
***KOOL-AID** (General Foods):			
Unsweetened	8 fl. oz.	100	25.0
Sweetened	8 fl. oz.	90	23.0

(USDA): United States Department of Agriculture
(HEW/FAO): Health, Education and Welfare/Food and Agriculture Organization
* Prepared as Package Directs

Food and Description	Measure or Quantity	Calories	Carbo- hydrates (grams)
KOTTBULLAR (Hormel)	1 oz. (1-lb. can)	48	.9
KRIMPETS (Tastykake):			
Apple spice	1 cake (.9 oz.)	135	25.2
Butterscotch	1 cake (.9 oz.)	123	22.9
Chocolate	1 cake (.9 oz.)	119	21.6
Jelly	1 cake (.9 oz.)	103	21.0
Lemon	1 cake (.9 oz.)	113	21.4
Orange	1 cake (.9 oz.)	114	21.5
KUMMEL LIQUEUR:			
(Garnier) 70 proof	1 fl. oz.	75	4.3
(Hiram Walker) 70 proof	1 fl. oz.	71	3.2
(Leroux) 70 proof	1 fl. oz.	75	4.1
KUMQUAT, fresh (USDA):			
Whole	1 lb. (weighed with seeds)	274	72.1
Flesh & skin	4 oz.	74	19.4
Flesh only	5-6 med. kumquats	65	17.1

L

Food and Description	Measure or Quantity	Calories	Carbo- hydrates (grams)
LAKE COUNTRY WINE (Taylor):			
Gold, 12% alcohol	3 fl. oz.	78	5.4
Pink, 12.5% alcohol	3 fl. oz.	78	4.8
Red, 12.5% alcohol	3 fl. oz.	81	4.8
White, 12.5% alcohol	3 fl. oz.	81	4.2
LAKE HERRING, raw (USDA):			
Whole	1 lb.	226	0.
Meat only	4 oz.	109	0.
LAKE TROUT, raw (USDA):			
Drawn	1 lb. (weighed with head, fins & bones)	282	0.
Meat only	4 oz.	191	0.

Food and Description	Measure or Quantity	Calories	Carbo-hydrates (grams)
LAKE TROUT or SISCOWET, raw (USDA):			
Less than 6.5 lb. whole	1 lb. (weighed whole)	404	0.
Less than 6.5 lb. whole	4 oz. (meat only)	273	0.
More than 6.5 lb. whole	1 lb. (weighed whole)	856	0.
More than 6.5 lb. whole	4 oz. (meat only)	594	0.
LAMB, choice grade (USDA):			
Chop, broiled:			
Loin. One 5-oz. chop (weighed before cooking with bone) will give you:			
Lean & fat	2.8 oz.	280	0.
Lean only	2.3 oz.	122	0.
Rib. One 5-oz. chop (weighed before cooking with bone) will give you:			
Lean & fat	2.9 oz.	334	0.
Lean only	2 oz.	118	0.
Fat, separable, cooked	1 oz.	201	0.
Leg:			
Raw, lean & fat	1 lb. (weighed with bone)	845	0.
Roasted, lean & fat	4 oz.	316	0.
Roasted, lean only	4 oz.	211	0.
Shoulder:			
Raw, lean & fat	1 lb. (weighed with bone)	1082	0.
Roasted, lean & fat	4 oz.	383	0.
Roasted, lean only	4 oz.	232	0.
LAMB'S-QUARTERS (USDA):			
Raw, trimmed	1 lb.	195	33.1
Boiled, drained	4 oz.	36	5.7

(USDA): United States Department of Agriculture
(HEW/FAO): Health, Education and Welfare/Food and Agriculture
             Organization
* Prepared as Package Directs

Food and Description	Measure or Quantity	Calories	Carbo-hydrates (grams)
LAMB STEW, canned, dietetic (Featherweight)	7¼-oz. can	230	23.0
LARD:			
(USDA)	1 cup (7.2 oz.)	1849	0.
(USDA)	1 T. (.5 oz.)	117	0.
LASAGNE:			
Canned (Nalley's)	8 oz.	213	27.2
Frozen:			
(Buitoni) with meat sauce	½ of 15-oz. pkg.	255	24.9
(Green Giant) with meat sauce, boil-in-bag	9-oz. serving	310	33.0
(Green Giant) with meat sauce, oven bake	7-oz. entree	300	28.0
(Ronzoni)	⅛ of 26-oz. pkg.	160	22.0
(Swanson) *Hungry Man*	12¾-oz. entree	540	51.0
(Swanson) *Hungry Man*, with meat	17¾-oz. dinner	740	86.0
(Weight Watchers) 1-compartment casserole	13-oz. meal	368	35.1
Mix (Golden Grain) *Stir-n-Serv*	⅙ of 7-oz. pkg.	140	26.3
Seasoning mix (Lawry's)	1.1-oz. pkg.	86	19.6
LAZY BONE (Drake's)	1 cake (.9 oz.)	94	15.2
LEEKS, raw (USDA):			
Whole	1 lb. (weighed untrimmed)	123	26.4
Trimmed	4 oz.	59	12.7
LEMON, fresh, peeled (USDA)	1 med. (2⅛″ dia.)	20	6.1
LEMONADE:			
Chilled (Sealtest)	½ cup (4.4 oz.)	55	13.4
Frozen, concentrate, sweetened:			
(USDA)	6-fl.-oz. can	427	112.0
*(USDA) diluted with 4⅓ parts water	½ cup (4.4 oz.)	55	14.1
*(Minute Maid)	6 fl. oz.	74	19.6

Food and Description	Measure or Quantity	Calories	Carbo-hydrates (grams)
(ReaLemon)	6-oz. can	414	108.0
*(Seneca)	½ cup (4.3 oz.)	56	14.0
Mix:			
*Country Time, regular & pink	8 fl. oz.	90	22.0
*(Salada)	6 fl. oz.	79	19.2
*(Wyler's) regular & pink	6 fl. oz.	64	15.8
LEMON EXTRACT:			
Pure (Ehlers)	1 tsp.	30	
(Virginia Dare) 77% alcohol	1 tsp.	22	0.
LEMON JUICE:			
Fresh:			
(USDA)	1 cup (8.6 oz.)	61	19.5
(USDA)	1 T. (.5 oz.)	4	1.2
(Sunkist)	1 lemon (3.9 oz.)	11	4.0
(Sunkist)	1 T. (.5 oz.)	4	1.0
Canned, unsweetened:			
(USDA)	1 cup (8.6 oz.)	56	18.6
(USDA)	1 T. (.5 oz.)	3	1.1
Plastic container (USDA)	¼ cup (2 oz.)	13	4.3
Plastic container, *ReaLemon*	1 T. (.5 oz.)	3	.8
Frozen, unsweetened:			
(USDA) concentrate	½ cup (5.1 oz.)	169	54.6
(USDA) single strength	½ cup (4.3 oz.)	27	8.8
(Minute Maid) full strength, already reconstituted	6 fl. oz.	74	19.6
*LEMON-LIMEADE, sweetened, concentrate, frozen (Minute Maid)	6 fl. oz.	75	19.6
LEMON PEEL, CANDIED:			
(USDA)	1 oz.	90	22.9
(Liberty)	1 oz.	93	22.6

(USDA): United States Department of Agriculture
(HEW/FAO): Health, Education and Welfare/Food and Agriculture Organization
* Prepared as Package Directs

Food and Description	Measure or Quantity	Calories	Carbo-hydrates (grams)
LEMON PIE:			
(USDA) chiffon, home recipe	⅙ of 9″ pie (3.8 oz.)	338	47.3
(USDA) meringue, home recipe	⅙ of 9″ pie (4.9 oz.)	357	52.8
(Hostess)	4½-oz. pie	415	52.4
(Tastykake)	4-oz. pie	366	52.0
Frozen:			
(Banquet) cream	⅙ of 14-oz. pie	168	21.8
(Morton) cream	⅙ of 16-oz. pie	182	22.0
(Morton) cream, mini	3½-oz. pie	240	28.9
Tart (Pepperidge Farm)	3-oz. pie tart	317	36.4
LEMON PIE FILLING:			
(Comstock)	1-lb. 5-oz. can	864	191.8
(Lucky Leaf)	8 oz.	412	95.4
(Wilderness)	22-oz. can	1104	230.2
LEMON PUDDING, canned			
(Hunt's) *Snack Pack*	5-oz. can	140	31.0
LEMON PUDDING or PIE FILLING MIX:			
Sweetened:			
(Ann Page) regular	¼ of 3-oz. pkg.	80	20.0
(Ann Page) instant	¼ of 3¾-oz. pkg.	100	25.0
*(Jell-O) regular	½ cup (5.1 oz.)	189	38.0
*(Jell-O) instant	½ cup (5.3 oz.)	180	31.0
*(My-T-Fine) regular	½ cup (5 oz.)	164	30.0
*(Royal) regular	⅛ of 9″ pie (including crust, 4.6 oz.)	224	39.8
*(Royal) instant	½ cup (5.1 oz.)	178	28.7
*Dietetic (Dia-Mel)	½ cup	53	8.2
LEMON RENNET CUSTARD MIX (Junket):			
Powder	1 oz.	116	28.1
*Powder	4 oz.	109	14.7
Tablet	1 tablet	1	.2
*Tablet, with sugar	4 oz.	101	13.5

Food and Description	Measure or Quantity	Calories	Carbo-hydrates (grams)
LEMON TURNOVER, frozen			
(Pepperidge Farm)	1 turnover (3.3 oz.)	341	33.1
LENTIL:			
Whole:			
Dry:			
(USDA)	½ lb.	771	136.3
(USDA)	1 cup (6.7 oz.)	649	114.8
(Sinsheimer)	1 oz.	05	17.0
Cooked, drained (USDA)	½ cup (3.6 oz.)	107	19.5
Split, dry (USDA)	½ lb.	782	140.2
LENTIL SOUP, canned:			
(Crosse & Blackwell) with ham	6½ oz. (½ can)	123	17.0
*(Manischewitz)	8-oz. (by wt.)	166	29.3
LETTUCE (USDA):			
Bibb, untrimmed	1 lb. (weighed untrimmed)	47	8.4
Bibb, untrimmed	7.8-oz. head (4″ dia.)	23	4.1
Boston, untrimmed	1 lb. (weighed untrimmed)	47	8.4
Boston, untrimmed	7.8-oz. head (4″ dia.)	23	4.1
Butterhead varieties (See Bibb & Boston)			
Cos (See Romaine)			
Dark green (See Romaine)			
Grand Rapids	1 lb. (weighed untrimmed)	52	10.2
Grand Rapids	2 large leaves (1.8 oz.)	9	1.8
Great Lakes	1 lb. (weighed untrimmed)	56	12.5
Great Lakes, trimmed	1-lb. head (4¾″ dia.)	59	13.2

(USDA): United States Department of Agriculture
(HEW/FAO): Health, Education and Welfare/Food and Agriculture Organization
* Prepared as Package Directs

Food and Description	Measure or Quantity	Calories	Carbo-hydrates (grams)
Iceberg:			
Untrimmed	1 lb. (weighed untrimmed)	56	12.5
Trimmed	1-lb. head (4¾″ dia.)	59	13.2
Leaves	1 cup (2.3 oz.)	9	1.9
Chopped	1 cup (2 oz.)	8	1.7
Chunks	1 cup (2.6 oz.)	10	2.1
Looseleaf varieties (See Salad Bowl)			
New York	1 lb. (weighed untrimmed)	56	12.5
New York	1-lb. head (4¾″ dia.)	59	13.2
Romaine:			
Untrimmed	1 lb. (weighed untrimmed)	52	10.2
Trimmed, shredded & broken into pieces	½ cup (.8 oz.)	4	.8
Salad Bowl	1 lb. (weighed untrimmed	52	10.2
Salad Bowl	2 large leaves (1.8 oz.)	9	1.8
Simpson	1 lb. (weighed untrimmed)	52	10.2
Simpson	2 large leaves (1.8 oz.)	9	1.8
White Paris (See Romaine)			
LIEBFRAUMILCH WINE:			
(Anheuser) 10% alcohol	3 fl. oz.	63	0.
(Deinhard) 11% alcohol	3 fl. oz.	60	3.6
(Deinhard) *Hans Christof*, 11% alcohol	3 fl. oz.	60	3.6
(Julius Kayser) Glockenspiel, 10% alcohol	3 fl. oz.	57	1.8
LIFE, cereal (Quaker)	⅔ cup (1 oz.)	105	19.7
LIMA BEAN (See BEAN, LIMA)			

Food and Description	Measure or Quantity	Calories	Carbohydrates (grams)
LIME, fresh, whole:			
(USDA)	1 lb. (weighed with skin & seeds)	107	36.2
(USDA)	1 med. (2″ dia., 2.4 oz.)	15	4.9
LIMEADE, concentrate, sweetened, frozen:			
(USDA)	6-fl.-oz. can	408	107.9
*(USDA) diluted with 4⅓ parts water	½ cup (4.4 oz.)	51	13.6
*(Minute Maid)	6 fl. oz.	75	20.1
(ReaLemon)	6-oz. can	414	108.0
*LIMEADE MIX (Wyler's)	6 fl. oz.	64	15.8
LIME JUICE:			
Fresh (USDA)	1 cup (8.7 oz.)	64	22.1
Home recipe (USDA)	8 oz. (by wt.)	177	73.9
Canned or bottled, unsweetened:			
(USDA)	1 cup (8.7 oz.)	64	22.1
(USDA)	1 fl. oz. (1.1 oz.)	8	2.8
Plastic container, *ReaLime*	1 T. (.5 oz.)	2	.5
LINGCOD, raw (USDA):			
Whole	1 lb. (weighed whole)	130	0.
Meat only	4 oz.	95	0.
LINGUINI IN CLAM SAUCE, frozen (Ronzoni)	4-oz. serving	120	16.0
LIQUEUR (See individual kinds)			
LITCHI NUT (USDA):			
Fresh:			
Whole	4 oz. (weighed in shell with seeds)	44	11.2

(USDA): United States Department of Agriculture
(HEW/FAO): Health, Education and Welfare/Food and Agriculture Organization
* Prepared as Package Directs

Food and Description	Measure or Quantity	Calories	Carbo- hydrates (grams)
Flesh only	4 oz.	73	18.6
Dried:			
Whole	4 oz. (weighed in shell with seeds)	145	36.9
Flesh only	2 oz.	157	40.1
LIVER:			
Beef, raw (USDA)	1 lb.	635	24.0
Beef, cooked (Swift) sliced	⅕ of 1 lb. (3.2 oz.)	141	3.1
Beef, fried (USDA)	4 oz.	260	6.0
Calf, raw	1 lb.	635	18.6
Calf, fried	4 oz.	296	4.5
Chicken, raw	1 lb.	585	13.2
Chicken, simmered	4 oz.	187	3.5
Goose, raw	1 lb.	826	24.5
Hog, raw	1 lb.	594	11.8
Hog, fried	4 oz.	273	2.8
Lamb, raw	1 lb.	617	13.2
Lamb, broiled	4 oz.	296	3.2
Turkey, raw	1 lb.	626	13.2
LIVER PÂTÉ (See PÂTÉ)			
LIVER SAUSAGE or LIVERWURST, spread (Underwood)	1 oz.	92	1.1
LOBSTER:			
Raw:			
Whole (USDA)	1 lb. (weighed whole)	107	.6
Meat only	4 oz.	103	.6
Cooked, meat only (USDA)	4 oz.	108	.3
Canned, meat only (USDA)	4 oz.	108	.3
Frozen, South African rock lobster tail	2-oz. tail	65	.1
LOBSTER NEWBURG, home recipe (USDA)	4 oz.	220	5.8
LOBSTER PASTE, canned (USDA)	1 oz.	51	.4

Food and Description	Measure or Quantity	Calories	Carbo-hydrates (grams)
LOBSTER SALAD, home recipe (USDA)	4 oz.	125	2.6
LOBSTER SOUP, canned, cream of (Crosse & Blackwell)	6½ oz. (½ can)	92	6.5
LOCHON ORA, Scottish liqueur (Leroux) 70 proof	1 fl. oz.	89	7.4
LOGANBERRY (USDA):			
Fresh:			
Untrimmed	1 lb. (weighed with caps)	267	64.2
Trimmed	1 cup (5.1 oz.)	89	21.5
Canned, solids & liq.:			
Water pack	4 oz.	45	10.7
Juice pack	4 oz.	61	14.4
Light syrup	4 oz.	79	19.5
Heavy syrup	4 oz.	101	25.2
Extra heavy syrup	4 oz.	122	30.8
LOG CABIN, syrup:			
Regular	1 T. (.7 oz.)	52	13.1
Buttered	1 T. (.7 oz.)	55	13.0
Maple-honey	1 T.	56	13.9
LONGAN (USDA):			
Fresh:			
Whole	1 lb. (weighed with shell & seeds)	147	38.0
Flesh only	4 oz.	69	17.9
Dried:			
Whole	1 lb. (weighed with shell & seeds)	467	120.8
Flesh only	4 oz.	324	83.9

(USDA): United States Department of Agriculture
(HEW/FAO): Health, Education and Welfare/Food and Agriculture
         Organization
* Prepared as Package Directs

Food and Description	Measure or Quantity	Calories	Carbo-hydrates (grams)
LOQUAT, fresh (USDA):			
Whole	1 lb. (weighed with seeds)	168	43.3
Flesh only	4 oz.	54	14.1
LOVE BIRD COCKTAIL, dry mix (Holland House)	1 serving (.6-oz. pkg.)	69	17.0
LUCKY CHARMS, cereal	1 cup (1 oz.)	110	24.0
LUMBERJACK, syrup (Nalley's)	1 oz.	78	19.6
LUNCHEON MEAT (See also individual listings, e.g., **BOLOGNA**):			
All meat (Oscar Mayer)	1-oz. slice	98	.7
Bar-B-Q-Loaf (Oscar Mayer)	1-oz. slice	47	1.7
Ham & cheese (See **HAM & CHEESE**)			
Honey loaf (Oscar Mayer)	1-oz. slice	35	1.1
Liver cheese (Oscar Mayer)	1.3-oz. slice	112	.5
Meat loaf (USDA)	1 oz.	57	.9
New England Brand sliced sausage (Oscar Mayer)	.8-oz. slice	34	.3
Old-fashioned Loaf (Oscar Mayer)	1-oz. slice	61	2.3
Olive loaf (Oscar Mayer)	1-oz. slice	65	2.6
Peppered beef (Vienna)	1 oz.	50	.4
Pickle & pimiento:			
(Hormel)	1 oz.	81	.3
(Oscar Mayer)	1-oz. slice	65	2.9
Spiced (Hormel)	1 oz.	70	<1.0
LUNG, raw (USDA):			
Beef	1 lb.	435	0.
Calf	1 lb.	481	0.
Lamb	1 lb.	467	0.
MACADAMIA NUT:			
Whole (USDA)	1 lb. (weighed in shell)	972	22.4
Shelled (Royal Hawaiian)	¼ cup (2 oz.)	394	9.1

Food and Description	Measure or Quantity	Calories	Carbo-hydrates (grams)

M

MACARONI. Plain macaroni products are essentially the same in caloric value and carbohydrate content on the same weight basis. The longer they are cooked, the more water is absorbed and this affects the nutritive values. (USDA):

Food and Description	Measure or Quantity	Calories	Carbo-hydrates (grams)
Dry:			
Elbow-type	1 cup (4.8 oz.)	502	102.3
1-inch pieces	1 cup (3.8 oz.)	406	82.7
2-inch pieces	1 cup (3 oz.)	317	64.7
Cooked:			
8-10 minutes, firm	1 cup (4.6 oz.)	192	39.1
8-10 minutes, firm	4 oz.	168	34.1
14-20 minutes, tender	1 cup (4.9 oz.)	155	32.2
14-20 minutes, tender	4 oz.	126	26.1
MACARONI & BEEF:			
Canned:			
(Bounty) in tomato sauce, *Chili Mac*	7¾-oz. can	255	29.7
(Buitoni) tiny meatballs & sauce	4 oz. serving	111	12.3
(Franco-American) in tomato sauce, *Beefy Mac*	7½-oz. can	220	28.0
Frozen:			
(Banquet)	12-oz. dinner	394	55.1
(Banquet) buffet	2-lb. pkg.	1000	106.4

(USDA): United States Department of Agriculture
(HEW/FAO): Health, Education and Welfare/Food and Agriculture Organization
* Prepared as Package Directs

Food and Description	Measure or Quantity	Calories	Carbohydrates (grams)
(Green Giant) with tomato sauce	9-oz. entree	240	31.0
(Swanson)	12-oz. dinner	400	56.0
MACARONI & CHEESE:			
Home recipe (USDA), baked	1 cup (7.1 oz.)	430	40.2
Canned:			
(USDA)	1 cup	228	25.7
(Franco-American)	½ of 14¾-oz. can	184	23.5
(Franco-American) elbow	7½-oz. can	186	23.8
Frozen:			
(Banquet) buffet	2-lb. pkg.	1027	110.9
(Banquet) cooking bag	8-oz. bag	261	28.6
(Banquet) dinner	12-oz. dinner	326	45.6
(Banquet) entree	8-oz. entree	279	35.9
(Green Giant) boil-in-bag	9-oz. entree	330	36.0
(Green Giant) oven bake	7-oz. entree	290	14.0
(Morton) casserole	8-oz. casserole	284	34.1
(Swanson)	12½-oz. dinner	390	55.0
MACARONI & CHEESE MIX:			
(USDA) dry	1 oz.	113	17.8
(Ann Page) dinner	¼ of 7¼-oz. pkg.	189	37.5
(Betty Crocker)	¼ of pkg.	200	37.0
*(Betty Crocker)	¼ of pkg.	310	38.0
(Golden Grain) dinner, deluxe	¼ of 7½-oz. pkg.	200	38.1
*(Kraft)	¾ cup	290	32.0
*(Kraft) deluxe	4 oz. serving	202	27.9
(Pennsylvania Dutch Brand)	½ cup serving	160	25.0
*(Prince)	¾ cup serving	268	34.6
MACARONI DINNER or ENTREE, frozen:			
(Morton) & beef	10-oz. dinner	267	45.5
(Morton)	11-oz.-dinner	334	53.1
(Weight Watchers) ziti	13-oz. meal	363	39.1
MACARONI SALAD, canned			
(Nalley's)	4 oz.	203	13.9

Food and Description	Measure or Quantity	Calories	Carbo-hydrates (grams)
MACE (French's)	1 tsp. (1.8 grams)	10	.8
MACKEREL (USDA):			
Atlantic:			
Raw:			
Whole	1 lb. (weighed whole)	468	0.
Meat only	4 oz.	217	0.
Broiled with butter	4 oz.	268	0.
Canned, solids & liq.	4 oz.	208	0.
Pacific:			
Raw:			
Dressed	1 lb. (weighed with bones & skin)	519	0.
Meat only	4 oz.	180	0.
Canned, solids & liq.	4 oz.	204	0.
Salted	4 oz.	346	0.
Smoked	4 oz.	248	0.
MACKEREL, JACK (See JACK MACKEREL)			
MADEIRA WINE (Leacock) 19% alcohol	3 fl. oz.	120	6.3
MAI TAI COCKTAIL:			
(Lemon Hart) 48 proof	3 fl. oz.	180	15.6
(National Distillers) *Duet,* 12.5% alcohol	8-fl.-oz. can	288	28.8
(Party Tyme) 12.5% alcohol	2 fl. oz.	65	5.7
Dry mix (Bar-Tender's)	1 serving (5.8 oz.)	69	17.0
Dry mix (Holland House)	1 serving (.6-oz. pkg.)	69	17.0
Dry mix (Party Tyme)	1 serving (½ oz.)	50	11.8
Liquid mix (Holland House)	1½ fl. oz.	50	12.0
Liquid mix (Party Tyme)	2 fl. oz.	44	11.2
MALT, dry (USDA)	1 oz.	104	21.9

(USDA): United States Department of Agriculture
(HEW/FAO): Health, Education and Welfare/Food and Agriculture
         Organization
* Prepared as Package Directs

Food and Description	Measure or Quantity	Calories	Carbohydrates (grams)
MALTED MILK MIX:			
(USDA) Dry powder	1 oz.	116	20.1
(Borden) chocolate, instant	2 heaping tsps. (.7 oz.)	77	16.0
(Borden) natural, instant	2 heaping tsps. (.7 oz.)	80	13.4
(Carnation) chocolate	3 heaping tsps. (.7 oz.)	85	18.0
(Carnation) natural	3 heaping tsps. (.7 oz.)	90	15.6
(Horlicks) chocolate	3 heaping tsps. (1.1 oz.)	124	26.0
(Horlicks) natural	3 heaping tsps. (1.1 oz.)	127	22.3
(Kraft) chocolate	2 heaping tsps. (.4 oz.)	51	10.0
*(Kraft) chocolate	1 cup (8.7 oz.)	241	29.8
(Kraft) natural	2 heaping tsps. (.4 oz.)	52	9.2
*(Kraft) natural	1 cup (8.6 oz.)	240	27.7
MALT EXTRACT, dried (USDA)	1 oz.	104	25.3
MALT LIQUOR:			
Big Cat	12 fl. oz.	155	
Champale, 6.25% alcohol	12 fl. oz.	173	11.5
Country Club, 6.8% alcohol	12 fl. oz.	183	2.8
Schlitz	12 fl. oz.	177	13.7
MAMEY or MAMMEE APPLE, fresh (USDA)	1 lb. (weighed with skin & seeds)	143	35.2
MANDARIN ORANGE (See **TANGERINE**)			
MANGO, fresh (USDA):			
Whole	1 lb. (weighed with seeds & skin)	201	51.1
Whole	1 med. (7 oz.)	88	22.5
Flesh only, diced or sliced	½ cup (2.9 oz.)	54	13.8

Food and Description	Measure or Quantity	Calories	Carbohydrates (grams)
MANGO & PINEAPPLE FRUIT DRINK (Alegre)	8 fl. oz.	186	45.0
MANHATTAN COCKTAIL:			
(Hiram Walker) 55 proof	3 fl. oz.	147	3.0
(National Distillers) *Duet*, 20% alcohol	8-fl.-oz. can	576	11.2
(Party Tyme) 20% alcohol	2 fl. oz.	74	1.5
Dry Mix (Bar-Tender's)	1 serving (⅛ oz.)	24	5.6
MANICOTTI, without sauce, frozen (Buitoni)	4 oz.	218	19.9
MAPLE RENNET CUSTARD MIX:			
Powder:			
(Junket)	1 oz.	117	27.9
*(Junket)	4 oz.	109	14.7
Tablet:			
(Junket)	1 tablet	1	.2
*(Junket) & sugar	4 oz.	101	13.5
MAPLE SYRUP (See also individual brand names):			
(USDA)	1 T. (.7 oz.)	50	13.0
(Cary's)	1 T. (.8 oz.)	63	15.7
MARASCHINO LIQUEUR:			
(Garnier) 60 proof	1 fl. oz.	94	11.1
(Leroux) 60 proof	1 fl. oz.	88	9.7
MARGARINE, salted or unsalted:			
(USDA)	1 lb.	3266	1.8
(USDA)	1 cup (8 oz.)	1633	.9
(USDA)	1 T. (.5 oz.)	101	<.1
(Blue Bonnet) regular or soft	1 T. (.5 oz.)	101	.1

(USDA): United States Department of Agriculture
(HEW/FAO): Health, Education and Welfare/Food and Agriculture Organization
* Prepared as Package Directs

Food and Description	Measure or Quantity	Calories	Carbo-hydrates (grams)
(Borden) Danish flavor	1 T. (.5 oz.)	101	<.1
(Fleishmann's) regular or soft	1 T. (.5 oz.)	101	.1
(Golden Glow)	1 T. (.4 oz.)	89	.1
(Holiday)	1 T. (.5 oz.)	103	0.
(Imperial) soft or stick	1 T. (.5 oz.)	102	<.1
(Mazola)	1 T. (.5 oz.)	104	.1
(Miracle) corn oil	1 T. (9 grams)	67	<.1
(Nucoa)	1 T. (.5 oz.)	103	0.
(Nucoa) soft	1 T. (.4 oz.)	82	0.
(Parkay) regular	1 T. (.5 oz.)	102	.1
(Parkay) soft	1 T. (.5 oz.)	101	.1
(Parkay) *Squeeze*	1 T. (.5 oz.)	101	.2
(Phenix)	1 T. (.5 oz.)	101	.1
(Promise) soft or stick	1 T. (.5 oz.)	102	<.1
(Saffola) regular or soft	1 T. (.5 oz.)	101	<.1
Imitation, or dietetic:			
(Fleishmann's)	1 T. (.5 oz.)	50	0.
(Imperial) soft	1 T. (.5 oz.)	50	0.
(Mazola)	1 T. (.5 oz.)	50	0.
(Parkay) soft	1 T.	55	0.
Whipped:			
(Blue Bonnet)	1 T. (9 grams)	67	<.1
(Imperial)	1 T. (9 grams)	65	0.
(Miracle)	1 T. (9 grams)	67	<.1
(Parkay) cup	1 T.	67	<.1
MARGARITA COCKTAIL:			
(National Distillers) *Duet,* 12.5% alcohol	8-fl.-oz. can	248	20.0
(Party Tyme) 12.5% alcohol	2 fl. oz.	66	5.7
Dry mix (Bar-Tender's)	1 serving (⅝ oz.)	70	17.3
MARGAUX, French red Bordeaux (Barton & Guestier) 12% alcohol	3 fl. oz.	62	.4
MARINADE MIX:			
(Adolph's) chicken	1-oz. pkg.	64	14.4
(Adolph's) meat	.8-oz. pkg.	38	8.5
(Durkee) meat	1-oz. pkg.	47	9.0
(French's) meat	1-oz. pkg.	80	16.0

Food and Description	Measure or Quantity	Calories	Carbo-hydrates (grams)
(Lawry's) beef	1.6-oz. pkg.	69	15.1
(Lawry's) lemon pepper	2.7-oz. pkg.	159	29.7
MARJORAM (French's)	1 tsp. (1.2 grams)	4	.8
MARMALADE:			
Sweetened:			
(USDA)	1 T. (.7 oz.)	51	14.0
(Ann Page)	1 T. (.7 oz.)	59	14.8
(Bama)	1 T. (.7 oz.)	54	13.5
(Crosse & Blackwell)	1 T. (.6 oz.)	60	14.9
(Kraft)	1 oz.	78	19.3
(Ma Brown)	1 oz.	73	17.0
(Smucker's)	1 T. (.7 oz.)	54	13.9
Dietetic or low calorie:			
(Dia-Mel)	1 tsp.	2	0.
(Louis Sherry)	1 tsp.	2	0.
(S and W) *Nutradiet*	1 T. (.5 oz.)	11	2.6
(Tillie Lewis)	1 T. (.5 oz.)	12	3.0
MARMALADE PLUM (USDA):			
Fresh, whole	1 lb. (with skin & seeds)	431	108.9
Fresh, flesh only	4 oz.	142	35.8
MARSHMALLOW FLUFF	1 heaping T. (.7 oz.)	65	15.5
MARTINI COCKTAIL:			
Gin:			
(Hiram Walker) 65.5 proof	3 fl. oz.	168	.6
(National Distillers) *Duet*, 21% alcohol	8-fl.-oz. can	560	1.6
(Party Tyme) 24% alcohol	2 fl. oz.	82	0.
Liquid mix (Holland House)	1½ fl. oz.	15	3.8
Liquid mix (Party Tyme)	2 fl. oz.	12	3.2

(USDA): United States Department of Agriculture
(HEW/FAO): Health, Education and Welfare/Food and Agriculture Organization
* Prepared as Package Directs

Food and Description	Measure or Quantity	Calories	Carbo-hydrates (grams)
Vodka:			
(Hiram Walker) 60 proof	3 fl. oz.	147	Tr.
(National Distillers)			
Duet, 20% alcohol	8-fl.-oz. can	536	1.6
(Party Tyme) 21% alcohol	2 fl. oz.	72	0.
MASA HARINA (Quaker)	⅛ cup	137	27.4
MATZO:			
(Goodman's):			
Diet-10's	1 sq.	109	23.0
Midgetea	1 matzo (.4 oz.)	40	7.4
Round tea	1 matzo (.6 oz.)	70	12.9
Unsalted	1 matzo (1 oz.)	109	23.0
(Horowitz-Margareten)			
unsalted	1 matzo (1.2 oz.)	135	28.2
(Manischewitz):			
Regular	1 matzo (1.1 oz.)	114	28.1
American	1 matzo (1 oz.)	121	22.6
Diet-thins	1 matzo (1 oz.)	113	24.5
Egg	1 matzo (1.2 oz.)	133	26.6
Egg'n onion	1 matzo (1 oz.)	116	24.6
Onion Tams	1 piece (3 grams)	13	1.9
Tam Tams	1 piece (3 grams)	14	1.7
Tasteas	1 matzo (1 oz.)	119	24.2
Thin tea	1 matzo (1 oz.)	114	24.8
Whole wheat	1 matzo (1.2 oz.)	124	24.2
MATZO MEAL (Manischewitz)	1 cup (4.1 oz.)	438	96.2
MAYONNAISE:			
(USDA)	1 cup (7.8 oz.)	1587	4.9
(USDA)	1 T. (.5 oz.)	101	.3
(Ann Page)	1 T. (.5 oz.)	105	.1
(Bama)	1 T. (.5 oz.)	95	.3
(Bennett's)	1 T. (.5 oz.)	113	.3
(Best Foods) *Real*	1 T. (.5 oz.)	103	<.1
(Cellu) *Soyamaise,* low sodium	1 T.	100	0.
(Dia-Mel)	1 T. (.5 oz.)	106	.2
(Hellmann's) *Real*	1 T. (.5 oz.)	103	<.1
(Kraft)	1 T. (.5 oz.)	102	.1

Food and Description	Measure or Quantity	Calories	Carbo-hydrates (grams)
(Kraft) *Salad Bowl*	1 T. (.5 oz.)	102	.2
(Nalley's)	1 oz.	214	.9
(Saffola)	1 T. (.5 oz.)	95	.3
(Sultana)	1 T. (.5 oz.)	103	.2
MAYPO, cereal, dry:			
30-second	¼ cup (.8 oz.)	89	16.4
Vermont style	¼ cup	121	22.0
MAY WINE (Deinhard) 11% alcohol	3 fl. oz.	60	1.0
McDONALD'S:			
Big Mac	1 hamburger (6.6 oz.)	541	39.0
Cheeseburger	1 cheeseburger (4.0 oz.)	306	30.8
Cookie, *McDonaldland*	1 package (2.2 oz.)	294	45.4
Egg McMuffin	1 serving	352	26.0
English muffin, buttered	1 muffin (2.2 oz.)	186	28.3
Filet-o-Fish	1 sandwich	402	34.3
French fries, regular	1 serving	211	25.8
Hamburger	1 hamburger	257	30.2
Hot cakes with butter & syrup	1 serving	471	89.0
Pie:			
Apple	1 pie (3.2 oz.)	300	31.1
Cherry	1 pie (3.3 oz.)	298	32.5
Quarter Pounder, regular	1 burger	418	33.0
Quarter Pounder, with cheese	1 burger with cheese	514	33.1
Sausage, pork	1 serving (1.7 oz.)	184	.5
Scrambled eggs	1 serving	161	1.9
Shake:			
Chocolate	1 serving (10.2 oz.)	363	59.8

(USDA): United States Department of Agriculture
(HEW/FAO): Health, Education and Welfare/Food and Agriculture Organization
* Prepared as Package Directs

Food and Description	Measure or Quantity	Calories	Carbo-hydrates (grams)
Strawberry	1 serving (10.3 oz.)	347	57.3
Vanilla	1 serving (10.2 oz.)	322	51.7
MEAL (See CORNMEAL or CRACKER MEAL or MATZO MEAL)			
MEATBALL DINNER or ENTREE, frozen:			
(Swanson)	11¾-oz. dinner	400	35.0
(Swanson) with brown gravy & whipped potatoes	9½-oz. entree	330	26.0
(Tom Thumb) with Kluski noodles	3 lb.-8-oz. tray	2362	140.5
MEATBALL SEASONING MIX:			
(Durkee) Italian	1-oz. pkg.	22	9.0
*(Durkee) Italian	¼ of 1-oz. pkg.	285	2.3
(Durkee) Italian with cheese	1-oz. pkg.	85	9.0
*(Durkee) Italian with cheese	¼ of 1-oz. pkg.	325	2.3
(French's)	1½-oz. pkg.	140	28.0
MEATBALL STEW, canned:			
(Libby's)	⅓ of 24-oz. can	275	24.5
(Morton House)	⅓ of 24-oz. can	290	18.0
MEAT LOAF DINNER or ENTREE, frozen:			
(Banquet) buffet	2-lb. pkg.	1445	46.4
(Banquet) cooking bag	5-oz. bag	224	13.6
(Banquet) dinner	11-oz. dinner	412	29.0
(Banquet) dinner, *Man-Pleaser*	19-oz. dinner	916	63.6
(Kraft)	5-oz. serving	332	16.0
(Morton) dinner	11-oz. dinner	342	28.1
(Morton) dinner, *Country Table*	15-oz. dinner	477	59.7

Food and Description	Measure or Quantity	Calories	Carbo-hydrates (grams)
(Morton) entree, *Country Table*	12½-oz. entree	433	32.1
(Swanson) dinner	10¾-oz. dinner	530	48.0
(Swanson) entree, with tomato sauce & whipped potatoes	9-oz. entree	330	27.0
MEAT LOAF SEASONING MIX:			
(Contadina)	3¾-oz. pkg.	363	72.8
(French's)	1½-oz. pkg.	160	40.0
(Lawry's)	3½-oz. pkg.	333	65.2
MEAT, POTTED:			
(Armour Star)	3-oz. can	181	0.
(Hormel)	3-oz. can	158	1.0
(Libby's)	1 oz.	59	.3
MEAT TENDERIZER:			
(Adolph's):			
Unseasoned	1 tsp. (5 grams)	2	.5
Seasoned	1 tsp. (5 grams)	1	.3
(French's) unseasoned or seasoned	1 tsp. (5 grams)	2	<.5
MELBA TOAST:			
Garlic (Keebler)	1 piece (2 grams)	9	1.5
Garlic, rounds (Old London)	1 piece (2 grams)	10	1.8
Onion, rounds (Old London)	1 piece (2 grams)	10	1.8
Plain (Keebler)	1 piece (2 grams)	9	1.5
Pumpernickel (Old London)	1 piece (5 grams)	17	3.4
Rye:			
(Keebler)	1 piece (2 grams)	8	1.7
(Old London)	1 piece (5 grams)	17	3.4
Unsalted (Old London)	1 piece (5 grams)	18	3.5
Sesame (Keebler)	1 piece (2 grams)	11	1.4
Sesame, rounds (Old London)	1 piece (2 grams)	11	1.6

(USDA): United States Department of Agriculture
(HEW/FAO): Health, Education and Welfare/Food and Agriculture Organization
● Prepared as Package Directs

Food and Description	Measure or Quantity	Calories	Carbo-hydrates (grams)
Wheat (Old London)	1 piece (5 grams)	17	3.4
Wheat, unsalted (Old London)	1 piece (5 grams)	18	3.5
White:			
(Keebler)	1 piece (4 grams)	16	3.3
(Old London)	1 piece (5 grams)	17	3.4
Rounds (Old London)	1 piece (2 grams)	10	1.8
Unsalted (Old London)	1 piece (5 grams)	18	3.5
MELLORINE (Sealtest)	¼ pt. (2.3 oz.)	132	15.8
MELON (See individual listings, eg. **CANTALOUPE**, **WATERMELON**, etc.)			
MELON BALL, cantaloupe & honeydew, in syrup, frozen (USDA)	½ cup (4.1 oz.)	72	18.2
MENHADEN, Atlantic, canned, solids & liq. (USDA)	4 oz.	195	0.
MEXICAN DINNER, frozen:			
(Banquet) Mexican style	16-oz. dinner	608	73.5
(Banquet) combination	12-oz. dinner	571	72.1
(Patio) 3-compartment	12-oz. dinner	270	30.0
(Swanson) combination	16-oz. dinner	600	72.0
MILK, CONDENSED, sweetened, canned:			
(USDA)	1 cup (10.8 oz.)	982	166.2
Dime Brand	1 fl. oz. (1.3 oz.)	125	21.1
Eagle Brand	1 cup (10.6 oz.)	942	150.0
Magnolia Brand	1 T. (.7 oz.)	60	9.5
MILK, DRY:			
Whole (USDA) packed cup	1 cup (5.1 oz.)	728	55.4
Nonfat, instant:			
(USDA) ⅞ cup makes 1 qt.	⅞ cup (3.2 oz.)	330	47.6
*(Carnation)	8 fl. oz.	80	12.0

Food and Description	Measure or Quantity	Calories	Carbo-hydrates (grams)
(Featherweight) low sodium	⅔ oz.	70	10.0
*(Pet)	1 cup	80	12.0
*(Sanalac)	1 cup	80	11.5
MILK, EVAPORATED, canned:			
Regular:			
(USDA) unsweetened	1 cup (8.9 oz.)	345	24.4
(Borden)	14.5-oz. can	563	39.9
(Carnation)	1 fl. oz.	42	3.0
(Pet)	½ cup	170	12.0
Filled (Pet)	½ cup (4 oz.)	150	12.0
Skimmed:			
(Carnation)	1 fl. oz.	25	3.5
(Pet)	½ cup	100	14.0
(Sunshine)	1 cup (8.9 oz.)	200	28.8
MILK, FRESH:			
Whole:			
(Borden) 3.25% fat, homogenized	1 cup	152	11.8
(Dean) 3.5% fat	1 cup	151	11.0
(Meadow Gold) Vitamin D₃ added	1 cup	150	11.0
(Sealtest):			
3.25% fat	1 cup (8.6 oz.)	144	10.8
3.5% fat	1 cup (8.6 oz.)	151	11.0
3.7% fat	1 cup (8.6 oz.)	157	11.1
Extra rich, Vitamin D	1 cup	170	11.0
Skim:			
(Borden):			
Regular	1 cup	99	13.6
Lite Line	1 cup (8.6 oz.)	119	14.2
Pro-Line, 2% fat	1 cup	140	14.2
Skim-Line	1 cup (8.6 oz.)	99	13.6
(Dean):			
.5% fat	1 cup (8.2 oz.)	91	11.7

(USDA): United States Department of Agriculture
(HEW/FAO): Health, Education and Welfare/Food and Agriculture
Organization
* Prepared as Package Directs

Food and Description	Measure or Quantity	Calories	Carbo-hydrates (grams)
2% fat	1 cup (8.7 oz.)	133	12.5
(Meadow gold):			
Vitamin A & D	1 cup	90	11.0
Viva, 2% fat, vitamins A & D	1 cup	130	12.0
(Sealtest):			
Regular	1 cup (8.6 oz.)	79	11.3
Protein fortified, vitamins A & D	1 cup	100	10.0
Protein fortified, 1% fat, vitamins A & D	1 cup	110	14.0
Protein fortified, 1.5% fat, vitamins A & D	1 cup	130	13.0
Vitamins A & D	1 cup	90	11.0
Buttermilk, cultured, fresh:			
(Borden):			
.1% fat	1 cup (8.6 oz.)	88	12.4
1.0% fat	1 cup (8.6 oz.)	107	12.4
3.5% fat	1 cup (8.6 oz.)	159	12.0
(Dean)	1 cup (8.6 oz.)	95	11.5
(Meadow Gold) .5% fat	1 cup	105	12.0
(Sealtest):			
Regular	1 cup	90	11.0
With golden nugget flakes	1 cup	90	11.0
Protein-fortified	1 cup	110	12.0
Protein fortified, *Light 'n Lively*	1 cup	110	14.0
Whole	1 cup	150	11.0
Chocolate milk drink, fresh:			
With whole milk:			
(Dean) 1% fat	1 cup (8.9 oz.)	166	27.9
(Dean) 3.5% fat	1 cup	212	25.5
(Sealtest) 3.4% fat	1 cup (8.6 oz.)	207	25.9
With skim milk (Sealtest):			
.5% fat	1 cup (8.6 oz.)	146	26.2
1% fat	1 cup (8.6 oz.)	180	28.0
MILK, HUMAN (USDA)	1 oz. (by wt.)	22	2.7
MILLET, whole-grain (USDA)	1 lb.	1482	330.7

Food and Description	Measure or Quantity	Calories	Carbo-hydrates (grams)
MINCEMEAT:			
(Comstock) pie filling	½ cup	222	49.5
(Crosse & Blackwell)	½ cup	480	114.4
(None Such) with brandy & rum	½ cup (5.3 oz.)	338	75.8
(None Such) condensed	9-oz. pkg.	950	224.3
(None Such) ready-to-use	⅓ cup	232	52.5
(Wilderness) pie filling	¼ of 22-oz. can	323	65.1
MINCE PIE:			
Home recipe (USDA) 2-crust	⅛ of 9″ pie	428	65.1
(Tastykake)	4-oz. pie	373	50.8
Frozen:			
(Banquet)	⅛ of 20-oz. pie	252	38.5
(Morton)	⅙ of 24-oz. pie	314	45.5
(Morton) mini	8-oz. pie	616	93.2
MINESTRONE SOUP:			
(USDA) condensed	8 oz. (by wt.)	197	26.3
*(USDA) prepared with equal volume water	1 cup (8.6 oz.)	105	14.2
*(Ann Page) with beef stock	1 cup	82	12.8
(Campbell) *Chunky*	19-oz. can	320	50.0
*(Campbell) condensed	10-oz. serving	110	15.0
(Crosse & Blackwell)	½ of 13-oz. can	107	17.0
MINI-WHEATS, cereal (Kelloggs):			
Frosted	4 biscuits (1 oz.)	110	24.0
Toasted	5 biscuits (1 oz.)	100	22.0
MOLASSES:			
(USDA):			
Barbados	1 T. (.7 oz.)	51	13.3
Blackstrap	1 T. (.7 oz.)	40	10.4
Light	1 T. (.7 oz.)	48	12.4
Dark	1 T. (.7 oz.)	48	12.4
Medium	1 T. (.7 oz.)	44	11.4

(USDA): United States Department of Agriculture
(HEW/FAO): Health, Education and Welfare/Food and Agriculture
Organization
* Prepared as Package Directs

Food and Description	Measure or Quantity	Calories	Carbo-hydrates (grams)
(Brer Rabbit) dark, Green Label	1 T.	53	13.3
(Brer Rabbit) light, Gold Label	1 T.	60	14.6
(Grandma's) unsulphured	1 T.	60	15.0
MORTADELLA, sausage (USDA)	1 oz.	89	.2
MOSELLE WINE (Great Western) Delaware, 12% alcohol	3 fl. oz.	73	2.9
MOSELMAID, German Moselle wine (Deinhard) 11% alcohol	3 fl. oz.	60	1.0
MOUNTAIN WINE (Louis M. Martini) 12% alcohol	3 fl. oz.	90	.2
MUFFIN (See also MUFFIN MIX):			
Blueberry:			
Home recipe (USDA)	3" muffin (1.4 oz.)	112	16.8
Frozen (Morton)	1.6-oz. muffin	125	22.9
Frozen (Morton) rounds	1.6-oz. muffin round	115	20.9
Bran:			
Home recipe (USDA)	3" muffin (1.4 oz.)	104	17.2
(Arnold) *Oroweat, bran'nola*	2.3-oz. muffin	160	30.0
Corn:			
Home recipe (USDA) prepared with whole-ground cornmeal	1.4-oz. muffin	115	17.0
(Drake's)	7/8-oz. muffin	107	15.8
(Morton) frozen	1.7-oz. muffin	129	20.3
(Morton) frozen, rounds	1.5-oz. muffin round	127	20.9
(Thomas')	2-oz. muffin	184	25.8

Food and Description	Measure or Quantity	Calories	Carbohydrates (grams)
English:			
(Arnold)	2-oz. muffin	130	25.0
(Arnold) *Oroweat* sourdough	2.2-oz. muffin	150	30.0
(Pepperidge Farm)	1 muffin	140	27.0
(Pepperidge Farm) cinnamon raisin	1 muffin	140	28.0
(Thomas')	2-oz. muffin	133	26.6
(Thomas') onion	2-oz. muffin	129	26.3
(Wonder)	2-oz. muffin	130	26.0
Honey butter (Arnold) *Oroweat*	2.2-oz. muffin	150	30.0
Honey wheat berry (Arnold) *Oroweat*	2.5-oz. muffin	160	30.0
Plain, home recipe (USDA)	1.4-oz. muffin (3″ dia.)	118	16.9
Raisin (Arnold) *Oroweat*	2.5-oz. muffin	160	30.0
Raisin (Wonder) rounds	2-oz. muffin round	150	28.0
Sourdough (Wonder)	2-oz. muffin	130	27.0
MUFFIN MIX:			
*Apple cinnamon (Betty Crocker)	1 muffin	160	26.0
*Banana, *Chiquita* (Betty Crocker)	1 muffin	180	25.0
Blueberry:			
*(Betty Crocker) wild	1 muffin	120	19.0
(Duncan Hines)	1 muffin	99	17.0
*Butter pecan (Betty Crocker)	1 muffin	160	21.0
*Cinnamon nut (Betty Crocker)	1 muffin	150	21.0
Corn:			
Home recipe (USDA) prepared with egg & milk	1.4-oz. muffin	92	14.2

(USDA): United States Department of Agriculture
(HEW/FAO): Health, Education and Welfare/Food and Agriculture Organization
* Prepared as Package Directs

Food and Description	Measure or Quantity	Calories	Carbo-hydrates (grams)
Home recipe (USDA) prepared with egg & water	1.4-oz. muffin	119	20.8
*(Betty Crocker)	1 muffin	160	25.0
*(Dromedary)	1 muffin	130	20.0
*(Flako)	1 muffin	140	23.0
*Orange, *Sunkist* (Betty Crocker)	1 muffin	160	26.0
*Pineapple (Betty Crocker)	1 muffin	120	20.0
MUG-O-LUNCH (General Mills):			
Macaroni & cheese sauce	1 pouch (1.5 oz.)	240	40.0
Noodles & beef-flavored sauce	1 pouch (1.5 oz.)	170	29.0
Spaghetti & tomato sauce	1 pouch (1.5 oz.)	170	29.0
MULLET, raw (USDA):			
Whole	1 lb. (weighed whole)	351	0.
Meat only	4 oz.	166	0.
MUNG BEAN SPROUT (See BEAN SPROUT)			
MUSCATEL WINE:			
(Gallo) 20% alcohol	3 fl. oz.	111	8.3
(Gold Seal) 19% alcohol	3 fl. oz.	159	9.4
MUSHROOM:			
Raw, whole (USDA)	½ lb. (weighed untrimmed)	62	9.7
Raw, trimmed slices (USDA)	½ cup (1.2 oz.)	10	1.5
Raw, slices (Shady Oak)	½ cup	10	1.5
Canned, solids & liq.:			
(USDA)	½ cup (4.3 oz.)	21	2.9
(Green Giant)	2 oz.	14	2.0
(Shady Oak)	4-oz. can	19	2.0
Dried (HEW/FAO)	1 oz.	72	10.5
Frozen (Green Giant) in butter sauce	2 oz.	30	2.0
MUSHROOM, CHINESE:			
Dried (HEW/FAO)	1 oz.	81	18.9

Food and Description	Measure or Quantity	Calories	Carbo- hydrates (grams)
Dried, soaked, drained (HEW/FAO)	1 oz.	12	2.4
MUSHROOM SOUP:			
(USDA):			
Cream of, condensed	8 oz. (by wt.)	252	19.1
*Cream of, prepared with equal volume water	1 cup (8.5 oz.)	134	10.1
*Cream of, prepared with equal volume milk	1 cup (8.6 oz.)	216	16.2
*(Ann Page) cream of, condensed	1 cup	126	10.2
(Campbell):			
*Cream of, condensed	8-oz. serving	120	8.8
Cream of, with wine, *Soup For One*	7½-oz. can	160	12.0
*Golden, condensed	8-oz. serving	88	8.8
(Crosse & Blackwell) bisque	½ of 13-oz. can	103	8.3
*(Manischewitz) barley	8 fl. oz.	72	12.2
Dietetic:			
(Campbell) cream of, low sodium	7¼-oz. can	140	10.0
(Dia-Mel) cream of, condensed	8-oz. serving	45	9.0
(Featherweight) cream of, low sodium	8-oz. can	120	18.0
Mix:			
(Lipton):			
*Beef mushroom	1 cup	45	7.0
Cream of, *Cup-a-Soup*	6 fl. oz.	80	11.0
*(Nestlé's) *Souptime*	6 fl. oz.	80	9.0
(Wyler's) cream of	.7-oz. pkg.	78	10.3
MUSKELLUNGE, raw			
(USDA):			
Whole	1 lb. (weighed whole)	242	0.
Meat only	4 oz.	124	0.

(USDA): United States Department of Agriculture
(HEW/FAO): Health, Education and Welfare/Food and Agriculture Organization
* Prepared as Package Directs

Food and Description	Measure or Quantity	Calories	Carbohydrates (grams)
MUSKMELON (See **CANTALOUPE, CASABA** or **HONEYDEW**)			
MUSKRAT, roasted (USDA)	4 oz.	174	0.
MUSSEL (USDA):			
Atlantic & Pacific, raw, in shell	1 lb. (weighed in shell)	153	7.2
Atlantic & Pacific, raw, meat only	4 oz.	108	3.7
Pacific, canned, drained	4 oz.	129	1.7
MUSTARD POWDER (French's)	1 tsp.	9	.3
MUSTARD, PREPARED:			
Brown:			
(USDA)	1 tsp.	8	.5
(French's) *'N Spicy*	1 tsp.	5	.3
(Gulden's)	1 scant tsp.	6	.4
Cream sauce (French's)	1 tsp.	3	.3
German style (Kraft)	1 oz.	30	1.7
Grey Poupon	1 tsp.	6	.2
Horseradish (French's)	1 tsp.	5	.3
Horseradish (Kraft)	1 oz.	29	1.6
Hot, *Mr. Mustard*	1 tsp.	11	.4
Medford (French's)	1 tsp.	5	.3
Onion (French's)	1 tsp.	8	1.7
Salad (Kraft)	1 oz.	23	1.7
Yellow:			
(USDA)	1 tsp.	7	.6
(Gulden's)	1 scant tsp.	5	.4
MUSTARD GREENS:			
Raw, whole (USDA)	1 lb. (weighed untrimmed)	98	17.8
Boiled, drained (USDA)	1 cup (7.8 oz.)	51	8.8
Frozen (USDA) boiled, drained	½ cup (3.8 oz.)	21	3.3
Frozen (Birds Eye) chopped	⅓ pkg. (3.3 oz.)	18	3.0

Food and Description	Measure or Quantity	Calories	Carbo-hydrates (grams)
MUSTARD SPINACH (USDA):			
Raw	1 lb.	100	17.7
Boiled, drained solids	4 oz.	18	3.2

N

NATURAL CEREAL:			
Heartland:			
Coconut	½ cup (1 oz.)	122	18.1
Coconut, hot	¼ cup (1 oz.)	126	19.0
Plain, oat	¼ cup (1 oz.)	122	18.7
Raisin	¼ cup (1 oz.)	122	18.7
Regular, hot	¼ cup (1 oz.)	121	19.0
Hot, spice	¼ cup (1 oz.)	121	19.1
Toasted corn	¼ cup (1 oz.)	114	21.1
Toasted wheat	¼ cup (1 oz.)	120	20.7
(Quaker):			
100%	¼ cup (1 oz.)	139	17.0
100%, with apples & cinnamon	¼ cup (1 oz.)	135	18.0
100%, with raisins & dates	¼ cup (1 oz.)	134	17.8
Whole wheat, hot	⅛ cup (1 oz.)	100	20.6
NEAR BEER (See **BEER, NEAR**)			
NECTARINE, fresh (USDA):			
Whole	1 lb. (weighed with pits)	267	71.4
Flesh only	4 oz.	73	19.4
NEAPOLITAN CREAM PIE, frozen (Morton)	⅙ of 16-oz. pie	192	22.7
NEAPOLITAN ICE CREAM (Sealtest)	¼ pt.	130	18.0

(USDA): United States Department of Agriculture
(HEW/FAO): Health, Education and Welfare/Food and Agriculture Organization
* Prepared as Package Directs

Food and Description	Measure or Quantity	Calories	Carbo- hydrates (grams)
NEW ZEALAND SPINACH (USDA):			
Raw	1 lb.	86	14.1
Boiled, drained solids	4 oz.	15	2.4
NOODLE. Plain noodle products are essentially the same in caloric value and carbohydrate content on the same weight basis. The longer they are cooked, the more water is absorbed and this affects the nutritive values. (USDA):			
Dry, 1½" strips	1 cup (2.6 oz.)	283	52.6
Dry	1 oz.	110	20.4
Cooked	1 cup (5.6 oz.)	200	37.3
Cooked	1 oz.	35	6.6
NOODLE & BEEF, frozen (Banquet)	2-lb. pkg.	754	83.6
NOODLE, CHOW MEIN, canned:			
(USDA)	1 cup (1.6 oz.)	220	26.1
(Chun King)	1 cup	211	23.2
(Hung's)	1 oz.	148	16.1
(La Choy)	1 cup	258	29.0
NOODLE MIX:			
*(Betty Crocker):			
Almondine	¼ pkg.	260	27.0
Romanoff	¼ pkg.	230	23.0
Stroganoff	¼ pkg.	230	26.0
Noodle Roni, parmesano	⅙ of 6-oz. pkg.	130	23.2
*(Pennsylvania Dutch Brand) *Noodles Plus Sauce:*			
Beef	½ cup	130	24.0
Butter	½ cup	150	23.0
Cheese	½ cup	150	24.0
Chicken	½ cup	150	25.0

Food and Description	Measure or Quantity	Calories	Carbo-hydrates (grams)
NUITS ST. GEORGE, French red Burgundy (Barton & Guestier) 13.5% alcohol	3 fl. oz.	70	.5
NUT, MIX (See also individual kinds):			
Dry roasted:			
(A&P)	1 oz.	179	6.6
(Flavor House) salted	1 oz.	172	5.4
(Planters)	1 oz.	176	6.2
(Skippy)	1 oz.	183	5.4
Oil roasted:			
(A&P) Fancy, without peanuts	1 oz.	190	5.9
(Excel) with peanuts	1 oz.	187	5.4
(Planters) with peanuts	1 oz.	176	6.2
(Planters) without peanuts	1 oz.	178	6.0
NUT ICE CREAM (Dean) 14% fat	1 cup (5.6 oz.)	376	36.3
NUT LOAF (See **BREAD, CANNED**)			
NUTMEG (French's)	1 tsp.	11	.9
NUTRIMATO (Mott's)	6 fl. oz.	70	17.0

O

OAK FLAKES, cereal (Post)	⅔ cup (1 oz.)	110	20.0
OATMEAL:			
Instant, dry:			
(H-O)			
Regular	1 T. (4 grams)	16	2.8
Regular	1 cup (2.4 oz.)	258	44.3

(USDA): United States Department of Agriculture
(HEW/FAO): Health, Education and Welfare/Food and Agriculture Organization
* Prepared as Package Directs

Food and Description	Measure or Quantity	Calories	Carbo-hydrates (grams)
With maple & brown sugar flavor	1.5-oz. packet	160	31.7
With raisins & spices	1.6-oz. packet	165	32.9
Sweet & mellow	1.4-oz. packet	150	28.9
(Quaker):			
Regular	1-oz. packet	105	18.1
Apple & cinnamon	1¼-oz. packet	134	26.0
Bran & raisins	1½-oz. packet	153	29.2
Cinnamon & spice	1⅝-oz. packet	176	34.8
Maple & brown sugar	1½-oz. packet	163	31.9
Raisins & spice	1½-oz. packet	159	31.4
Quick, dry:			
(H-O)	1 T. (4 grams)	16	2.8
(H-O)	1 cup (2.5 oz.)	269	46.3
(Ralston Purina)	⅓ cup (1 oz.)	110	19.0
Regular, dry:			
(USDA)	1 T.	18	3.1
(H-O) old fashioned	1 T. (5 grams)	17	3.0
(H-O) old fashioned	1 cup (2.6 oz.)	278	48.0
(Ralston Purina)	⅓ cup (1 oz.)	110	19.0
Regular, cooked (USDA)	1 cup (8.5 oz.)	132	23.3
OCEAN PERCH (USDA):			
Atlantic:			
Raw, whole	1 lb. (weighed whole)	124	0.
Fried	4 oz.	257	7.7
Frozen, breaded, fried, reheated	4 oz.	362	18.7
Pacific, raw:			
Whole	1 lb. (weighed whole)	116	0.
Meat only	4 oz.	108	0.
OCTOPUS, raw, meat only (USDA)	4 oz.	83	0.
OESTRICHLER LENCHEN RIESLING, German Rhine wine (Deinhard) 11% alcohol	3 fl. oz.	72	4.5
OIL, SALAD or COOKING:			
(USDA) all, including olive	1 T. (.5 oz.)	124	0.

Food and Description	Measure or Quantity	Calories	Carbo-hydrates (grams)
(USDA) all, including olive	½ cup (3.9 oz.)	972	0.
Corn:			
(Fleischmann's)	1 T. (.5 oz.)	126	0.
(Kraft)	1 oz.	251	0.
(Mazola)	1 T.	128	0.
(Mazola)	½ cup (3.9 oz.)	997	0.
Crisco	1 T.	126	0.
Peanut (Planters)	1 T.	126	0.
Puriton	1 T.	126	0.
Safflower (Kraft)	1 oz.	251	0.
Saffola	1 T. (.5 oz.)	124	0.
Saffola	½ cup (3.9 oz.)	972	0.
Vegetable (Kraft)	1 oz.	251	0.
Wesson	1 T.	120	0.
OKRA:			
Raw, whole (USDA)	1 lb. (weighed untrimmed)	140	29.6
Boiled, drained (USDA):			
Whole	½ cup (3.1 oz.)	26	5.3
Pods	8 pods 3″ x ⅝″ (3 oz.)	25	5.1
Slices	½ cup (2.8 oz.)	23	4.8
Canned (King Pharr) with tomatoes	½ cup	26	5.0
Frozen:			
(USDA) cut, boiled, drained	½ cup (3.2 oz.)	35	8.1
(USDA) whole, boiled, drained	½ cup (2.4 z.)	26	6.1
(Birds Eye) cut	⅓ pkg. (3.3 oz.)	25	5.0
(Birds Eye) whole	⅓ pkg. (3.3 oz.)	35	7.0
(Green Giant) gumbo	½ cup	110	6.0
OLD-FASHIONED COCKTAIL:			
(Hiram Walker) 62 proof	3 fl. oz.	165	3.0

(USDA): United States Department of Agriculture
(HEW/FAO): Health, Education and Welfare/Food and Agriculture Organization
* Prepared as Package Directs

Food and Description	Measure or Quantity	Calories	Carbohydrates (grams)
Mix:			
Dry (Bar-Tender's)	1 serving (⅛ oz.)	20	4.7
Liquid (Holland House)	1 fl. oz.	36	9.0
OLEOMARGARINE (See MARGARINE)			
OLIVE:			
Green style (USDA):			
With pits, drained	1 oz.	77	2.0
Pitted, drained	1 oz.	96	2.5
Green (USDA)	1 oz.	33	.4
Ripe, by variety (USDA):			
Ascalano, any size, pitted & drained	1 oz.	37	.7
Manzanilla, any size	1 oz.	37	.7
Mission, any size	1 oz.	52	.9
Mission	3 small or 2 large	18	.3
Mission, slices	½ cup (2.2 oz.)	114	2.0
Sevillano, any size	1 oz.	26	6.1
Ripe, by size (Lindsay):			
Colossal	1 olive	13	.3
Extra large	1 olive	5	.1
Giant	1 olive	8	.2
Jumbo	1 olive	10	.2
Large	1 olive	5	.1
Mammoth	1 olive	6	.1
Medium	1 olive	4	.1
Select	1 olive	3	.1
Supercolossal	1 olive	16	.3
Super supreme	1 olive	18	.3
ONION (See also ONION, GREEN and ONION, WELCH)			
Raw (USDA):			
Whole	1 lb. (weighed untrimmed)	157	35.9
Whole	3.9-oz. onion (2½" dia.)	38	8.7
Chopped	½ cup (3 oz.)	33	7.5
Chopped	1 T. (.4 oz.)	4	1.0
Grated	1 T. (.5 oz.)	5	1.2

Food and Description	Measure or Quantity	Calories	Carbo-hydrates (grams)
Slices	½ cup (2 oz.)	21	4.9
Boiled, drained (USDA):			
Whole	½ cup (3.7 oz.)	30	6.8
Whole, pearl onions	½ cup (3.2 oz.)	27	6.0
Halves or pieces	½ cup (3.2 oz.)	26	5.8
Canned:			
(Comstock-Greenwood) boiled, solids & liq.	4 oz.	33	7.4
O & C, boiled	¼ of 16-oz. jar	32	8.0
O & C, in cream sauce	¼ of 15½-oz. can	554	65.9
O & C, french-fried	3-oz. can	534	30.0
Dehydrated:			
Flakes (USDA)	1 tsp. (1.3 grams)	5	1.1
Flakes (Gilroy)	1 tsp.	5	1.2
Powder (Gilroy)	1 tsp.	9	2.0
Frozen:			
(Birds Eye):			
Chopped	1 oz.	8	2.0
Small, whole	⅓ pkg.	40	10.0
Small, with cream sauce	⅓ pkg.	100	11.0
(Commodore)			
French-fried rings	1 oz.	55	2.9
(Mrs. Paul's) batter fried rings	½ of 5-oz. pkg.	156	21.2
Pickled (Crosse & Blackwell) cocktail	1 T. (.5 oz.)	1	.3
ONION BOUILLON:			
(Croyden House)	1 tsp.	11	2.3
(Herb-Ox)	1 cube	10	1.4
(Herb-Ox) instant	1 packet	5	2.0
MBT	1 packet	16	2.0
(Steero)	1 cube	7	1.5
(Wyler's) cube	1 cube	10	1.2
ONION, GREEN, raw (USDA):			
Whole	1 lb. (weighed untrimmed)	157	35.7

(USDA): United States Department of Agriculture
(HEW/FAO): Health, Education and Welfare/Food and Agriculture Organization
* Prepared as Package Directs

Food and Description	Measure or Quantity	Calories	Carbohydrates (grams)
Bulb & entire top	1 oz.	10	2.3
Bulb without green top	3 small onions (.9 oz.)	11	2.6
Slices, bulb & white portion of top	½ cup (1.8 oz.)	22	5.2
Tops only	1 oz.	8	1.6
ONION SOUP:			
(USDA) Condensed	8 oz. (by wt.)	131	9.8
*(USDA) prepared with equal volume water	1 cup (8.5 oz.)	65	5.3
*(Campbell) condensed	10-oz. serving	80	9.0
*(Campbell) cream of, condensed	10-oz. serving	180	20.0
(Crosse & Blackwell)	½ of 13-oz. can	46	4.8
(Hormel)	½ of 15-oz. can	72	2.8
Mix:			
*(USDA)	1 cup (8.1 oz.)	34	5.3
(Ann Page)	1¾-oz. pkg.	115	21.1
*(Lipton)	1 cup (8 oz.)	40	6.0
*(Lipton) beefy onion	1 cup (8 oz.)	30	4.0
*(Lipton) Cup-a-Soup	6 fl. oz.	30	5.0
*(Lipton) onion mushroom	1 cup (8 oz.)	35	5.0
*(Nestle's) Souptime, French	6 fl. oz.	20	4.0
*(Wyler's)	6 fl. oz.	28	5.3
ONION, WELCH, raw (USDA):			
Whole	1 lb. (weighed untrimmed	100	19.2
Trimmed	4 oz.	39	7.4
OPOSSUM, roasted, meat only (USDA)	4 oz.	251	0.
ORANGE, fresh:			
All varieties:			
Whole, medium (USDA)	5.5-oz. orange (3" dia.)	77	19.0
Sections (USDA)	1 cup (8.5 oz.)	118	29.4

Food and Description	Measure or Quantity	Calories	Carbohydrates (grams)
Sections (Kraft) sweetened, chilled, bottled	4 oz.	61	14.1
California Navel:			
Whole (USDA)	1 lb. (weighed with rind & seeds)	157	39.2
Whole (USDA)	6.3-oz. orange (2⅝" dia.)	62	15.5
Sections (USDA)	1 cup (8.5 oz.)	123	30.6
Wedge, unpeeled (Sunkist)	⅛ orange	10	4.0
Cut, bite-size (Sunkist)	½ cup	62	16.0
California Valencia (USDA):			
Whole	1 lb. (weighed with rind & seeds)	174	42.2
Fruit including peel	6.3-oz. orange (2⅝" dia.)	72	27.9
Sections	1 cup (8.5 oz.)	123	29.9
Florida, all varieties (USDA):			
Whole	1 lb. (weighed with rind & seeds)	158	40.3
Whole	7.4-oz. orange (3" dia.)	73	18.6
Sections	1 cup (8.5 oz.)	113	28.9
ORANGEADE:			
Chilled (Sealtest)	½ cup	60	8.0
*Frozen (Minute Maid)	6 fl. oz.	94	22.7
ORANGE-APRICOT JUICE DRINK, canned:			
(USDA) 40% fruit juices	1 cup (8.8 oz.)	124	31.6
(Ann Page)	1 cup (8.7 oz.)	125	31.2
ORANGE CREAM BAR			
(Sealtest)	2½-fl.-oz. bar	100	18.0

(USDA): United States Department of Agriculture
(HEW/FAO): Health, Education and Welfare/Food and Agriculture Organization
* Prepared as Package Directs

Food and Description	Measure or Quantity	Calories	Carbo- hydrates (grams)
ORANGE DRINK:			
Canned:			
(Alegre) Island orange	8 fl. oz. (8.7 oz.)	136	33.1
(Ann Page)	1 cup (8.7 oz.)	121	30.2
(Hi-C)	6 fl. oz.	92	23.0
Chilled (Sealtest)	6 fl. oz.	87	21.3
*Mix (Wagner) crystals	6 fl. oz.	90	22.5
ORANGE EXTRACT			
(Virginia Dare) 79% alcohol	1 tsp.	22	0.
ORANGE-GRAPEFRUIT JUICE:			
Canned, unsweetened:			
(USDA)	1 cup (8.7 oz.)	106	24.8
(Del Monte)	6 fl. oz. (6.5 oz.)	79	18.3
Canned, sweetened:			
(USDA)	1 cup (8.9 oz.)	126	30.6
(Del Monte)	6 fl. oz. (6.5 oz.)	91	21.1
Frozen:			
*(USDA) unsweetened	½ cup (4.4 oz.)	55	13.0
*(Minute Maid) unsweetened	6 fl. oz.	76	19.1
ORANGE ICE (Sealtest)	¼ pt. (3.2 oz.)	130	33.0
ORANGE JUICE:			
Fresh:			
(USDA) all varieties	½ cup (4.4 oz.)	56	12.9
(USDA) California Navel	½ cup (4.4 oz.)	60	14.0
(USDA) California Valencia	½ cup (4.4 oz.)	58	13.0
(USDA) Florida, early or midseason	½ cup (4.4 oz.)	50	11.5
(USDA) Florida Temple	½ cup (4.4 oz.)	67	16.0
(USDA) Florida Valencia	½ cup (4.4 oz.)	56	13.0
(Kraft) chilled	½ cup (4.4 oz.)	60	13.8
(Sunkist) California Navel or Valencia	6 fl. oz.	78	19.5
Canned, unsweetened:			
(USDA)	½ cup (4.4 oz.)	60	13.9
(Del Monte)	6 fl. oz. (6.5 oz.)	82	18.5

Food and Description	Measure or Quantity	Calories	Carbohydrates (grams)
(Featherweight) low sodium	½ cup	53	12.0
Canned, sweetened:			
(USDA)	½ cup (4.4 oz.)	66	15.4
(Del Monte)	6 fl. oz.	76	17.4
*Dehydrated crystals (USDA)	½ cup (4.4 oz.)	57	13.4
Frozen:			
*(USDA)	½ cup (4.4 oz.)	56	13.3
*(Lake Hamilton)	½ cup (4.4 oz.)	58	13.3
*(Minute Maid) unsweetened	6 fl. oz.	90	21.4
*(Snow Crop) unsweetened	6 fl. oz.	90	21.4
ORANGE, MANDARIN (See TANGERINE)			
ORANGE PEEL, CANDIED (Liberty)	1 oz.	93	22.6
ORANGE-PINEAPPLE DRINK, canned:			
(Ann Page)	1 cup (8.7 oz.)	126	31.5
(Hi-C)	6 fl. oz.	94	23.0
(Kraft) chilled	½ cup (4.4 oz.)	64	14.9
(Wagner) sweetened	6 fl. oz.	86	21.6
ORANGE PINEAPPLE PIE (Tastykake)	4-oz. pie	374	56.2
***ORANGE PLUS** (Birds Eye) frozen	6 fl. oz.	100	24.0
ORANGE PUDDING, canned (Royal) *Creamerino*	5-oz. container	225	33.0
ORANGE RENNET CUSTARD MIX (Junket): Powder	1 oz.	116	27.7

(USDA): United States Department of Agriculture
(HEW/FAO): Health, Education and Welfare/Food and Agriculture Organization
* Prepared as Package Directs

Food and Description	Measure or Quantity	Calories	Carbo-hydrates (grams)
*Powder	4 oz.	108	14.6
Tablet	1 tablet	1	.2
*Tablet, with sugar	4 oz.	101	13.5
ORANGE SHERBET (See SHERBET)			
OREGANO, dried (French's)	1 tsp.	6	1.0
ORGEAT SYRUP (Julius Wile)	1 fl. oz.	103	26.0
ORVIETO WINE, Italian white (Antinori):			
12% alcohol	3 fl. oz.	84	6.3
Castello La Scala, 12½% alcohol	3 fl. oz.	87	6.3
OVALTINE, dry:			
Chocolate flavor	¾ oz. (4 heaping tsps.)	77	16.0
Malt flavor	¾ oz. (4 heaping tsps.)	85	17.0
*OXTAIL CONSOMME MIX (Knorr swiss)	6 fl. oz.	11	
OXTAIL SOUP (Crosse & Blackwell)	½ of 13-oz. can	136	7.5
OYSTER:			
Raw, Eastern (USDA) meat only	13-19 med. oysters (1 cup, 8.5 oz.)	158	8.2
Raw, Eastern (USDA) meat only	4 oz.	75	3.9
Raw, Pacific (USDA) meat only	4 oz.	103	7.3
Canned, solids & liq.:			
(USDA)	4 oz.	86	5.6
(Bumble Bee) whole	½ of 8-oz. can	86	5.5
Fried (USDA) dipped in egg, milk & breadcrumbs	4 oz.	271	21.1

Food and Description	Measure or Quantity	Calories	Carbo-hydrates (grams)
OYSTER CRACKER (See **CRACKER**)			
OYSTER STEW:			
Home recipe (USDA) 1 part oysters to 1 part milk by volume	1 cup (8.5 oz., 6-8 oysters)	245	14.2
Home recipe (USDA) 1 part oysters to 2 parts milk by volume	1 cup (8.5 oz.)	233	10.8
Home recipe (USDA) 1 part oysters to 3 parts milk by volume	1 cup (8.5 oz.)	206	11.3
Frozen:			
*(USDA) prepared with equal volume water	1 cup (8.5 oz.)	122	8.2
*(USDA) prepared with equal volume milk	1 cup (8.5 oz.)	201	14.2
***OYSTER STEW SOUP** (Campbell) prepared with milk	10-oz. serving	70	5.0

P

PAGAN PINK WINE (Gallo) 11% alcohol	3 fl. oz.	81	6.8
PAISANO WINE (Gallo) 13% alcohol	3 fl. oz.	53	1.3
PANCAKE, home recipe (USDA)	4" pancake (1 oz.)	62	9.2
PANCAKE & SAUSAGE, frozen (Swanson)	6-oz. breakfast	500	50.0

(USDA): United States Department of Agriculture
(HEW/FAO): Health, Education and Welfare/Food and Agriculture
Organization
* Prepared as Package Directs

Food and Description	Measure or Quantity	Calories	Carbo-hydrates (grams)
*PANCAKE & WAFFLE			
BATTER, frozen:			
Plain (Aunt Jemima)	4″ pancake	70	14.1
Plain (Rich's)	1 pancake	113	17.9
Blueberry (Aunt Jemima)	4″ pancake	68	13.8
Blueberry (Rich's)	1.6-oz. pancake		
	(⅒ of pkg.)	102	16.5
Buttermilk (Aunt Jemima)	4″ pancake	71	14.2
Buttermilk (Rich's)	1 pancake		
	(⅒ of pkg.)	109	16.9
PANCAKE & WAFFLE MIX:			
Plain:			
(USDA)	1 oz.	101	21.5
(USDA)	1 cup (4.8 oz.)	481	102.2
*(USDA), prepared with			
milk	4″ pancake (1 oz.)	55	8.6
*(USDA) prepared with			
egg & milk	4″ pancake	61	8.7
(Aunt Jemima):			
Complete	⅛ cup (1.9 oz.)	198	38.2
*Complete	4″ pancake	66	12.7
Original	1¼ cups (1.1 oz.)	108	22.5
*Original	4″ pancake	73	8.7
*(Log Cabin) complete	4″ pancake	60	8.7
*(Pillsbury):			
Complete, *Hungry Jack*	4″ pancake	73	14.0
Hungry Jack Extra			
Lights	4″ pancake	60	8.7
*Blueberry (Pillsbury)			
Hungry Jack	4″ pancake	113	14.3
Buckwheat:			
(USDA)	1 cup (4.8 oz.)	443	94.9
*(USDA) prepared with			
egg & milk	4″ pancake	54	6.4
(Aunt Jemima)	¼ cup (1.1 oz.)	110	21.3
*(Aunt Jemima)	4″ pancake	67	8.3
Buttermilk:			
(USDA)	1 cup (4.8 oz.)	481	102.2
*(USDA) prepared with			
egg & milk	4″ pancake	61	8.7
(Aunt Jemima)	⅓ cup (1.8 oz.)	175	36.5
*(Aunt Jemima)	4″ pancake	100	13.3

Food and Description	Measure or Quantity	Calories	Carbohydrates (grams)
(Aunt Jemima) complete	⅓ cup (2.3 oz.)	236	46.2
*(Aunt Jemima) complete	4″ pancake	79	15.4
*(Betty Crocker)	4″ pancake	90	13.0
*(Betty Crocker) complete	4″ pancake	70	13.7
*(Log Cabin)	4″ pancake	77	10.7
*(Pillsbury) *Hungry Jack*	4″ pancake	80	9.7
*(Pillsbury) *Hungry Jack*, complete	4″ pancake	113	11.3
Whole wheat (Aunt Jemima)	⅓ cup (1.5 oz.)	142	28.5
*Whole wheat (Aunt Jemima)	4″ pancake	83	10.7
*Dietetic or low calorie (Tillie Lewis) complete	4″ pancake (.5 oz. dry)	45	8.6
PANCAKE & WAFFLE SYRUP:			
Sweetened:			
(USDA) cane & maple	1 T. (.7 oz.)	50	13.0
(USDA) chiefly corn, light & dark	1 T. (.7 oz.)	58	15.0
(Bama)	1 T. (.7 oz.)	53	13.2
(Golden Griddle)	1 T. (.7 oz.)	54	13.4
Mrs. Butterworth's	1 T. (.7 oz.)	52	13.0
(Polaner)	1 T.	54	13.5
(Smucker's)	1 T. (.8 oz.)	62	16.0
Dietetic or low calorie:			
(Diet Delight)	1 T. (.6 oz.)	4	.9
(Featherweight)	1 T.	12	3.0
(Tillie Lewis)	1 T. (.5 oz.)	4	1.1
PANCREAS, raw (USDA):			
Beef, lean only	4 oz.	160	0.
Calf	4 oz.	183	0.
Hog or hog sweetbread	4 oz.	274	0.

(USDA): United States Department of Agriculture
(HEW/FAO): Health, Education and Welfare/Food and Agriculture
Organization
* Prepared as Package Directs

Food and Description	Measure or Quantity	Calories	Carbohydrates (grams)
PAPAW, fresh (USDA):			
Whole	1 lb. (weighed with rind & seeds)	289	57.2
Flesh only	4 oz.	96	19.1
PAPAYA, fresh (USDA):			
Whole	1 lb. (weighed with skin & seeds)	119	30.4
Cubed	1 cup (6.4 oz.)	71	18.2
PAPAYA JUICE, canned (HEW/FAO)	4 oz.	77	19.6
PAPRIKA, domestic (French's)	1 tsp.	7	1.1
PARSLEY, fresh (USDA):			
Whole	½ lb.	100	19.3
Chopped	1 T. (4 grams)	2	.3
PARSLEY FLAKES, dehydrated (French's)	1 tsp. (1.1 grams)	4	.6
PARSNIP (USDA):			
Raw, whole	1 lb. (weighed unprepared)	293	67.5
Boiled, drained, cut in pieces	½ cup (3.7 oz.)	70	15.8
PARTY PUNCH WINE, undiluted (Mogen David) 12% alcohol	3 fl. oz.	156	21.4
PASHA TURKISH COFFEE LIQUEUR (Leroux) 53 proof	1 fl. oz.	97	13.3
PASSION FRUIT, fresh (USDA):			
Whole	1 lb. (weighed with shell)	212	50.0
Pulp & seeds	4 oz.	102	24.0
PASSION FRUIT JUICE, fresh (HEW/FAO)	4 oz.	50	11.5

Food and Description	Measure or Quantity	Calories	Carbohydrates (grams)
PASTINA, dry:			
(USDA):			
Carrot	1 oz.	105	21.5
Egg	1 oz.	109	20.4
Spinach	1 oz.	104	21.2
(Ann Page) regular	1 oz.	108	20.5
PASTOSO (Petri) 12% alcohol	3 fl. oz.	71	1.2
PASTRAMI, packaged			
(Vienna)	1 oz.	86	0.
PASTRY SHELL (See also PIE CRUST):			
Home recipe (USDA) baked	1 shell (1.5 oz.)	212	18.6
(Keebler):			
Pot pie, bland	4" shell (1.7 oz.)	236	29.6
Tart, sweet	3" tart (1 oz.)	158	16.6
(Stella D'oro)	1 shell (1 oz.)	143	16.2
(Stella D'oro) pot, bland	1 shell (1.6 oz.)	205	22.8
Frozen (Pepperidge Farm)			
patty	1 shell (1.8 oz.)	232	14.5
PÂTÉ, canned:			
(USDA) de foie gras	1 T. (.5 oz.)	69	.7
(USDA) de foie gras	1 oz.	131	1.4
(Hormel) liver	1 oz.	78	1.1
(Sell's) liver	1 T. (.5 oz.)	45	.5
PDQ:			
Chocolate flavor	1 T. (.6 oz.)	64	14.6
Egg nog flavor	2 heaping T. (.9 oz.)	113	27.5
Strawberry flavor	1 T. (.5 oz.)	60	15.1
PEA, GREEN:			
Raw (USDA):			
In pod	1 lb. (weighed in pod)	145	24.8

(USDA): United States Department of Agriculture
(HEW/FAO): Health, Education and Welfare/Food and Agriculture Organization
• Prepared as Package Directs

Food and Description	Measure or Quantity	Calories	Carbohydrates (grams)
Shelled	1 lb.	381	65.3
Shelled	½ cup (2.4 oz.)	58	9.9
Boiled, drained (USDA)	½ cup (2.9 oz.)	58	9.9
Canned, regular pack:			
(USDA):			
Alaska, early or June, solids & liq.	½ cup (4.4 oz.)	82	15.5
Alaska, early or June, drained solids	½ cup (3 oz.)	76	14.4
Sweet, solids & liq.	½ cup (4.4 oz.)	71	12.9
Sweet, drained solids	½ cup (3 oz.)	69	12.9
Sweet, drained liq.	4 oz.	25	4.9
(April Showers) Early, solids & liq.	½ cup	60	11.0
(Butter Kernel):			
Alaska, drained solids	½ cup (4.1 oz.)	69	12.8
Sweet, drained solids	½ cup (4.1 oz.)	60	10.4
(Del Monte):			
Early Garden, solids & liq.	½ cup (4. oz.)	52	9.9
Early Garden, drained solids	½ cup (4 oz.)	72	12.5
Seasoned, solids & liq.	½ cup	54	9.8
Seasoned, drained solids	½ cup	53	9.2
Sweet, tiny size, solids & liq.	½ cup	50	9.0
Sweet, tiny size, drained solids	½ cup	62	10.7
(Diamond A) solids & liq.	½ cup	65	12.4
(Green Giant):			
Early, with onion, solids & liq.	½ cup	60	11.0
Sweet, solids & liq.	½ cup	55	8.5
Sweet, small, *Sweetlets*, solids & liq.	½ cup	60	8.5
Sweet, with onion, solids & liq.	½ cup	55	8.5
(Jack and the Bean Stalk) solids & liq.	½ cup (4.3 oz.)	65	12.4
(Kounty Kist):			
Early, solids & liq.	½ cup	70	13.5
Sweet, solids & liq.	½ cup	65	11.0

Food and Description	Measure or Quantity	Calories	Carbohydrates (grams)
(Le Sueur):			
Early, small, solids & liq.	½ cup	55	9.5
Sweet, small, solids & liq.	½ cup	50	8.5
(Libby's) Sweet, solids & liq.	½ cup (4.2 oz.)	60	11.6
(Lindy):			
Early, solids & liq.	½ cup	70	12.5
Sweet, solids & liq.	½ cup	65	11.0
(Minnesota Valley) Early, small, solids & liq.	½ cup	55	9.5
(Stokely-Van Camp):			
Early, solids & liq.	½ cup (4.4 oz.)	65	12.5
Sweet, solids & liq.	½ cup (4.4 oz.)	65	12.0
Canned, dietetic or low calorie:			
(USDA):			
Alaska, Early or June, solids & liq.	4 oz.	62	11.1
Alaska, Early or June, drained solids	4 oz.	88	16.2
Sweet, solids & liq.	4 oz.	53	9.3
Sweet, drained solids	4 oz.	82	14.7
(Blue Boy) sweet, solids & liq.	4 oz.	49	8.0
(Diet Delight) solids & liq.	½ cup (4.3 oz.)	50	7.0
(Featherweight) sweet, solids & liq.	½ cup	50	10.0
(S and W) *Nutradiet,* unseasoned	4 oz.	40	7.6
(Tillie Lewis) solids & liq.	½ cup (4.4 oz.)	40	7.5
Frozen:			
(USDA) boiled, drained	½ cup (3 oz.)	57	9.9
(Birds Eye):			
With cream sauce	⅓ pkg. (2.6 oz.)	120	14.0
With sliced mushrooms	⅓ pkg.	70	11.0

(USDA): United States Department of Agriculture
(HEW/FAO): Health, Education and Welfare/Food and Agriculture Organization
* Prepared as Package Directs

Food and Description	Measure or Quantity	Calories	Carbo- hydrates (grams)
Sweet, 5-minute style	⅛ pkg.	70	11.0
Tender tiny, deluxe	⅛ pkg.	60	9.0
(Green Giant):			
Creamed with bread crumb topping, *Bake 'n Serve*	1 cup	300	33.0
Early, small	½ cup	50	8.0
Sweet	½ cup	50	8.0
(Kounty Kist)	½ cup	60	10.0
(Le Sueur):			
Early, in butter sauce	½ cup	75	10.0
Sweet, in butter sauce	½ cup	75	9.0
PEA, MATURE SEED, dry (USDA):			
Whole	1 lb.	1542	273.5
Whole	1 cup	680	120.6
Split	1 lb.	1579	284.4
Split	1 cup (7.2 oz.)	706	127.3
Cooked, split, drained solids	½ cup (3.4 oz.)	112	20.2
PEA POD, edible-podded or Chinese (USDA):			
Raw	1 lb. (weighed untrimmed)	228	51.7
Boiled, drained solids	4 oz.	49	10.8
PEA & CARROT:			
Canned, regular pack:			
(Del Monte) solids & liq.	½ cup (4 oz.)	49	9.4
(Del Monte) drained solids	½ cup (2.8 oz.)	44	8.2
(Libby's) solids & liq.	½ cup (4.2 oz.)	52	10.3
Canned, dietetic or low calorie, solids & liq.:			
(Blue Boy)	4 oz.	26	5.9
(Diet Delight)	½ cup (4.3 oz.)	40	6.0
(S and W) *Nutradiet*	4 oz.	36	7.4
Frozen:			
(USDA) boiled, without salt, drained	½ cup (3.1 oz.)	46	8.8
(Birds Eye)	⅓ pkg.	50	9.0
(Kounty Kist)	½ cup	45	6.5

Food and Description	Measure or Quantity	Calories	Carbohydrates (grams)
PEA & CAULIFLOWER, frozen (Birds Eye) with cream sauce	⅓ of 10-oz. pkg.	100	12.0
PEA & ONION, frozen (Birds Eye)	⅓ pkg.	60	12.0
PEA & POTATO, frozen (Birds Eye) with cream sauce	⅓ of 8-oz. pkg.	140	16.0
PEA SOUP, GREEN (See also **PEA SOUP, SPLIT**)			
Canned, regular pack:			
(USDA) condensed	8 oz. (by wt.)	240	41.7
*(USDA) condensed, prepared with equal volume water	1 cup (8.6 oz.)	130	22.5
*(USDA) condensed, prepared with equal volume milk	1 cup (8.6 oz.)	208	28.7
*(Campbell) condensed	8-oz. serving	144	23.2
Canned, dietetic or low calorie:			
(Campbell) low sodium	7½-oz. can	150	24.0
*(Claybourne) low sodium	8 oz.	98	19.1
*(Dia-Mel)	8-oz. serving	110	18.0
(Featherweight)	8-oz. can	180	32.0
Mix:			
*(USDA)	1 cup (8.5 oz.)	121	20.3
*(Lipton)	1 cup	130	22.0
*(Lipton) *Cup-a-Soup*	6 fl. oz.	120	20.0
*(Nestlé's) *Souptime*	6 fl. oz.	70	14.0
*Frozen (USDA) condensed, with ham, prepared with equal volume water	8 oz. serving	129	18.1

(USDA): United States Department of Agriculture
(HEW/FAO): Health, Education and Welfare/Food and Agriculture Organization
* Prepared as Package Directs

Food and Description	Measure or Quantity	Calories	Carbohydrates (grams)
PEA SOUP, SPLIT, canned, regular pack:			
*(USDA) condensed, prepared with equal volume water	1 cup (8.6 oz.)	145	20.6
*(Ann Page) with ham	1 cup	180	26.9
*(Campbell) with ham & bacon	8-oz. serving	168	24.0
(Campbell) with ham, *Chunky*	19-oz. can	440	60.0
*(Manischewitz)	8 fl. oz.	133	22.6
PEACH:			
Fresh:			
Whole (USDA) without skin	1 lb. (weighed unpeeled)	150	38.3
Whole (USDA)	4-oz. peach (2″ dia.)	38	9.6
Diced (USDA)	½ cup (4.7 oz.)	51	12.9
Sliced (USDA)	½ cup (3 oz.)	32	8.2
Canned, regular pack, solids & liq.: (USDA):			
Extra heavy syrup	4 oz.	110	28.5
Heavy syrup	2 med. halves & 2 T. syrup (4.1 oz.)	91	23.5
Juice pack	4 oz.	51	13.2
Light syrup	4 oz.	66	17.1
(Del Monte):			
Cling halves or slices	½ cup	95	22.8
Freestone, halves or slices	½ cup	93	22.4
Spiced	½ of 7¼-oz. can	85	20.6
(Libby's):			
Halves, heavy syrup	½ cup (4.5 oz.)	94	25.4
Sliced, heavy syrup	½ cup (4.5 oz.)	92	24.7
(Stokely-Van Camp):			
Halves	½ cup (4.4 oz.)	95	24.5
Slices	½ cup (4.5 oz.)	90	24.0
Canned, dietetic or low calorie, unsweetened or			

Food and Description	Measure or Quantity	Calories	Carbo-hydrates (grams)
water pack:			
(USDA) water pack	½ cup (4.3 oz.)	38	9.9
(Blue Boy) sliced, solids & liq.	4 oz.	32	7.4
(Cellu) water pack, Cling halves & slices, solids & liq.	½ cup	30	7.0
(Diet Delight):			
Unsweetened, Cling halves or slices, solids & liq.	½ cup (4.4 oz.)	61	14.5
Unsweetened, Freestone, halves or slices, solids & liq.	½ cup (4.4 oz.)	59	13.9
Water pack, Cling halves, solids & liq.	½ cup (4.3 oz.)	30	7.0
Water pack, Cling slices, solids & liq.	½ cup (4.3 oz.)	30	8.0
(Featherweight) unsweetened, Cling halves or slices, solids & liq.	½ cup	50	14.0
(Libby's) water pack, sliced, solids & liq.	½ cup (4.3 oz.)	29	7.5
(Tillie Lewis) unsweetened, Cling, solids & liq.	½ cup (4.3 oz.)	49	12.2
Dehydrated (USDA):			
Uncooked	1 oz.	96	24.9
Cooked, with added sugar, solids & liq.	½ cup (5.4 oz.)	184	47.6
Dried:			
(USDA) uncooked	½ cup	231	60.1
(USDA) cooked, unsweetened	½ cup	111	28.9
(USDA) cooked, sweetened	½ cup (5.4 oz.)	181	46.8

(USDA): United States Department of Agriculture
(HEW/FAO): Health, Education and Welfare/Food and Agriculture Organization
* Prepared as Package Directs

Food and Description	Measure or Quantity	Calories	Carbo-hydrates (grams)
Canned (Del Monte) uncooked	2 oz.	153	35.2
Frozen:			
(USDA) unthawed, slices, sweetened	½ cup	104	26.7
(Birds Eye) quick thaw	5 oz.	130	34.0
PEACH BRANDY			
(DeKuyper) 70 proof	1 fl. oz.	85	6.9
PEACH BUTTER			
(Smucker's)	1 T. (.7 oz.)	48	12.1
PEACH CREEK (Annie Green Springs) 8% alcohol	3 fl. oz.	63	6.8
PEACH DUMPLING, frozen (Pepperidge Farm)	3.3-oz. dumpling	293	34.6
PEACH FRUIT DRINK, canned:			
(Alegre) Paradise Peach	6 fl. oz.	93	22.9
(Hi-C)	6 fl. oz.	90	23.0
PEACH ICE CREAM:			
(Breyer's)	¼ pt.	130	18.0
(Sealtest) old-fashioned	¼ pt.	130	19.0
PEACH LIQUEUR:			
(Bols) 60 proof	1 fl. oz.	96	8.9
(DeKuyper) 60 proof	1 fl. oz.	82	8.3
(Hiram Walker) 60 proof	1 fl. oz.	81	8.0
(Leroux) 60 proof	1 fl. oz.	85	8.9
PEACH NECTAR, canned (USDA), 40% fruit juice	1 cup (8.8 oz.)	120	31.0
PEACH & PEAR, canned, dietetic (Featherweight) sliced, solids & liq.	½ cup	50	14.0
PEACH PIE:			
Home recipe (USDA) 2-crust	⅛ of 9″ pie (5.6 oz.)	403	60.4

Food and Description	Measure or Quantity	Calories	Carbo-hydrates (grams)
(Hostess)	4½-oz. pie	409	52.4
(Tastykake)	4-oz. pie	360	52.8
Frozen:			
(Banquet)	⅛ of 20-oz. pie	263	35.8
(Morton)	⅙ of 24-oz. pie	286	38.7
(Morton) mini	8-oz. pie	570	81.8
(Sara Lee)	⅛ of 31-oz. pie	395	54.3
PEACH PIE FILLING:			
(Comstock)	½ cup	150	34.7
(Lucky Leaf)	8 oz.	300	74.0
PEACH PRESERVE:			
Sweetened (Smucker's)	1 T. (.7 oz.)	51	13.1
Low calorie:			
(Dia-Mel)	1 T.	6	1.4
(Featherweight)	1 T.	14	3.0
(Louis Sherry)	1 tsp.	2	0.
(Tillie Lewis)	1 tsp.	4	1.0
PEACH TURNOVER, frozen (Pepperidge Farm)	3.3-oz. turnover	323	33.4
PEANUT:			
Raw:			
In shell (USDA)	1 lb. (weighed in shell)	1868	61.6
In shell (A&P) fancy	1 oz.	171	5.3
With skins	1 oz.	160	5.3
Without skins	1 oz.	161	5.0
Roasted:			
(USDA):			
Whole	1 lb. (weighed in shell)	1769	62.6
With skins, unsalted	1 oz.	165	5.8
Chopped	½ cup	404	13.0
Halves	½ cup	421	13.5
(A&P):			
Dry roasted	1 oz.	176	5.7

(USDA): United States Department of Agriculture
(HEW/FAO): Health, Education and Welfare/Food and Agriculture Organization
* Prepared as Package Directs

Food and Description	Measure or Quantity	Calories	Carbo-hydrates (grams)
In shell	1 oz.	178	5.8
Oil roasted	1 oz.	181	4.7
(Excel) halves	1 oz.	185	4.8
(Frito-Lay's)	1 oz.	172	6.2
(Frito-Lay's) salted-in-the-shell	1-oz. shelled	163	5.7
(Planters):			
Dry roasted	1-oz. (jar)	170	5.4
Oil roasted	¾-oz. bag	133	3.7
(Skippy) dry roasted	1 oz.	179	4.1
(Tom Houston) toasted	2 T. (1.1 oz.)	176	5.6
Spanish:			
(Ann Page) oil roasted	1 oz.	180	5.2
Freshnut, oil roasted	1 oz.	170	5.1
(Frito-Lay's)	1 oz.	168	6.6
(Planters):			
Dry roasted	1 oz. (jar)	175	3.4
Oil roasted	1 oz. (can)	182	3.4
PEANUT BUTTER:			
(Ann Page):			
Creamy smooth	1 T. (.6 oz.)	107	3.6
Krunchy	1 T. (.6 oz.)	105	3.6
(Bama):			
Crunchy	1 T. (.6 oz.)	100	3.4
Smooth	1 T. (.6 oz.)	103	2.9
(Cellu) low sodium	1 T. (.6 oz.)	101	2.2
(Jif) creamy	1 T.	93	2.7
(Peter Pan):			
Crunchy	1 T.	101	3.0
Smooth	1 T. (.6 oz.)	94	3.1
Low sodium	1 T.	106	2.3
(Planters)	1 T. (.6 oz.)	100	2.7
(Skippy):			
Creamy	1 T. (.6 oz.)	108	2.2
Old-fashioned	1 T.	107	1.8
Super chunk	1 T. (.6 oz.)	109	2.0
(Sultana):			
Regular grind	1 T. (.6 oz.)	107	3.6
Krunchy	1 T. (.6 oz.)	105	3.9
PEANUT BUTTER BAKING CHIPS (Reese's)	3 T. (1 oz.)	151	12.8

Food and Description	Measure or Quantity	Calories	Carbohydrates (grams)
PEANUT BUTTER			
PUDDING, refrigerated (Sanna)	4¼-oz. container	203	26.4
PEAR:			
Fresh (USDA):			
Whole	1 lb. (weighed with stems & core)	252	63.2
Whole	6.4-oz. pear (3″ x 2½″ dia.)	101	25.4
Quartered	1 cup (6.8 oz.)	117	29.4
Slices	½ cup (6.8 oz.)	50	12.5
Canned, regular pack, solids & liq.:			
(USDA):			
Extra heavy syrup	4 oz.	104	26.8
Heavy syrup	½ cup	87	22.3
Juice pack	4 oz.	52	13.4
Light syrup	4 oz.	69	17.7
(Del Monte) Bartlett halves or slices	½ cup (4 oz.)	88	21.3
(Libby's) halves, heavy syrup	½ cup (4.5 oz.)	94	25.1
(Stokely-Van Camp):			
Halves	½ cup (4.5 oz.)	105	25.0
Slices	½ cup (4.5 oz.)	100	23.5
Canned, unsweetened or dietetic, solids & liq.:			
(USDA) water pack	½ cup (4.3 oz.)	39	10.1
(Cellu) Bartlett halves, water pack	½ cup	37	9.0
(Diet Delight) unsweetened	½ cup (4.4 oz.)	65	15.5
(Diet Delight) water pack	½ cup (4.3 oz.)	35	9.0
(Featherweight) Bartlett halves, unsweetened	½ cup	57	14.0

(USDA): United States Department of Agriculture
(HEW/FAO): Health, Education and Welfare/Food and Agriculture Organization
* Prepared as Package Directs

Food and Description	Measure or Quantity	Calories	Carbo-hydrates (grams)
(Libby's) halves, water pack	½ cup (4.3 oz.)	36	9.8
(Tillie Lewis)	½ cup (4.3 oz.)	49	12.2
Dried:			
Uncooked (USDA)	1 lb.	1216	305.3
Cooked (USDA) without added sugar	4 oz.	143	36.0
Cooked (USDA) with added sugar, solids & liq.	4 oz.	171	43.1
PEAR, CANDIED (USDA)	1 oz.	86	21.5
PEAR NECTAR, canned (Del Monte)	6 fl. oz.	122	30.3
PEBBLES, cereal (Post) cocoa & fruity	⅞ cup (1 oz.)	120	25.0
PECAN:			
In shell (USDA)	1 lb. (weighed in shell)	1652	35.1
Shelled:			
Whole (USDA)	1 lb.	3116	66.2
Chopped (USDA)	½ cup (1.8 oz.)	357	7.6
Chopped (USDA)	1 T. (7 grams)	48	1.0
Chopped & pieces (Ann Page)	1 oz.	205	4.2
Halves (USDA)	12-14 (.5 oz.)	96	2.0
Halves (USDA)	½ cup (1.9 oz.)	371	7.9
Dry roasted (Flavor House)	1 oz.	195	4.1
Dry roasted (Planters)	1 oz.	206	3.5
PECAN PIE:			
Home recipe (USDA) 1 crust	⅛ of 9" pie	577	70.8
(Frito-Lay's)	3-oz. serving	353	53.5
Frozen (Morton) mini	6½-oz. pie	596	81.3
PEP, cereal (Kellogg's)	¾ cup (1 oz.)	100	24.0
PEPPER, BLACK:			
(French's)	1 tsp. (2.3 grams)	9	1.5

Food and Description	Measure or Quantity	Calories	Carbo-hydrates (grams)
(French's) seasoned	1 tsp. (2.9 grams)	8	1.0
(Lawry's) seasoned	1 tsp. (2.4 grams)	8	1.6
PEPPER, HOT CHILI:			
Green:			
(USDA):			
Raw, whole	4 oz.	31	7.5
Raw, without seeds	4 oz.	42	10.3
Canned, chili sauce	1 oz.	6	1.4
Canned pods, without seeds, solids & liq.	4 oz.	28	6.9
(Ortega) canned, diced, strips or whole	1 oz.	8	1.6
Red:			
(USDA):			
Raw, whole	4 oz. (weighed with seeds)	105	20.5
Raw, trimmed, pods only	4 oz.	54	13.1
Canned, chili sauce	1 oz.	6	1.1
(Ortega) canned	1 oz.	8	1.6
PEPPERMINT PIE, pink, frozen (Kraft)	¼ of 13-oz. pie	328	40.3
PEPPERONI:			
(Hormel) sliced	1 oz.	140	4.0
(Swift)	1 oz.	152	1.0
⁕PEPPER POT SOUP, canned (Campbell) condensed	8-oz. serving	104	9.6
PEPPER, STUFFED:			
Home recipe (USDA) with beef & crumbs	2¾″ x 2½″ pepper with 1⅛ cups stuffing (6.5 oz.)	314	31.1
Frozen (Green Giant) with beef, in Creole sauce	7-oz. entree	200	18.0

(USDA): United States Department of Agriculture
(HEW/FAO): Health, Education and Welfare/Food and Agriculture Organization
⁕ Prepared as Package Directs

Food and Description	Measure or Quantity	Calories	Carbo-hydrates (grams)
Frozen (Weight Watchers) with veal stuffing	13-oz. meal	366	51.0
PEPPER, SWEET (USDA):			
Green:			
Raw:			
Whole	1 lb. (weighed untrimmed)	82	17.9
Without stems & seeds	1 med. pepper (2.6 oz.)	13	2.9
Chopped	½ cup (2.6 oz.)	16	3.6
Slices	½ cup (1.4 oz.)	9	2.0
Strips	½ cup (1.7 oz.)	11	2.4
Boiled strips, drained	½ cup (2.4 oz.)	12	2.6
Boiled, drained	1 med. pepper (2.6 oz.)	13	2.8
Red:			
Raw, whole	1 lb. (weighed with stems & seeds)	112	25.8
Raw, without stems & seeds	1 med. pepper (2.2 oz.)	19	2.4
PERCH, raw (USDA):			
White, whole	1 lb. (weighed whole)	193	0.
White, meat only	4 oz.	134	0.
Yellow, whole	1 lb. (weighed whole)	161	0.
Yellow, meat only	4 oz.	103	0.
PERCH DINNER or LUNCHEON, frozen:			
(Banquet)	8¾-oz. dinner	434	49.8
(Weight Watchers) 2-compartment meal	8.5-oz. meal	206	13.0
(Weight Watchers) 3-compartment meal	16-oz. meal	294	15.0
PERNOD (Julius Wile) 40 proof	1 fl. oz.	79	1.1

Food and Description	Measure or Quantity	Calories	Carbohydrates (grams)
PERSIMMON (USDA):			
Japanese or Kaki, fresh:			
With seeds	1 lb. (weighed with skin, calyx & seeds)	286	78.3
With seeds	4.4-oz. persimmon	79	20.1
Seedless	1 lb. (weighed with skin & calyx)	293	75.1
Seedless	4.4-oz. persimmon (2½" dia.)	81	20.7
Native, fresh, whole	1 lb. (weighed with seeds & calyx)	472	124.6
Native, fresh, flesh only	4 oz.	144	38.0
PHEASANT, raw (USDA):			
Ready-to-cook	1 lb. (weighed ready-to-cook)	596	0.
Meat & skin	4 oz.	172	0.
Meat only	4 oz.	184	0.
PICKEREL, chain, raw (USDA):			
Whole	1 lb. (weighed whole)	194	0.
Meat only	4 oz.	95	0.
PICKLE:			
Chowchow (See **CHOWCHOW**)			
Cucumber, fresh or bread & butter:			
(USDA)	3 slices (¼" x 1½")	15	3.8
(Aunt Jane's)	4 slices or sticks (1 oz.)	21	5.1
(Aunt Jane's)	1 spear (1 oz.)	4	.3
(Bond's)	3 pieces	23	5.0
(Fanning's)	14-fl.-oz. jar	196	45.7

(USDA): United States Department of Agriculture
(HEW/FAO): Health, Education and Welfare/Food and Agriculture Organization

* Prepared as Package Directs

Food and Description	Measure or Quantity	Calories	Carbo hydrate (gram.
(Featherweight) dietetic, slices or whole	1 oz.	12	2.
Dill:			
(USDA)	4.8-oz. pickle	15	3.
(Aunt Jane's)	2-oz. pickle	6	1.
(Bond's)	1 pickle	1	
(Bond's) fresh-pack	1 spear	2	
L & S Dills	1 large pickle	15	2.
(Smucker's) baby, fresh pack	2¾″ pickle (.8 oz.)	3	
(Smucker's) candied stick	4″ pickle (.8 oz.)	46	11.
(Smucker's) hamburger	3 slices (.4 oz.)	2	.
Hot, mixed (Smucker's)	4 pieces (.7 oz.)	5	1.
Hot peppers (Smucker's)	4″ pepper (1 oz.)	10	2.
Kosher dill:			
(Bond's)	1 pickle	2	.
(Featherweight) dietetic	1 oz.	5	.
(Smucker's)	3½″ pickle (.5 oz.)	8	1.
Sour:			
(USDA) cucumber	1¾″ x 4″ (4.8 oz.)	14	2.
(Aunt Jane's)	2-oz. pickle	6	1.
Sweet:			
(USDA) cucumber, whole	1 oz. whole	41	10.
(USDA) cucumber, chopped	1 T. (9 grams)	13	3.
(Aunt Jane's)	1.5-oz. pickle	62	15.
(Smucker's)	.4-oz. pickle	17	4.
Gherkins (Bond's)	1 pickle	19	3.
PIE CRUST (See also **PASTRY SHELL**):			
Home recipe (USDA) baked	1 9″ pie crust (6.3 oz.)	900	78.
Home recipe (USDA) baked	2 9″ pie crusts (12.7 oz.)	1800	157.
Mix:			
(USDA) Dry	10-oz. pkg.	1482	140.
(USDA) prepared with water, baked	4 oz.	526	49.
(Betty Crocker)	⅟₁₆ pkg.	120	10.
(Betty Crocker)	⅛ stick	120	10.
*(Flako)	⅛ of 9″ pie shell	260	29.

Food and Description	Measure or Quantity	Calories	Carbo-hydrates (grams)
*(Pillsbury) double crust	⅛ of 2 crusts	290	27.0
*(Pillsbury) sticks	⅙ of 2-crust pie	290	27.0
PIE FILLING (See individual kinds)			
PIESPORTER RIESLING (Julius Kayser) 10% alcohol	3 fl. oz.	57	1.7
PIGEON (See **SQUAB**)			
PIGEONPEA (USDA):			
Raw, immature seeds in pods	1 lb.	207	37.7
Dry seeds	1 lb.	1551	288.9
PIGNOLIA (See **PINE NUT**)			
PIGS FEET, pickled:			
(USDA)	4 oz.	226	0.
(Hormel)	1-pt. can	442	.2
PIKE, raw (USDA):			
Blue, whole	1 lb. (weighed whole)	180	0.
Blue, meat only	4 oz.	102	0.
Northern, whole	1 lb. (weighed whole)	104	0.
Northern, meat only	4 oz.	100	0.
Walleye, whole	1 lb. (weighed whole)	240	0.
Walleye, meat only	4 oz.	105	0.
PILI NUT (USDA):			
In shell	1 lb. (weighed in shell)	546	6.9
Shelled	4 oz.	759	9.5
PIMIENTO, canned:			
(USDA) solids & liq.	4 oz.	31	6.6
(Ortega) drained	¼ cup (1.7 oz.)	6	1.3

(USDA): United States Department of Agriculture
(HEW/FAO): Health, Education and Welfare/Food and Agriculture Organization

* Prepared as Package Directs

Food and Description	Measure or Quantity	Calories	Carbo-hydrates (grams)
PIÑA COLADA:			
Canned (Party Tyme) 12½ % alcohol	2 fl. oz.	63	5.1
Mix:			
Dry (Holland House)	1 serving (.6 oz.)	66	16.0
Dry (Party Tyme)	½-oz. pkg.	50	13.2
Liquid (Holland House)	1½ fl. oz.	90	22.5
PINCH OF HERBS (Lawry's)	1 tsp. (2.7 grams)	9	1.0
PINEAPPLE:			
Fresh:			
Whole (USDA)	1 lb. (weighed untrimmed)	123	32.3
Diced (USDA)	½ cup (2.8 oz.)	41	10.7
Sliced (USDA)	¾" x 3½" slice (3 oz.)	44	11.5
(Dole) cut in chunks	½ cup (3.5 oz.)	52	13.7
Canned, regular pack, solids & liq.:			
(USDA):			
Heavy syrup, crushed	½ cup (4.6 oz.)	97	25.4
Heavy syrup, slices	1 large slice & 2 T. syrup (4.3 oz.)	90	23.7
Heavy syrup, tidbits	½ cup (4.6 oz.)	95	25.0
Juice pack	4 oz.	66	17.1
Light syrup	4 oz.	67	17.5
(Del Monte):			
Crushed	½ cup (4 oz.)	94	22.7
Chunks	½ cup (4 oz.)	91	22.2
Slices, medium	½ cup (4 oz.)	92	22.4
Slices, large	½ cup (4 oz.)	103	25.2
Tidbits	½ cup (4 oz.)	95	22.9
(Dole):			
Heavy syrup, chunks	½ cup	84	22.0
Juice pack, chunks or crushed	½ cup	64	16.5
Heavy syrup, crushed or tidbits	½ cup	84	21.7
Heavy syrup, slices	2 med. slices & 2½ T. syrup (4 oz.)	84	21.7
Juice pack, sliced	2 med. slices & 2½ T. syrup	66	15.5

Food and Description	Measure or Quantity	Calories	Carbohydrates (grams)
Canned, unsweetened or water pack, dietetic or low calorie, solids & liq.:			
(USDA)	4 oz.	44	11.6
(Del Monte):			
Unsweetened	½ cup	77	18.5
Unsweetened, chunks	½ cup	70	16.8
Unsweetened, slices	½ cup	81	19.6
(Cellu) water pack, slices	½ cup	60	15.0
(Diet Delight) unsweetened, chunks, slices or tidbits	½ cup	70	18.0
(Featherweight) unsweetened, chunks, crushed or sliced	½ cup	70	18.0
(Tillie Lewis)	½ cup	70	17.5
PINEAPPLE, CANDIED			
(Liberty)	1 oz.	93	22.6
PINEAPPLE & GRAPEFRUIT JUICE DRINK, canned:			
(USDA) 40% fruit juices	½ cup (4.4 oz.)	68	17.0
(Del Monte) pink	6 fl. oz. (6.6 oz.)	97	23.9
(Dole) regular or pink	6 fl. oz.	91	23.0
(Wagner)	6 fl. oz.	86	21.6
PINEAPPLE JUICE:			
Canned, unsweetened:			
(Del Monte)	6 fl. oz.	98	23.7
(Del Monte) with vitamin C	6 fl. oz.	108	26.2
(Dole) with vitamin C	6 fl. oz.	93	22.8
Frozen, unsweetened:			
*(USDA)	½ cup (4.4 oz.)	64	15.9
*(Minute Maid)	6 fl. oz.	92	22.7

(USDA): United States Department of Agriculture
(HEW/FAO): Health, Education and Welfare/Food and Agriculture Organization
* Prepared as Package Directs

Food and Description	Measure or Quantity	Calories	Carbohydrates (grams)
PINEAPPLE & ORANGE JUICE DRINK:			
Canned:			
(USDA) 40% fruit juices	½ cup (4.4 oz.)	67	16.7
(Del Monte)	6 fl. oz.	97	24.0
*Frozen (Minute Maid)	6 fl. oz.	94	23.0
PINEAPPLE PIE:			
Home recipe (USDA)	⅛ of 9″ pie (5.6 oz.)	400	60.2
Home recipe, chiffon (USDA)	⅛ of 9″ pie (3.8 oz.)	311	42.2
Home recipe, custard (USDA)	⅛ of 9″ pie (5.4 oz.)	334	48.8
(Tastykake)	4-oz. pie	389	57.8
(Tastykake) with cheese	4-oz. pie	436	59.4
PINEAPPLE PIE FILLING (Comstock)	½ cup	150	35.2
PINEAPPLE PRESERVE, sweetened:			
(Bama)	1 T. (.7 oz.)	54	13.5
(Smucker's)	1 T. (.7 oz.)	53	13.7
*PINEAPPLE PUDDING MIX, sweetened (Jell-O) instant, cream	½ cup	180	31.0
PINE NUT (USDA):			
Pignolias, shelled	4 oz.	626	13.2
Piñon, whole	4 oz. (weighed in shell)	418	13.5
Piñon, shelled	4 oz.	720	23.2
PINK SQUIRREL COCKTAIL MIX, dry (Holland House)	.6-oz. pkg.	69	17.0
PINOT CHARDONNAY WINE (Louis M. Martini) 12.5% alcohol	3 fl. oz.	90	.2

Food and Description	Measure or Quantity	Calories	Carbo-hydrates (grams)
PINOT NOIR WINE:			
(Inglenook) Estate, 12% alcohol	3 fl. oz.	58	.3
(Louis M. Martini) 12½% alcohol	3 fl. oz.	90	.2
PISTACHIO NUT:			
(USDA) in shell	4 oz. (weighed in shell)	337	10.8
(USDA) shelled	½ cup (2.2 oz.)	368	11.8
(USDA) shelled	1 T. (8 grams)	46	1.5
Dry roasted (Flavor House)	1 oz.	168	5.4
(Frito-Lay's)	1 oz.	175	5.8
PISTACHIO PUDDING & PIE FILLING MIX, instant (Ann Page)	¼ of 3½-oz. pkg.	97	22.7
PITANGA, fresh (USDA):			
Whole	1 lb. (weighed whole)	187	45.9
Flesh only	4 oz.	58	14.2
PIZZA PIE (See also **PIZZA PIE MIX**):			
Regular (Pizza Hut):			
Beef	½ of 10″ pizza (7.6 oz.)	488	55.0
Cheese	½ of 10″ pie	436	53.2
Pepperoni	½ of 10″ pie	459	54.4
Pork	½ of 10″ pie	466	54.6
Supreme	½ of 10″ pie	475	54.4
Frozen:			
Cheese:			
(Buitoni)	4 oz.	270	36.6
(Celeste)	½ of 7-oz. pie	247	31.8
(Celeste)	¼ of 19-oz. pie	320	36.2

(USDA): United States Department of Agriculture
(HEW/FAO): Health, Education and Welfare/Food and Agriculture Organization
* Prepared as Package Directs

Food and Description	*Measure or Quantity*	*Calories*	*Carbo-hydrates (grams)*
(Jeno's)	½ of 13-oz. pie	420	54.0
(Jeno's) deluxe	⅓ of 20-oz. pie	490	57.0
(Kraft)	½ of 14-oz. pie	413	49.5
(Kraft) *Pee Wee*	2½-oz. pie	169	20.1
Tostino's	½ pie	440	53.0
(Weight Watchers)	6-oz. pie	386	37.2
(Weight Watchers)	7-oz. pie	450	43.4
Cheese & mushroom (Celeste)	½ of 9-oz. pie	285	29.0
Cheese & mushroom (Celeste)	¼ of 21-oz. pie	298	30.1
Cheese, Sicilian style (Celeste)	¼ of 20-oz. pie	329	42.5
Combination:			
(Jeno's) deluxe	⅓ of 23-oz. pie	560	55.0
Tostino's, classic	⅓ of pie	520	48.0
Tostino's, deep crust	⅙ of pie	310	33.0
Deluxe (Celeste)	½ of 9-oz. pie	298	27.7
Deluxe (Celeste)	½ of 23½-oz. pie	367	33.9
Hamburger:			
(Jeno's)	½ of 13½-oz. pie	440	57.0
Tostino's	½ of pie	460	51.0
Pepperoni:			
(Buitoni)	4 oz.	288	38.7
(Celeste)	½ of 7½-oz. pie	264	25.9
(Celeste)	¼ of 20-oz. pie	356	31.7
(Jeno's)	½ of 12-oz. pie	450	57.0
Tostino's	½ of pie	460	52.0
Tostino's, deep crust	⅙ of pie	300	34.0
Sausage:			
(Buitoni)	4 oz.	281	34.1
(Celeste)	½ of 8-oz. pie	281	25.8
(Celeste)	¼ of 22-oz. pie	375	33.9
(Jeno's)	½ of 13½-oz. pie	450	57.0
(Jeno's) deluxe	⅓ of 21-oz. pie	500	53.0
(Kraft)	½ of 14½-oz. pie	500	49.8
(Kraft) *Pee Wee*	2½-oz. pie	191	19.7
Tostino's	½ of pie	470	54.0
Tostino's, classic	⅓ of pie	500	50.0
Tostino's, deep crust	⅙ of pie	300	33.0
(Weight Watchers)	6-oz. pie	330	30.7
(Weight Watchers)	7-oz. pie	385	35.8

Food and Description	Measure or Quantity	Calories	Carbo- hydrates (grams)
Sausage & mushroom (Celeste)	½ of 9-oz. pie	285	29.0
Sausage & mushroom (Celeste)	¼ of 24-oz. pie	379	34.3
PIZZA PIE MIX:			
Regular (Jeno's)	½ of pkg.	420	67.0
Cheese:			
(Jeno's)	½ of mix	420	62.0
*(Kraft)	4 oz.	265	26.1
Skillet Pizza (General Mills)	¼ pkg.	210	30.0
Pepperoni:			
(Jeno's)	½ pkg.	510	67.0
Skillet Pizza (General Mills)	¼ pkg.	220	31.0
Sausage:			
(Jeno's)	½ of pkg.	530	66.0
*(Kraft)	4 oz.	274	23.9
Skillet Pizza (General Mills)	¼ pkg.	230	29.0
PIZZA ROLL (Jeno's) frozen, 12 to pkg.:			
Cheeseburger	½-oz. roll	45	4.5
Pepperoni & cheese	½-oz. roll	43	4.2
Sausage & cheese	½-oz. roll	43	4.2
Shrimp & cheese	½-oz. roll	37	3.8
PIZZA SAUCE, canned:			
(Buitoni)	4 oz.	76	10.0
(Contadina)	8 oz.	140	23.0
(Ragu)	5 oz.	120	15.0
PIZZA SAUCE MIX:			
(French's)	1-oz. pkg.	77	17.2
*(French's)	2 T.	18	4.1

(USDA): United States Department of Agriculture
(HEW/FAO): Health, Education and Welfare/Food and Agriculture
        Organization
* Prepared as Package Directs

Food and Description	Measure or Quantity	Calories	Carbo-hydrates (grams)
PLANTAIN, raw (USDA):			
Whole	1 lb. (weighed with skin)	389	101.9
Flesh only	4 oz.	135	35.4
PLUM:			
Damson, fresh (USDA):			
Whole	1 lb. (weighed with pits)	272	73.5
Flesh only	4 oz.	75	20.2
Japanese & hybrid, fresh (USDA):			
Whole	1 lb. (weighed with pits)	205	52.4
Whole	2.1-oz. plum (2″ dia.)	27	6.9
Diced	½ cup (2.9 oz.)	39	10.1
Halves	½ cup (3.1 oz.)	42	10.8
Slices	½ cup (3 oz.)	40	10.3
Prune type, fresh (USDA):			
Whole	1 lb. (weighed with pits)	310	84.0
Halves	½ cup (2.8 oz.)	60	15.8
Canned, purple, regular, solids & liq. (USDA):			
Light syrup	4 oz.	71	18.8
Heavy syrup, with pits	½ cup (4.5 oz.)	106	27.6
Heavy syrup, without pits	½ cup (4.2 oz.)	100	25.9
Extra heavy syrup	4 oz.	116	30.3
Canned, unsweetened or low calorie, solids & liq.:			
(Cellu) purple, water pack	½ cup	39	9.0
(Diet Delight) purple	½ cup	70	19.0
(Diamond A) purple, whole	½ cup (4.4 oz.)	47	12.4
(Featherweight) purple	½ cup	67	18.0
(Tillie Lewis)	½ cup (4.3 oz.)	73	18.2
PLUM HOLLOW WINE			
(Annie Green Springs) 8% alcohol	3 fl. oz.	63	6.8
PLUM JELLY:			
Sweetened (Smucker's)	1 T. (.7 oz.)	52	13.3

Food and Description	Measure or Quantity	Calories	Carbo-hydrates (grams)
Dietetic or low calorie (Featherweight)	1 T.	16	4.0
PLUM PIE (Tastykake)	4-oz. pie	364	53.8
PLUM PRESERVE OR JAM, sweetened (Smucker's)	1 T. (.7 oz.)	50	12.9
PLUM PUDDING:			
(Crosse & Blackwell)	4 oz.	340	62.4
(R&R)	¼ of 14½-oz. can	272	61.6
P.M. FRUIT DRINK (Mott's)	6 fl. oz.	90	22.0
POLISH-STYLE SAUSAGE:			
(USDA)	1 oz.	86	.3
(Frito-Lay's) smoked beef	1 oz.	73	.6
(Hormel) *Kolbase*	1 oz.	80	.4
(Vienna) beef	3-oz. piece	240	1.3
(Wilson)	1 oz.	82	.3
POMEGRANATE, raw (USDA):			
Whole	1 lb. (weighed whole)	160	41.7
Pulp only	4 oz.	71	18.6
POMMARD WINE, French red Burgundy:			
(Barton & Guestier) 13% alcohol	3 fl. oz.	67	.4
(Chanson) *St. Vincent,* 11½% alcohol	3 fl. oz.	60	6.3
POMPANO, raw (USDA):			
Whole	1 lb. (weighed whole)	422	0.
Meat only	4 oz.	188	0.
POPCORN:			
Unpopped (USDA)	1 oz.	103	20.4

(USDA): United States Department of Agriculture
(HEW/FAO): Health, Education and Welfare/Food and Agriculture
Organization

* Prepared as Package Directs

Food and Description	Measure or Quantity	Calories	Carbohydrates (grams)
Popped:			
(USDA):			
Plain	1 oz.	109	21.7
Plain, large kernel	1 cup (6 grams)	23	4.6
Butter or oil & salt added	1 oz.	129	16.8
Butter or oil & salt added	1 cup (9 grams)	41	5.3
Sugar-coated	1 cup (1.2 oz.)	134	29.9
(Bachman):			
Plain	1 oz.	160	13.0
Caramel-coated	1 oz.	130	23.0
Cheese-flavored	1 oz.	150	16.0
Cracker Jack	¾-oz. bag	90	16.7
Cracker Jack	3-oz. box	350	65.5
(Jiffy Pop):			
Plain	½ pkg. (2½ oz.)	244	29.8
Buttered	½ pkg. (2½ oz.)	247	29.4
(Old London):			
Buttered	1 cup	57	6.4
Without peanuts	1¾-oz. bag	195	43.6
With peanuts	1 cup	142	30.2
Cheese-flavored	1 cup	74	6.6
Seasoned	1¼-oz. bag	174	22.4
(Tom Houston)	1 cup (.5 oz.)	68	8.9
(Wise):			
Buttered	1 cup	57	6.4
Cheese-flavored	1 cup (.5 oz.)	74	6.6
POPOVER			
Home recipe (USDA)	1 average popover (2 oz.)	128	14.7
Mix *(Flako)	1 popover	170	25.0
POPPY SEED (French's)	1 tsp.	13	.8
POP TARTS (Kellogg's):			
Regular:			
Blueberry, concord grape, raspberry and strawberry	1.8 oz. tart	210	36.0
Brown sugar cinnamon	1¾-oz. tart	210	34.0
Cherry	1.8-oz. tart	210	35.0
Frosted:			
Blueberry, concord grape, raspberry	1.8-oz. tart	210	37.0

Food and Description	Measure or Quantity	Calories	Carbo-hydrates (grams)
Brown sugar cinnamon	1¾-oz. tart	210	33.0
Cherry, Dutch apple, strawberry	1.8-oz. tart	210	36.0
Chocolate fudge, chocolate peppermint	1.8-oz. tart	210	35.0
Chocolate-vanilla creme	1.8-oz. tart	210	34.0
PORK, medium-fat:			
Fresh (USDA):			
Boston butt:			
Raw	1 lb. (weighed with bone & skin)	1220	0.
Roasted, lean & fat	4 oz.	400	0.
Roasted, lean only	4 oz.	277	0.
Chop:			
Broiled, lean & fat	1 chop (4 oz., weighed with bone)	295	0.
Broiled, lean & fat	1 chop (3 oz., weighed with bone)	332	0.
Broiled, lean only	1 chop (3 oz., weighed without bone)	230	0.
Fat, separable, cooked	1 oz.	219	0.
Ham (See also HAM):			
Raw	1 lb. (weighed with bone & skin)	1188	0.
Roasted, lean & fat	4 oz.	424	0.
Roasted, lean only	4 oz.	246	0.
Loin:			
Raw	1 lb. (weighed with bone)	1065	0.
Roasted, lean & fat	4 oz.	411	0.
Roasted, lean only	4 oz.	288	0.

(USDA): United States Department of Agriculture
(HEW/FAO): Health, Education and Welfare/Food and Agriculture
            Organization
* Prepared as Package Directs

Food and Description	Measure or Quantity	Calories	Carbohydrates (grams)
Picnic:			
Raw	1 lb. (weighed with bone & skin)	1083	0.
Simmered, lean & fat	4 oz.	424	0.
Simmered, lean only	4 oz.	240	0.
Spareribs:			
Raw, with bone	1 lb. (weighed with bone)	976	0.
Braised, lean & fat	4 oz.	499	0.
Cured, light commercial cure:			
Bacon (See BACON)			
Bacon butt (USDA):			
Raw	1 lb. (weighed with bone & skin)	1227	0.
Roasted, lean & fat	4 oz.	374	0.
Roasted, lean only	4 oz.	276	0.
Ham (See also HAM):			
Raw (USDA)	1 lb. (weighed with bone & skin)	1100	0.
Roasted, lean & fat (USDA)	4 oz.	328	0.
Roasted, lean only (USDA)	4 oz.	212	0.
Fully cooked, boneless:			
Parti-Style (Armour Star)	4 oz.	167	.1
(Wilson) rolled	4 oz.	222	0.
Picnic:			
Raw (USDA)	1 lb. (weighed with bone & skin)	1060	0.
Raw (Wilson) smoked	4 oz.	279	0.
Roasted, lean & fat (USDA)	4 oz.	366	0.
Roasted, lean only (USDA)	4 oz.	239	0.
Canned (Hormel)	4 oz. (3-lb. can)	206	.2

Food and Description	Measure or Quantity	Calories	Carbo- hydrates (grams)
Cured, long-cure, country-style **Virginia** ham, raw:			
(USDA)	1 lb. (weighed with bone & skin)	1535	1.2
(USDA)	1 lb. (weighed without bone & skin)	1765	1.4
PORK & BEANS (See **BEAN, BAKED**)			
PORK, CANNED, chopped luncheon meat:			
(USDA)	1 oz.	83	.4
(USDA) chopped	1 cup (4.8 oz.)	400	1.8
(USDA) diced	1 cup (5 oz.)	415	1.8
(Hormel)	1 oz.	70	.3
PORK DINNER, frozen			
(Swanson) loin or pork	11¼-oz. dinner	470	48.0
PORK RINDS, fried:			
Baken-Ets	1 oz.	140	.5
PORK SAUSAGE:			
Uncooked (USDA) links or bulk	1 oz.	141	Tr.
Cooked (USDA) links or bulk	1 oz.	135	Tr.
(Armour Star) uncooked	1-oz. sausage	133	0.
(Hormel):			
Country style	1 oz.	107	.4
Little Sizzlers	.8-oz. sausage	105	.2
Midget	.8-oz. link	90	.2
Smoked	1 oz.	97	.3
(Oscar Mayer) *Little Friers,* cooked	.6-oz. link	61	.5

(USDA): United States Department of Agriculture
(HEW/FAO): Health, Education and Welfare/Food and Agriculture Organization
* Prepared as Package Directs

Food and Description	Measure or Quantity	Calories	Carbo-hydrates (grams)
(Wilson) uncooked	1 oz.	135	.3
Canned (USDA) solids & liq.	1 oz.	118	.7
Canned (USDA) drained	1 oz.	108	.5
PORK, sweet & sour, frozen (Chun King)	7½-oz. serving	220	26.0
PORT WINE:			
(Gallo) 16% alcohol	3 fl. oz.	94	7.8
(Gallo) ruby, 20% alcohol	3 fl. oz.	112	8.7
(Gallo) tawny, Old Decanter, 20% alcohol	3 fl. oz.	112	8.4
(Gallo) white, 20% alcohol	3 fl. oz.	111	8.4
(Gold Seal) 19% alcohol	3 fl. oz.	158	9.4
(Great Western) Solera, 18% alcohol	3 fl. oz.	138	11.5
(Great Western) Solera, tawny, 18% alcohol	3 fl. oz.	136	11.4
(Italian Swiss Colony-Gold Medal) 19.7% alcohol	3 fl. oz.	130	8.7
(Louis M. Martini) 19½% alcohol	3 fl. oz.	165	2.0
(Louis M. Martini) tawny, 19½% alcohol	3 fl. oz.	165	2.0
(Robertson's) ruby, 20% alcohol	3 fl. oz.	138	9.9
(Robertson's) tawny, *Dry Humour*, 21% alcohol	3 fl. oz.	145	9.9
(Robertson's) tawny, *Game Bird*, 21% alcohol	3 fl. oz.	145	9.9
(Robertson's) *Rebello Valente*, 20½% alcohol	3 fl. oz.	141	9.9
(Taylor) 18.5% alcohol	3 fl. oz.	144	13.2
(Taylor) tawny, 18.5% alcohol	3 fl. oz.	138	12.0
POSTUM, cereal	6 fl. oz.	10	2.0
POTATO (See also **POTATO CHIP, POTATO MIX, POTATO SALAD,**			

Food and Description	Measure or Quantity	Calories	Carbo-hydrates (grams)
POTATO STICK, and others):			
Raw (USDA):			
Whole	1 lb. (weighed unpared)	279	62.8
Pared, chopped	1 cup (5.2 oz.)	112	25.1
Pared, diced	1 cup (5.5 oz.)	119	26.8
Pared, sliced	1 cup (5.2 oz.)	113	25.5
Cooked (USDA):			
Au gratin or scalloped, with cheese	½ cup (4.3 oz.)	127	17.9
Au gratin or scalloped, without cheese	½ cup (4.3 oz.)	177	16.6
Baked, peeled after baking	2½″ dia. potato (3 raw to 1 lb.)	92	20.9
Boiled, peeled after boiling	1 med. (3 raw to 1 lb.)	103	23.2
Boiled, peeled before boiling:			
Whole	1 med. (3 raw to 1 lb.)	79	17.7
Diced	½ cup (2.8 oz.)	51	11.3
Mashed	½ cup (3.7 oz.)	68	15.1
Riced	½ cup (4 oz.)	74	16.5
Sliced	½ cup (2.8 oz.)	52	11.6
French fried in deep fat	10 pieces (2″ x ½″ x ½″, 2 oz.)	156	20.5
Hash browned, after holding overnight	½ cup (3.4 oz.)	223	28.4
Mashed, milk added	½ cup (3.5 oz.)	64	12.7
Mashed, milk & butter added	½ cup (3.5 oz.)	92	12.1
Pan-fried from raw	½ cup (3 oz.)	228	27.7
Scalloped (See Au Gratin)			
Canned:			
(USDA) solids & liq.	1 cup (8.8 oz.)	110	24.5
(Butter Kernel) white	3-4 small potatoes (4.1 oz.)	96	22.0

(USDA): United States Department of Agriculture
(HEW/FAO): Health, Education and Welfare/Food and Agriculture
            Organization
* Prepared as Package Directs

Food and Description	Measure or Quantity	Calories	Carbo-hydrates (grams)
(Del Monte):			
White, solids & liq.	1 cup	84	19.8
White, drained solids	1 cup	265	28.4
(Stokely-Van Camp) whole, solids & liq.	½ cup (4.4 oz.)	50	11.0
Dehydrated, mashed:			
(USDA) flakes, without milk, dry	½ cup (.8 oz.)	84	19.3
*(USDA) flakes, prepared with water, milk & fat	½ cup (3.8 oz.)	100	15.5
(Borden) Country Store, flakes	¼ cup (1.1 oz.)	60	13.3
(USDA) granules, without milk, dry	½ cup	352	80.4
*(USDA) granules, prepared with water, milk & butter	½ cup (3.7 oz.)	101	15.1
Frozen:			
(USDA):			
French-fried, heated	10 pieces (2″ x ½″) (2 oz.)	125	19.2
Mashed, heated	4 oz.	105	17.8
(Birds Eye):			
Cottage fries	⅛ of 14-oz. pkg.	120	17.0
Crinkle cuts	⅛ of 9-oz. pkg.	110	18.0
Deep Gold	3-oz. serving	160	24.0
Deep Gold, crinkle cut	3-oz. serving	140	25.0
French fries	3-oz. serving	110	17.0
French fries, Tasti Fries	2.5-oz. serving	140	17.0
Hash browns	4-oz. serving	70	17.0
Hash browns O'Brien	4-oz. serving	60	14.0
Hash browns, shredded	3-oz. serving	60	13.0
Shoestring	3.3-oz. serving	140	20.0
Steak fries	3-oz. serving	110	18.0
Tasti Puffs	2.5-oz. serving	190	19.0
Tiny Taters	3.2-oz. serving	200	22.0
Whole, peeled	⅒ of 32-oz. pkg.	60	13.0
(Green Giant):			
Au gratin, Bake 'n Serve	1 cup	390	32.0
Diced, in sour cream sauce	1 cup	270	36.0
& sweet peas in bacon cream sauce	1 cup	240	31.0

Food and Description	Measure or Quantity	Calories	Carbo-hydrates (grams)
Shoestring, in butter sauce	1 cup	310	37.0
Slices in butter sauce	1 cup	210	27.0
Stuffed, with cheese-flavored topping	5-oz. entree	240	30.0
Vermicelli, with mushrooms & cheese sauce	1 cup	390	42.0
POTATO CHIP:			
(USDA)	1 oz.	161	14.2
(Frito-Lay's) natural style	1 oz.	157	15.1
Lay's	1 oz.	158	14.0
Lay's, Bar-B-Q-flavored	1 oz.	157	14.2
Lay's, sour cream & onion flavor	1 oz.	155	14.7
(Nally's)	1 oz.	158	13.9
(Planters)	10 chips (.6 oz.)	90	8.0
Pringle's, regular and country style	1 oz.	156	15.1
Pringle's Newfangled, regular and rippled	1 oz.	156	15.1
Ruffles	1 oz.	155	15.4
(Tom Houston)	10 chips (.7 oz.)	114	10.0
(Wise):			
Regular	1 oz.	165	15.7
Barbecue	½-oz. pkg.	75	7.9
Light, blanched	1-oz. pkg.	166	13.5
Onion, garlic	½-oz. pkg.	77	7.6
Ridgies	1-oz. pkg.	156	15.2
Ridgies, sour cream & onion	1 oz.	150	15.5
Sour cream & onion	1 oz.	150	15.5
(Wonder)	1 oz.	158	13.9
(Wonder) barbecue	1 oz.	154	13.8

(USDA): United States Department of Agriculture
(HEW/FAO): Health, Education and Welfare/Food and Agriculture Organization
* Prepared as Package Directs

Food and Description	Measure or Quantity	Calories	Carbohydrates (grams)
POTATO MIX:			
Au gratin:			
*(Betty Crocker)	⅙ pkg.	150	20.0
*(French's)	½ cup	190	28.6
*Buds (Betty Crocker)	⅓ cup	130	15.0
*Creamed (Betty Crocker) made in saucepan	⅙ pkg.	160	21.0
Hash brown:			
*(Betty Crocker) with onion	⅙ pkg.	150	22.0
*(French's) *Big Tate,* with seasonings	½ cup	165	22.0
*Julienne (Betty Crocker)	⅙ pkg.	130	17.0
Mashed:			
*(French's) *Big Tate*	½ cup	140	16.0
*(French's) Idaho	½ cup	120	16.0
*(Pillsbury) *Hungry Jack*	½ cup	140	16.0
Scalloped:			
*(Betty Crocker)	⅙ pkg.	150	20.0
*(French's)	½ cup	190	30.0
*Sour cream & chives (Betty Crocker)	⅙ pkg.	140	18.0
*POTATO PANCAKE MIX (French's) *Big Tate*	3″ pancake	43	5.7
POTATO SALAD (USDA):			
Home recipe, with cooked salad dressing & seasonings	4 oz.	112	18.5
Home recipe, with mayonnaise & French dressing, hard-cooked eggs, seasonings	4 oz.	164	15.2
*POTATO SOUP, canned (Campbell) cream of, condensed	10-oz. serving	90	14.0
POTATO STICK:			
O & C	1½ oz. can	231	22.0
O & C, Snackin' Crisp	4-oz. can	620	60.0

Food and Description	Measure or Quantity	Calories	Carbo-hydrates (grams)
POUILLY-FUISSÉ WINE, French white Burgundy: (Barton & Guestier) 12½% alcohol	3 fl. oz.	64	.3
(Chanson) *St. Vincent,* 12% alcohol	3 fl. oz.	84	6.3
POUILLY-FUMÉ, French white Loire Valley (Barton & Guestier) 12% alcohol	3 fl. oz.	60	.1
POUND CAKE (See **CAKE,** Pound)			
PRESERVE: Sweetened (Ann Page) all flavors	2 tsps. (.5 oz.)	38	9.6
Sweetened (Kraft)	1 oz.	78	19.3
PRETZEL: (Bachman) *Nutzel*	1 oz.	110	21.0
(Bachman) thins	1 oz.	110	22.0
(Cellu) unsalted	1 piece	7	1.3
(Nabisco) *Mister Salty* pretzelette	1 piece (1.7 grams)	7	1.3
(Nabisco) *Mister Salty Veri-Thin*	1 piece (5 grams)	20	4.0
(Old London) rings	1½-oz. bag	156	32.9
(Wise) old fashioned	1 oz.	103	21.3
(Wise) rods	1 oz.	102	22.2
(Wise) sticks	1 oz.	108	22.7
PRODUCT 19, cereal (Kellogg's)	¾ cup (1 oz.)	110	24.0
PRUNE: Canned: (Del Monte) stewed, with pits, solids & liq.	1 cup (8 oz.)	262	62.5

(USDA): United States Department of Agriculture
(HEW/FAO): Health, Education and Welfare/Food and Agriculture
          Organization
* Prepared as Package Directs

Food and Description	Measure or Quantity	Calories	Carbo- hydrates (grams)
(Del Monte) *Moist Pak*, with pits	2 oz.	142	33.5
(Sunsweet) cooked, pitted, solids & liq.	5-6 prunes (1.8 oz.)	138	32.9
Dietetic (Featherweight) stewed, water pack, solids & liq.	½ cup	93	24.0
Dried:			
(USDA) dried, cooked, with sugar	1 cup (16-18 prunes & ⅔ cup liq.)	504	132.1
(Del Monte):			
Breakfast, with pits	2 oz.	152	35.4
Medium, with pits	2 oz.	152	35.6
Large, with pits	2 oz.	153	36.2
Extra large, with pits	2 oz.	150	35.3
Jumbo, with pits	2 oz.	157	37.0
Pitted	2 oz.	151	35.4
PRUNE JUICE, canned:			
(USDA)	½ cup (4.5 oz.)	99	24.3
(Ann Page)	½ cup (4.5 oz.)	92	22.4
(Del Monte)	6 fl. oz.	137	33.2
(Mott's)	6 fl. oz.	140	34.0
(Mott's) with prune pulp	6 fl. oz.	120	30.0
(Sunsweet)	6 fl. oz.	136	32.9
PRUNE NECTAR, canned			
(Mott's)	6 fl. oz.	100	25.0
PUFFED RICE, cereal:			
(Malt-O-Meal)	½ oz.	52	11.9
(Quaker)	1 cup (½ oz.)	55	12.7
PUFFED WHEAT, cereal:			
(Malt-O-Meal)	½ oz.	48	9.9
(Quaker)	1 cup (½ oz.)	54	10.8
PUFFS, frozen (Rich's) vanilla	1.8-oz. puff	167	23.4

Food and Description	Measure or Quantity	Calories	Carbo-hydrates (grams)
PUMPKIN:			
Fresh, whole (USDA)	1 lb. (weighed with rind & seeds)	83	20.5
Fresh, flesh only (USDA)	4 oz.	29	7.4
Canned:			
(Del Monte)	½ cup (4.3 oz.)	45	9.5
(Libby's) solid pack	¼ of 16-oz. can	41	9.9
(Stokely-Van Camp)	½ cup (4.3 oz.)	45	9.5
PUMPKIN PIE:			
Home recipe (USDA)			
1-crust	⅛ of 9″ pie (5.4 oz.)	321	37.2
(Tastykake)	4-oz. pie	368	50.5
Frozen:			
(Banquet)	⅙ of 20-oz. pie	206	32.2
(Morton)	⅙ of 24-oz. pie	325	36.4
(Morton) mini	8-oz. pie	450	72.7
Mix (Libby's)	¼ of 30-oz. can	194	51.6
PUMPKIN PIE FILLING			
(Comstock)	1 cup (10.8 oz.)	366	90.2
PUMPKIN SEED, dry (USDA):			
Whole	4 oz. (weighed in hull)	464	12.6
Hulled	4 oz.	627	17.0

Q

QUAIL, raw (USDA):			
Ready-to-cook	1 lb. (weighed with bones)	686	0.
Meat & skin only	4 oz.	195	0.

(USDA): United States Department of Agriculture
(HEW/FAO): Health, Education and Welfare/Food and Agriculture Organization

* Prepared as Package Directs

Food and Description	Measure or Quantity	Calories	Carbohydrates (grams)
QUINCE, fresh (USDA):			
Untrimmed	1 lb. (weighed with skin & seeds)	158	42.3
Flesh only	4 oz.	65	17.4
QUINCE JELLY (Smucker's)	1 T. (.7 oz.)	51	13.1
QUISP, cereal (Quaker)	1⅛ cups (1 oz.)	121	23.1

R

Food and Description	Measure or Quantity	Calories	Carbohydrates (grams)
RABBIT (USDA):			
Domesticated, ready-to-cook	1 lb. (weighed with bones)	581	0.
Domesticated, stewed, flesh only	4 oz.	245	0.
Wild, ready-to-cook	1 lb. (weighed with bones)	490	0.
RACCOON, roasted, meat only (USDA)	4 oz.	289	0.
RADISH (USDA):			
Common, raw:			
Without tops	½ lb. (weighed untrimmed)	34	7.4
Trimmed, whole	4 small radishes (1.4 oz.)	7	1.4
Trimmed, sliced	½ cup (2 oz.)	10	2.1
Oriental, raw, without tops	½ lb. (weighed unpared)	34	7.4
Oriental, raw, trimmed & pared	4 oz.	22	4.8
RAISIN:			
Dried:			
(USDA):			
Whole, pressed down	½ cup (2.9 oz.)	237	63.5
Chopped	½ cup (2.9 oz.)	234	62.7
Ground	½ cup (4.7 oz.)	387	103.7

Food and Description	Measure or Quantity	Calories	Carbohydrates (grams)
(Del Monte):			
Golden seedless	3 oz.	287	67.8
Thompson seedless	3 oz.	283	66.5
Cooked (USDA) added sugar, solids & liq.	½ cup (4.3 oz.)	260	68.8
RAISIN PIE:			
Home recipe (USDA) 2 crusts	⅛ of 9″ pie (5.6 oz.)	427	67.9
(Tastykake)	4-oz. pie	391	60.8
RAISIN PIE FILLING, canned (Comstock)	½ cup	206	44.5
RALSTON, cereal, instant and regular	¼ cup (1 oz.)	100	20.0
RASPBERRY:			
Black:			
Fresh (USDA)	1 lb. (weighed with caps & stems)	160	34.6
Fresh (USDA) without caps and stems	½ cup (2.4 oz.)	49	10.5
Canned, water pack, unsweetened, solids & liq. (USDA)	4 oz.	58	12.1
Red:			
Fresh (USDA)	1 lb. (weighed with caps & stems)	126	29.9
Fresh (USDA) without caps & stems	½ cup (2.5 oz.)	41	9.8
Canned, water pack, unsweetened or low calorie, solids & liq. (USDA)	4 oz.	40	10.0

(USDA): United States Department of Agriculture
(HEW/FAO): Health, Education and Welfare/Food and Agriculture Organization
• Prepared as Package Directs

Food and Description	Measure or Quantity	Calories	Carbo-hydrates (grams)
Frozen (Birds Eye) quick thaw	5 oz.	140	35.0
RASPBERRY BRANDY (DeKuyper) 70 proof	1 fl. oz.	85	6.9
RASPBERRY JELLY, sweetened (Smucker's) black	1 T. (.7 oz.)	52	13.3
RASPBERRY PIE FILLING (Comstock)	½ cup	212	51.8
RASPBERRY PRESERVE:			
Sweetened:			
(Bama) black	1 T. (.7 oz.)	54	13.5
(Smucker's) black	1 T. (.7 oz.)	54	13.7
(Smucker's) red	1 T. (.7 oz.)	53	13.5
Dietetic or low calorie:			
(Diet Delight) black	1 tsp.	2	0.
(Louis Sherry) black or red	1 tsp.	2	0.
RAVIOLI:			
Canned, regular pack:			
(Buitoni) with beef or meat	8 oz.	188	26.9
(Buitoni) with cheese	8 oz.	218	27.3
(Franco-American) beef, in meat sauce	½ of 15-oz. can	220	36.0
(Franco-American) beef, *Raviolios* in meat sauce	½ of 15-oz. can	220	32.0
Canned, dietetic or low calorie:			
(Dia-Mel) beef, in sauce	8-oz. can	230	35.0
(Featherweight) beef, low sodium	8-oz. can	230	35.0
Frozen:			
(Buitoni) cheese	4 oz.	313	48.6
(Buitoni) meat, without sauce	4 oz.	278	41.6

REDFISH (See DRUM, RED & OCEAN PERCH, Atlantic)

Food and Description	Measure or Quantity	Calories	Carbo-hydrates (grams)
RED & GREY SNAPPER, raw (USDA):			
Whole	1 lb. (weighed whole)	219	0.
Meat only	4 oz.	105	0.
RELISH:			
(Crosse & Blackwell):			
Barbecue	1 T. (.7 oz.)	22	5.4
Corn	1 T. (.6 oz.)	15	3.6
Hamburger	1 T. (.6 oz.)	20	4.7
Hot dog	1 T. (.7 oz.)	22	5.4
Sour (USDA)	1 T. (.5 oz.)	3	.4
Dietetic (Featherweight) cucumber	1 oz.	10.6	2.3
RHINE WINE:			
(Deinhard) Rheinritter, 11% alcohol	3 fl. oz.	60	3.6
(Gallo) 12% alcohol	3 fl. oz.	50	.8
(Gallo) Rhine Garten, 12% alcohol	3 fl. oz.	59	3.0
(Gold Seal) 12% alcohol	3 fl. oz.	82	.4
(Great Western) 12% alcohol	3 fl. oz.	73	2.9
(Great Western) Dutchess, 12% alcohol	3 fl. oz.	72	2.9
(Inglenook):			
Navalle, 12% alcohol	3 fl. oz.	76	4.3
Vintage, 12% alcohol	3 fl. oz.	63	1.7
(Italian Swiss Colony) 11% alcohol	3 fl. oz.	59	.6
(Louis M. Martini) 12.5% alcohol	3 fl. oz.	90	.2
(Taylor) 12.5% alcohol	3 fl. oz.	75	3.0
RHUBARB:			
Fresh:			
Partly trimmed (USDA)	1 lb. (weighed with part leaves, ends & trimmings)	54	12.6

(USDA): United States Department of Agriculture
(HEW/FAO): Health, Education and Welfare/Food and Agriculture Organization
* Prepared as Package Directs

Food and Description	Measure or Quantity	Calories	Carbo-hydrates (grams)
Trimmed (USDA)	4 oz.	18	4.2
Diced (USDA)	½ cup (2.2 oz.)	10	2.3
Cooked, sweetened, solids & liq. (USDA)	½ cup (4.2 oz.)	169	43.2
Frozen, sweetened, cooked, added sugar (USDA)	½ cup (4.4 oz.)	177	44.9
RHUBARB PIE, home recipe (USDA)	⅙ of 9″ pie (5.6 oz.)	400	60.4
RICE:			
Brown:			
Raw (USDA)	½ cup (3.7 oz.)	374	80.5
Parboiled (Uncle Ben's) dry, long-grain	1 oz.	107	21.2
Cooked (Uncle Ben's) parboiled, no added butter or salt	⅔ cup	133	26.4
Cooked (Uncle Ben's) parboiled, with butter & salt	⅔ cup (4.2 oz.)	152	26.4
White:			
Instant or precooked:			
Dry:			
(USDA) long-grain	1 oz.	106	23.4
(Uncle Ben's) long-grain	1 oz.	101	23.3
Cooked:			
(Minute Rice) no added butter or salt	⅔ cup	120	27.0
(Uncle Ben's Quick) long-grain, no added butter or salt	⅔ cup (4.2 oz.)	119	27.4
(Uncle Ben's Quick) long-grain, with butter & salt	⅔ cup (4.3 oz.)	143	27.4
(Uncle Ben's Converted) long-grain, no butter or salt	⅔ cup (4.6 oz.)	129	28.9
Regular:			
Dry (USDA)	½ cup (3.3 oz.)	336	74.4

Food and Description	Measure or Quantity	Calories	Carbo-hydrates (grams)
Cooked (USDA)	⅔ cup (4.8 oz.)	149	33.2
Cooked (Carolina) long-grain	½ cup	100	22.0
Cooked (Mahatma) long-grain	½ cup	100	22.0
Cooked (Success Rice) long-grain	½ cup (½ bag)	110	23.0
RICE BRAN (USDA)	1 oz.	78	14.4
RICE CHEX, cereal (Ralston Purina)	1⅛ cups (1 oz.)	110	23.0
RICE, FRIED:			
Canned (La Choy)	1 cup	274	55.0
Canned (La Choy) chicken	1 cup	274	51.0
Canned (Temple) shrimp	1 cup	297	51.0
*Seasoning Mix (Durkee)	1 cup	215	46.5
RICE KRINKLES, cereal (Post)	⅞ cup (1 oz.)	110	26.0
RICE KRISPIES, cereal (Kellogg's)	1 cup (1 oz.)	110	25.0
RICE MIX:			
Beef:			
(Ann Page) *Rice 'n Easy*	1.3 oz. dry	131	26.2
*(Carolina) *Bake-it-Easy*	⅙ of 6-oz. pkg.	110	23.0
Rice-A-Roni	1.6 of 8-oz. pkg.	130	27.0
(Uncle Ben's):			
*Without butter	½ cup (3.6 oz.)	98	20.4
*With butter	½ cup (3.7 oz.)	114	20.4
*Fast cooking, without butter	½ cup (4.1 oz.)	117	24.7
*Fast cooking, with added butter	½ cup	141	24.7

(USDA): United States Department of Agriculture
(HEW/FAO): Health, Education and Welfare/Food and Agriculture Organization

* Prepared as Package Directs

Food and Description	*Measure or Quantity*	*Calories*	*Carbo-hydrates (grams)*
*Brown & wild (Uncle Ben's):			
Without butter	½ cup	126	24.7
With butter	½ cup	150	24.7
Chicken:			
*(Ann Page) *Rice 'n Easy*	1.3-oz. serving	137	27.4
*(Carolina) *Bake-It-Easy*	⅙ of 6-oz. pkg.	110	23.0
Rice-A-Roni	⅙ of 8-oz. pkg.	160	33.2
*(Uncle Ben's):			
Without butter	½ cup	103	20.9
With butter	½ cup	136	21.0
Fast cooking, without butter	½ cup	119	24.7
Fast cooking, with butter	½ cup	143	24.7
*Curried (Uncle Ben's):			
Without butter	½ cup	99	20.9
With butter	½ cup	115	20.9
Fast cooking, without butter	½ cup	109	23.8
Fast cooking, with butter	½ cup	132	23.8
*Drumstick (Minute Rice)	½ cup	170	25.0
*Fried (Minute Rice)	½ cup	160	25.0
*Long grain & wild (Uncle Ben's):			
Without butter	½ cup	97	20.6
With butter	½ cup	113	20.6
Fast cooking, without butter	½ cup	95	20.1
Fast cooking, with butter	½ cup	127	20.1
*Oriental (Carolina) *Bake-It-Easy*	⅙ of 6-oz. pkg.	120	25.0
*Pilaf (Uncle Ben's):			
Without butter	½ cup	101	21.7
With butter	½ cup	135	21.7
Fast cooking, without butter	½ cup	118	25.6
Fast cooking, with butter	½ cup	142	25.6
*Rib roast (Minute Rice)	½ cup	150	25.0
Spanish:			
*(Carolina) *Bake-It-Easy*	⅙ of 6-oz. pkg.	110	24.0
*(Minute Rice)	½ cup	150	25.0
Rice-A-Roni	⅙ of 7½-oz. pkg.	120	25.9

Food and Description	Measure or Quantity	Calories	Carbo- hydrates (grams)
*(Uncle Ben's):			
Without butter	½ cup	106	22.0
With butter	½ cup	126	22.0
Fast cooking, without butter	½ cup	104	23.1
Fast cooking, with butter	½ cup	137	26.2
RICE PUDDING:			
Home recipe (USDA)	½ cup (4.7 oz.)	193	35.2
Canned:			
(Betty Crocker)	½ cup (4.3 oz.)	150	25.0
(Hunt's) *Snack Pack*	5 oz. can	190	30.0
RICE, SPANISH:			
Home recipe (USDA)	4 oz.	99	18.8
Canned, regular pack:			
(Libby's)	½ of 15-oz. can	120	27.5
(Van Camp)	½ cup	95	15.5
Canned, dietetic (Featherweight)	½ of 7¼-oz. can	70	14.0
*RICE, SPANISH, SEASONING MIX (Durkee)	1 cup	274	44.7
RICE & VEGETABLES, frozen (Green Giant):			
& broccoli in cheese sauce	1 cup	250	40.0
Continental, with green beans & almonds	1 cup	230	35.0
Medley, with sweet peas & mushrooms	1 cup	200	35.0
Pilaf, with mushrooms & onions	1 cup	230	45.0
Verdi, with bell peppers & parsley	1 cup	270	47.0

(USDA): United States Department of Agriculture
(HEW/FAO): Health, Education and Welfare/Food and Agriculture Organization
* Prepared as Package Directs

Food and Description	Measure or Quantity	Calories	Carbo-hydrates (grams)
White & wild medley, with peas, celery, mushrooms & almonds	1 cup	320	47.0
White & wild, oriental, with bean sprouts, pea pods & water chestnuts	1 cup	230	40.0
RICE WINE (HEW/FAO):			
Chinese, 20.7% alcohol	3 fl. oz.	114	3.3
Japanese, 10.6% alcohol	3 fl. oz.	215	39.4
RING DING (Drake's):			
Jr., dark chocolate:			
Twin pack	2.5-oz. piece	307	40.0
Family pack	2.7-oz. piece	334	43.1
Jr., milk chocolate:			
Twin pack	2.5-oz. piece	304	38.9
Family pack	2.7-oz. piece	331	42.3
Restaurant size	2-oz. piece	245	31.5
ROAST BEEF SPREAD, canned (Underwood)	1 oz.	58	.3
ROE (USDA):			
Raw, carl, cod, haddock, herring, pike or shad	4 oz.	147	1.7
Raw, salmon, sturgeon, turbot	4 oz.	235	1.6
Baked or broiled, cod & shad	4 oz.	143	2.2
Canned, cod, haddock or herring, solids & liq.	4 oz.	134	.3
ROLAIDS (Warner-Lambert)	1 piece	4	1.4
ROLL OR BUN (See also **ROLL DOUGH, ROLL MIX**):			
Apple crunch, frozen (Sara Lee)	1 roll (1 oz.)	102	13.5
Biscuit (Wonder)	2.5-oz. roll	210	34.0
Brown 'n Serve (Wonder):			
With buttermilk	1-oz. roll	83	13.1
French style	1-oz. roll	86	13.6
Gem style	1-oz. roll	86	13.6

Food and Description	Measure or Quantity	Calories	Carbo-hydrates (grams)
Half & Half	1 oz. roll	86	13.1
Home bake	1 oz. roll	86	13.1
Butter crescent (Pepperidge Farm)	1 roll	130	15.0
Caramel pecan, frozen (Sara Lee)	1.3-oz. roll	154	14.6
Caramel sticky, frozen (Sara Lee)	1-oz. bun	118	15.0
Cinnamon, frozen (Sara Lee)	.9-oz. roll	105	12.6
Club (Pepperidge Farm)	1 roll	120	23.0
Croissant, frozen (Sara Lee)	.9-oz. roll	109	11.2
Deli twist (Arnold)	1.3-oz. roll	110	17.0
Dinner:			
(Arnold)	.7-oz. roll	60	9.5
(Pepperidge Farm)	1 roll	65	10.0
(Wonder)	2.5-oz. roll	210	34.0
(Wonder) *Home Pride*	1-oz. roll	90	13.5
Dinner Party Rounds			
(Arnold)	.7-oz. roll	55	10.0
Finger:			
(Arnold)	.6-oz. roll	55	10.0
(Arnold) *Dinner Party*	.7-oz. roll	55	10.0
(Pepperidge Farm) poppyseed	1 roll	60	9.0
(Pepperidge Farm) sesame	1 roll	60	9.0
Frankfurter:			
(Arnold) hot dog	1.3-oz. bun	110	20.0
(Wonder)	2-oz. bun	160	29.0
French:			
(Arnold) *Francisco, sourdough*	1.2-oz. roll	100	19.0
(Pepperidge Farm) large	1 roll	380	76.0
(Pepperidge Farm) small	1 roll	260	50.0
Golden twist (Pepperidge Farm)	1 roll	120	15.0
Hamburger:			
(Arnold)	1.4-oz. bun	110	21.0

(USDA): United States Department of Agriculture
(HEW/FAO): Health, Education and Welfare/Food and Agriculture Organization
Prepared as Package Directs

Food and Description	Measure or Quantity	Calories	Carbo hydrate (grams
(Pepperidge Farm)	1 bun	110	20.
(Wonder)	2-oz. bun	160	29.
Hard (Levy's)	2½-oz. roll	130	37.
Hearth (Pepperidge Farm)	1 roll	60	11.
Honey:			
(Hostess)	4¾-oz. piece	579	63.
(Morton) frozen	2¼-oz. piece	231	30.
(Morton) frozen, mini	1-oz. piece	103	13.
(Sara Lee) frozen	1-oz. roll	112	14.
Kaiser-Hogie (Wonder)	6-oz. roll	460	82.
Old-fashioned (Pepperidge Farm)	1 roll	37	5.
Pan (Wonder)	2.5-oz. roll	210	34.
Parkerhouse:			
(Arnold) *Dinner Party*	.7-oz. roll	55	10.
(Pepperidge Farm)	1 roll	60	9.
(Sara Lee) frozen	.8-oz. roll	73	10.
Party, frozen (Sara Lee)	.6-oz. roll	55	7.
Party pan (Pepperidge Farm)	1 roll	35	5.
Poppy seed, frozen (Sara Lee)	.6-oz. roll	55	7.
Sandwich:			
(Arnold) *Dutch Egg*	1.6-oz. bun	130	22.
(Arnold) soft, plain or poppy seeds	1.3-oz. roll	110	18.
(Arnold) soft, sesame seeds	1.3-oz. roll	110	19.
Sesame crisp (Pepperidge Farm)	1 roll	70	12.
Sesame seeds, frozen (Sara Lee)	.6-oz. roll	55	7.
Tea (Arnold) *Dinner Party*	.4-oz. roll	35	6.
Variety (Arnold) *Francisco*	1.2-oz. roll	100	20.
ROLL DOUGH:			
Frozen (Rich's) onion	2½-oz. roll	196	36.7
Refrigerated (Pillsbury):			
Caramel bun	1 bun	120	19.
Cinnamon, *Ballard,* with icing	1 bun	10	17.

Food and Description	Measure or Quantity	Calories	Carbo-hydrates (grams)
Cinnamon, *Hungry Jack,* with icing, *Butter Tastin'*	1 roll	145	19.5
Danish, caramel, with nuts	1 roll	150	19.5
Danish, cinnamon & raisins	1 roll	135	21.0
Danish, orange	1 roll	130	21.0
Dinner, butterflake	1 roll	100	17.0
Dinner, crescent	1 roll	95	12.5
Dinner, *Oven Lovin'*	1 roll	55	9.5
*ROLL MIX (Pillsbury) hot roll	1 roll	95	15.5
ROSEMARY LEAVES (French's)	1 tsp.	5	.8
ROSÉ WINE:			
(Antinori) 12% alcohol	3 fl. oz.	84	6.3
Chateau Ste. Roseline, 11–14% alcohol	3 fl. oz.	84	6.3
(Chanson) *Rosé des Anges,* 12% alcohol	3 fl. oz.	84	6.3
(Cruse) 12% alcohol	3 fl. oz.	72	
(Gallo) 13% alcohol	3 fl. oz.	55	1.8
(Gallo) *Gypsy,* 20% alcohol	3 fl. oz.	112	12.0
(Great Western) 12% alcohol	3 fl. oz.	80	2.4
(Great Western) Isabella, 12% alcohol	3 fl. oz.	77	4.0
(Inglenook) Gamay, Estate, 12% alcohol	3 fl. oz. (2.9 oz.)	60	.5
(Inglenook) Navalle, 12% alcohol	3 fl. oz. (2.9 oz.)	62	1.3
(Inglenook) Vintage, 12% alcohol	3 fl. oz. (2.9 oz.)	61	.9
(Italian Swiss Colony-Gold Medal) Grenache, 12.4% alcohol	3 fl. oz.	69	2.2

(USDA): United States Department of Agriculture
(HEW/FAO): Health, Education and Welfare/Food and Agriculture Organization
* Prepared as Package Directs

Food and Description	Measure or Quantity	Calories	Carbo- hydrates (grams)
(Italian Swiss Colony) Grenache, 12% alcohol	3 fl. oz.	61	.5
(Louis M. Martini) Gamay, 12.5% alcohol	3 fl. oz.	90	.2
(Mogen David) 12% alcohol	3 fl. oz.	75	8.9
Nectarosé, vin rosé d' Anjou, 12% alcohol	3 fl. oz.	70	2.6
(Taylor) 12.5% alcohol	3 fl. oz.	72	3.0
ROSÉ WINE, SPARKLING (Chanson)	3 fl. oz.	72	3.6
ROTINI, canned (Franco-American):			
In tomato sauce	½ of 15-oz. can	200	36.0
& meatballs in tomato sauce	½ of 14¾-oz. can	235	27.6
RUM (See DISTILLED LIQUOR)			
RUM & COLA, canned (Party Tyme) 10% alcohol	2 fl. oz.	55	5.2
RUTABAGA:			
Raw, without tops (USDA)	1 lb. (weighed with skin)	177	42.4
Raw, diced (USDA)	½ cup (2.5 oz.)	32	7.7
Boiled, drained, diced (USDA)	½ cup (3 oz.)	30	7.1
Boiled, drained, mashed (USDA)	½ cup (4.3 oz.)	43	10.0
RYE, whole grain (USDA)	1 oz.	95	20.8
RYE FLOUR (See FLOUR)			
RYE WHISKEY (See DISTILLED LIQUOR)			

Food and Description	Measure or Quantity	Calories	Carbo- hydrates (grams)

S

SABLEFISH, raw (USDA):

Whole	1 lb. (weighed whole)	362	0.
Meat only	4 oz.	215	0.

SAFFLOWER SEED KERNELS, dry (USDA) — 1 oz. — 174 — 3.5

SAGE (French's) — 1 tsp. (.9 grams) — 4 — .6

SAINT-EMILION WINE, French Bordeaux (Barton & Guestier) 12% alcohol — 3 fl. oz. — 63 — .7

SAINT JOHN'S BREAD FLOUR (See **FLOUR,** Carob)

SAKE WINE, 19.8% alcohol (HEW/FAO) — 3 fl. oz. — 116 — 4.3

SALAD DRESSING (See also **SALAD DRESSING MIX**):
Regular:
Avocado Goddess

(Marie's)	1 T. (.5 oz.)	95	1.0
Bacon (Marie's)	1 T. (.5 oz.)	95	1.0

Bleu or blue cheese:

(Kraft)	1 T. (.5 oz.)	74	.8
(Kraft) *Imperial*	1 T. (.5 oz.)	68	.9
(Kraft) *Roka*	1 T. (.5 oz.)	55	.8
(Lawry's)	1 T. (.5 oz.)	57	.8
(Marie's)	1 T. (.5 oz.)	100	1.0
(Wish-Bone) chunky	1 T. (.5 oz.)	80	1.0

(USDA): United States Department of Agriculture
(HEW/FAO): Health, Education and Welfare/Food and Agriculture Organization
* Prepared as Package Directs

Food and Description	Measure or Quantity	Calories	Carbo-hydrates (grams)
Boiled, home recipe (USDA)	1 T. (.6 oz.)	26	2.4
Caesar:			
(Lawry's)	1 T. (.5 oz.)	70	.5
(Wish-Bone)	1 T.	80	1.0
Canadian (Lawry's)	1 T. (.5 oz.)	72	.6
Coleslaw (Kraft)	1 T. (.5 oz.)	66	3.6
French:			
(Bernstein's)	1 T. (.5 oz.)	56	1.5
(Bernstein's) New Orleans	1 T. (.5 oz.)	56	1.5
(Kraft)	1 T. (.5 oz.)	59	2.1
(Kraft) *Casino*	1 T. (.5 oz.)	60	3.0
(Kraft) *Catalina*	1 T. (.5 oz.)	64	3.7
(Kraft) herb & garlic	1 T. (.5 oz.)	92	.5
(Kraft) *Miracle*	1 T. (.5 oz.)	57	2.5
(Lawry's)	1 T. (.5 oz.)	60	1.8
(Lawry's) San Francisco	1 T. (.5 oz.)	53	.8
(Wish-Bone) deluxe	1 T.	50	2.0
(Wish-Bone) garlic	1 T. (.5 oz.)	70	3.0
(Wish-Bone) *Sweet 'n Spicy*	1 T.	70	3.0
Fruit (Kraft)	1 T. (.5 oz.)	52	3.0
Garlic (Wish-Bone) creamy	1 T.	80	1.0
German style (Marzetti)	1 T. (.5 oz.)	55	2.4
Green Goddess:			
(Bernstein's)	1 T. (.5 oz.)	45	1.1
(Kraft)	1 T. (.5 oz.)	79	.8
(Lawry's)	1 T. (.5 oz.)	59	.7
(Wish-Bone)	1 T.	70	1.0
Green onion (Kraft)	1 T. (.5 oz.)	75	1.1
Hawaiian (Lawry's)	1 T. (.6 oz.)	77	5.8
Italian:			
(Bernstein's)	1 T. (.5 oz.)	62	1.1
(Kraft)	1 T. (.5 oz.)	75	1.1
(Lawry's)	1 T. (.5 oz.)	80	.9
(Lawry's) with cheese	1 T. (.5 oz.)	60	4.7
(Marie's) with garlic	1 T. (.5 oz.)	100	1.0
(Wish-Bone)	1 T.	80	1.0
Mayonnaise-type (USDA)	1 T. (.5 oz.)	65	2.2
Miracle Whip (Kraft)	1 T. (.5 oz.)	69	1.8

Food and Description	Measure or Quantity	Calories	Carbo-hydrates (grams)
Oil & vinegar (Kraft)	1 T. (.5 oz.)	68	.6
Onion:			
(Marie's) creamy	1 T.	90	1.4
(Wish-Bone) *California*	1 T.	80	1.0
Potato Salad (Marzetti)	1 T. (.5 oz.)	62	2.9
Ranch (Marie's)	1 T.	105	1.3
Red wine vinegar & oil (Lawry's)	1 T. (.6 oz.)	61	4.8
Rich 'n Tangy (Dutch Pantry)	1 T. (.6 oz.)	68	4.4
Roquefort:			
(Bernstein's)	1 T. (.5 oz.)	50	.7
(Kraft)	1 T. (.5 oz.)	56	.8
(Marie's)	1 T. (.5 oz.)	105	1.1
Royal Scandia (Bernstein's)	1 T. (.5 oz.)	45	1.1
Russian:			
(Kraft)	1 T. (.5 oz.)	55	4.3
(Kraft) creamy	1 T. (.5 oz.)	68	2.1
(Kraft) with pure honey	1 T.	58	4.6
(Wish-Bone)	1 T.	60	7.0
(Saffola)	1 T. (.5 oz.)	51	2.2
Salad Bowl (Kraft)	1 T. (.5 oz.)	53	2.2
Salad 'n Sandwich (Kraft)	1 T. (.5 oz.)	53	2.8
Salad Secret (Kraft)	1 T. (.5 oz.)	56	1.8
Sesame (Sahadi) creamy	1 T. (.5 oz.)	60	2.0
Sesame (Sahadi) spice	1 T. (.5 oz.)	80	1.0
Sherry (Lawry's)	1 T. (.5 oz.)	55	1.6
Spin Blend (Hellmann's)	1 T. (.6 oz.)	56	2.7
Sweet 'n Sour (Dutch Pantry)	1 T. (.6 oz.)	76	3.9
Sweet & sour (Kraft)	1 T. (.5 oz.)	28	6.5
Thousand Island:			
(Bernstein's)	1 T. (.5 oz.)	48	1.4
(Kraft)	1 T. (.5 oz.)	59	2.5
(Lawry's)	1 T. (.5 oz.)	69	2.3
(Marie's)	1 T. (.5 oz.)	85	1.6

(USDA): United States Department of Agriculture
(HEW/FAO): Health, Education and Welfare/Food and Agriculture Organization
* Prepared as Package Directs

Food and Description	Measure or Quantity	Calories	Carbo-hydrates (grams)
(Marzetti)	1 T. (.5 oz.)	70	2.3
(Wish-Bone)	1 T.	70	2.0
Tomato 'n Spice (Dutch Pantry)	1 T. (.6 oz.)	66	3.6
Vinaigrette (Bernstein's)	1 T. (.5 oz.)	41	.8
Dietetic or low calorie:			
Bleu or blue cheese:			
(Ann Page)	1 T.	13	.5
(Dia-Mel)	1 T. (.5 oz.)	15	0.
(Featherweight)	1 T.	16	1.0
(Kraft)	1 T. (.5 oz.)	13	.5
(Marie's)	1 T. (.5 oz.)	30	3.3
(Tillie Lewis)	1 T. (.5 oz.)	14	1.0
Caesar (Dia-Mel)	1 T. (.5 oz.)	50	.5
Chef style (Ann Page)	1 T. (.5 oz.)	20	3.2
Chef's (Tillie Lewis)	1 T. (.5 oz.)	2	.4
French:			
(Ann Page)	1 T.	24	2.0
(Cellu) imitation, low sodium	1 T.	60	0.
(Dia-Mel)	1 T. (.5 oz.)	30	1.0
(Diet Delight)	1 T. (.5 oz.)	9	.8
(Featherweight)	1 T.	20	1.0
(Kraft)	1 T. (.5 oz.)	21	2.0
(Tillie Lewis)	1 T. (.5 oz.)	8	2.0
(Wish-Bone)	1 T.	25	4.0
Imitation (Featherweight)	1 T.	16	1.0
Italian:			
(Ann Page)	1 T.	12	.7
(Dia-Mel)	1 T.	2	.5
(Diet Delight)	1 T. (.5 oz.)	7	.6
(Featherweight)	1 T.	18	1.0
(Kraft)	1 T. (.5 oz.)	7	.6
(Tillie Lewis)	1 T. (.5 oz.)	2	.2
(Wish-Bone)	1 T.	20	1.0
May-Lo-Naise (Tillie Lewis)	1 T. (.5 oz.)	30	1.0
Mayolite (Diet Delight)	1 T. (.5 oz.)	25	.7
Mayonnaise, imitation (Kraft)	1 T. (.5 oz.)	45	0.
Russian:			
(Dia-Mel)	1 T. (.5 oz.)	9	.5
(Featherweight) creamy	1 T.	16	1.0

Food and Description	Measure or Quantity	Calories	Carbo-hydrates (grams)
(Kraft)	1 T. (.5 oz.)	30	4.3
(Wish-Bone)	1 T.	25	5.0
Soyamaise (Cellu) low sodium	1 T.	100	0.
Thousand Island:			
(Ann Page)	1 T. (.6 oz.)	22	2.1
(Diet Delight)	1 T. (.5 oz.)	16	.5
(Dia-Mel)	1 T. (.5 oz.)	30	1.0
(Featherweight)	1 T.	16	1.0
(Kraft)	1 T. (.5 oz.)	28	2.2
(Tillie Lewis)	1 T. (.5 oz.)	13	1.0
(Wish-Bone)	1 T.	25	3.0
2-Calorie Low Sodium (Featherweight)	1 T.	2	0.
Whipped (Tillie Lewis)	1 T. (.5 oz.)	20	1.0
SALAD DRESSING MIX:			
Regular:			
Bacon (Lawry's)	.8-oz. pkg.	69	11.9
Bleu or blue cheese:			
*(Good Seasons)	1 T.	85	.5
*(Good Seasons) *Thick 'n Creamy*	1 T.	80	.5
(Lawry's)	.7-oz. pkg.	79	4.5
Caesar garlic cheese (Lawry's)	.8-oz. pkg.	71	8.7
*Cheese garlic (Good Seasons)	1 T.	85	.5
French:			
*(Good Seasons) old-fashioned	1 T.	85	1.5
*(Good Seasons) *Riviera*	1 T.	90	2.5
*(Good Seasons) *Thick 'n Creamy*	1 T.	75	2.0
(Lawry's) old-fashioned	.8-oz. pkg.	72	16.8
*Garlic (Good Seasons)	1 T.	85	.5
Green Goddess (Lawry's)	.8-oz. pkg.	69	12.7

(USDA): United States Department of Agriculture
(HEW/FAO): Health, Education and Welfare/Food and Agriculture Organization
* Prepared as Package Directs

Food and Description	Measure or Quantity	Calories	Carbo- hydrates (grams)
Italian:			
*(Good Seasons)	1 T.	85	1.0
*(Good seasons) cheese	1 T.	85	1.0
*(Good Seasons) mild	1 T.	85	1.5
*(Good Seasons) *Thick 'n Creamy*	1 T.	85	1.0
(Lawry's)	.6-oz. pkg.	44	9.6
(Lawry's) with cheese	.8-oz. pkg.	69	9.4
*Onion (Good Seasons)	1 T.	85	1.0
*Thousand Island (Good Seasons) *Thick 'n Creamy*	1 T. (.6 oz.)	75	2.0
Dietetic or low calorie:			
French:			
(Dia-Mel)	½-oz. packet	18	0.
(Louis Sherry)	½-oz. packet	18	0.
Garlic (Dia-Mel) creamy	½-oz. packet	21	1.0
Italian:			
(Dia-Mel)	½-oz. packet	2	0.
*(Good Seasons)	1 T.	8	2.0
(Louis Sherry)	½-oz. packet	2	0.
Russian (Louis Sherry)	½-oz. packet	20	0.
Thousand Island			
(Dia-Mel)	½-oz. packet	20	0.
SALAD FIXIN'S (Arnold):			
Danish style bleu cheese	½ oz.	66	8.8
French onion	½ oz.	67	8.7
Spicy Italian	½ oz.	67	9.2
SALAD SEASONING			
(Durkee):			
Regular	1 tsp.	4	.7
With cheese	1 tsp.	10	.4
SALAMI:			
Dry (USDA)	1 oz.	128	.3
Cooked (USDA)	1 oz.	88	.4
(Hormel) Dilusso Genoa	1 oz.	120	<1.0
(Hormel) hard, dairy	1 oz.	120	<1.0
(Oscar Mayer):			
For beer	.8-oz. slice	54	.3
Cotto	.8-oz. slice	53	.6

Food and Description	Measure or Quantity	Calories	Carbohydrates (grams)
Cotto, beef	.8-oz. slice	51	.6
Hard, all meat	.3-oz. slice	33	.1
(Swift):			
Genoa	1 oz.	114	.3
Hard	1 oz.	115	.9
(Vienna) beef	1 oz.	79	.8
(Wilson) cotto	1 oz.	84	.4
SALISBURY STEAK:			
Canned (Morton House)	⅛ of 12½-oz. can	160	7.0
Frozen:			
(Banquet)	5-oz. cooking bag	246	7.8
(Banquet)	11-oz. dinner	390	24.0
(Banquet) & gravy	2-lb. pkg.	1454	48.2
(Banquet) *Man-Pleaser*	19-oz. dinner	873	71.7
(Green Giant) with gravy, oven bake	7-oz. entree	290	14.0
(Green Giant) with tomato sauce, boil-in-bag	9-oz. entree	390	22.0
(Morton)	11-oz. dinner	287	25.1
(Morton) *Country Table*	15-oz. dinner	405	51.1
(Morton) *Country Table*	10¼-oz. entree	466	34.9
(Swanson)	11½-oz. dinner	500	40.0
(Swanson), with crinkle cut potatoes	5½-oz. entree	370	28.0
(Swanson) *Hungry Man*	17-oz. dinner	870	65.0
(Swanson) *Hungry Man*	12½-oz. entree	640	39.0
(Swanson) 3-course	16-oz. dinner	490	48.0
SALMON:			
Atlantic (USDA):			
Raw, whole	1 lb. (weighed whole)	640	0.
Meat only	4 oz.	246	0.
Canned, solids & liq., including bones	4 oz.	230	0.

(USDA): United States Department of Agriculture
(HEW/FAO): Health, Education and Welfare/Food and Agriculture
        Organization
* Prepared as Package Directs

Food and Description	Measure or Quantity	Calories	Carbo hydrate (grams
Chinook or King (USDA):			
Raw, steak	1 lb. (weighed whole)	886	0.
Raw, meat only	4 oz.	252	0.
Canned, solids & liq., including bones	4 oz.	238	0.
Chum, canned, solids & liq., including bones	4 oz.	158	0.
Coho, canned, solids & liq., including bones (USDA)	4 oz.	174	0.
Pink or Humpback:			
Raw, steak (USDA)	1 lb. (weighed whole)	475	0.
Raw, meat only (USDA)	4 oz.	135	0.
Canned:			
(USDA) solids & liq., including bones	4 oz.	160	0.
(Del Monte) solids & liq.	7¾-oz. can	277	0.
(Icy Point), solids & liq.	7¾-oz. can	310	0.
(Pink Beauty) solids & liq.	7¾-oz. can	310	0.
Sockeye or Red or Blueback, canned, solids & liq. (USDA)	4 oz.	194	0.
Unspecified kind of salmon, baked or broiled (USDA)	4.2-oz. steak (approx. 4" x 3" x ½")	218	0.
SALMON, SMOKED:			
(USDA)	4 oz.	200	0.
(Vita) lox, drained	4-oz. jar	136	.2
(Vita) Nova, drained	4-oz. can	221	1.0
SALT:			
Butter-flavored (French's) imitation	1 tsp. (3.6 grams)	8	0.
Garlic (Lawry's)	1 tsp. (4 grams)	5	1.0
Hickory smoke (French's)	1 tsp. (4 grams)	2	<.5
Lite Salt (Morton) iodized	1 tsp. (6 grams)	0	0.
Onion (Lawry's)	1 tsp.	4	.9
Seasoned (Lawry's)	1 tsp.	1	.1

Food and Description	Measure or Quantity	Calories	Carbo-hydrates (grams)
Substitute:			
(Adolph's)	1 tsp. (6 grams)	1	Tr.
(Adolph's)	1 packet (8 grams)	<1	Tr.
(Adolph's) seasoned	1 tsp.	6	1.1
(Dia-Mel) Salt-It	⅛ tsp.	0	0.
(Morton)	1 tsp. (6 grams)	Tr.	Tr.
(Morton) seasoned	1 tsp. (6 grams)	3	.5
Table (USDA)	1 tsp. (6 grams)	0	0.
Table (Morton) iodized	1 tsp. (7 grams)	0	0.
SALT PORK, raw (USDA):			
With skin	1 lb. (weighed with skin)	3410	0.
Without skin	1 oz.	222	0.
SALT STICK (See BREAD STICK)			
SANDWICH SPREAD:			
Regular:			
(USDA)	1 T. (.5 oz.)	57	2.4
(Bennett's)	1 T. (.5 oz.)	44	3.7
(Best Foods/Hellmann's)	1 T. (.5 oz.)	62	2.2
(Kraft)	1 oz.	105	5.6
(Kraft) pimiento	1 oz.	117	.8
Dietetic or low calorie			
(USDA)	1 T. (.5 oz.)	17	1.2
SANGRIA:			
(Taylor) 11.6% alcohol	3 fl. oz.	99	10.8
Mix (Party Tyme)	½-oz. pkg.	53	13.7
SARDINE:			
Raw, whole (HEW/FAO)	1 lb. (weighed whole)	321	0.
Raw, meat only (HEW/FAO)	4 oz.	146	0.

(USDA): United States Department of Agriculture
(HEW/FAO): Health, Education and Welfare/Food and Agriculture Organization
* Prepared as Package Directs

Food and Description	Measure or Quantity	Calories	Carbo-hydrates (grams)
Canned:			
Atlantic:			
(USDA) in oil, solids & liq.	3¾-oz. can	330	.6
(USDA) in oil, drained solids, with skin & bones	3¾-oz. can	187	DNA
(Del Monte) in tomato sauce, solids & liq.	7½-oz. can	330	4.0
Norwegian:			
(Snow)	1 oz.	66	DNA
(Underwood) in mustard sauce	3¾-oz. can	195	2.3
(Underwood) in soya bean oil	3¾-oz. can	233	.4
(Underwood) in tomato sauce	3¾-oz. can	169	4.5
Pacific (USDA) in brine or mustard, solids & liq.	4 oz.	222	1.9
SAUCE (See also SAUCE MIX):			
A1	1 T. (.6 oz.)	12	2.8
Barbecue:			
Chris & Pitt's	1 T.	15	4.0
(French's) regular & smoky	1 T.	14	3.0
(Kraft)	1 oz.	34	7.9
(Kraft) hickory smoke	1 oz.	34	7.9
Open Pit	1 T. (.6 oz.)	15	3.6
Open Pit, hickory smoked flavor	1 T.	16	4.0
Open Pit, original flavor with minced onions	1 T.	18	4.0
Escoffier Sauce Diable	1 T. (.6 oz.)	20	4.2
Escoffier Sauce Robert	1 T.	19	4.5
Famous (Durkee)	1 T.	69	2.2
Hot, Frank's	1 tsp.	14	2.0
H. P. Steak Sauce (Lea & Perrins)	1 T. (1 oz.)	20	4.8
Italian (Carnation)	2 fl. oz.	43	7.0
Italian (Ragu) red cooking	3½ fl. oz.	45	6.0
Marinara (Buitoni)	4 oz.	67	8.0

Food and Description	Measure or Quantity	Calories	Carbohydrates (grams)
Marinara (Ragu)	5 oz.	120	15.0
Salad (Bernstein's)	1 T. (.5 oz.)	19	4.6
Seafood cocktail (Del Monte)	1 T. (.6 oz.)	22	4.9
Soy (Kikkoman)	1 T. (.7 oz.)	11	1.2
Steak (Dawn Fresh) with mushrooms	2 oz.	18	4.0
Steak Supreme	1 T. (.6 oz.)	20	4.8
Sweet 'n Sour (Carnation)	2 fl. oz.	79	16.0
Swiss steak (Carnation)	2 fl. oz.	24	5.0
Taco (Ortega)	1 T.	21	4.8
Tartar (Best Foods)	1 T. (.5 oz.)	74	.2
Tartar (Hellmann's)	1 T. (.5 oz.)	74	.2
Tartar (Kraft)	1 oz.	145	1.4
Teriyaki (Kikkoman)	1 T. (.7 oz.)	16	3.0
White (USDA) medium	1 cup (9 oz.)	413	22.4
Worcestershire (French's) regular or smoky	1 T.	10	2.0
Worcestershire (Lea & Perrins)	1 T. (.6 oz.)	12	3.0
SAUCE MIX:			
A la King (Durkee)	1.1-oz. pkg.	133	14.0
*Barbecue (Kraft)	1 oz.	32	7.9
Cheese:			
(Durkee)	1.1-oz. pkg.	175	7.0
*(Durkee)	1 cup	337	19.0
(French's)	1.2-oz. pkg.	163	14.0
*(Kraft) cheddar	1 oz.	52	1.9
Enchilada (Durkee)	1.1-oz. pkg.	89	18.0
*Enchilada (Durkee)	1 cup	57	12.5
Hollandaise:			
(Durkee)	1-oz. pkg.	173	11.0
(French's)	1.1-oz. pkg.	188	7.4
*(Kraft)	1 oz.	54	2.0
Sour cream:			
(Durkee)	1-oz. pkg.	135	9.0
*(Durkee)	⅔ cup	214	15.0

(USDA): United States Department of Agriculture
(HEW/FAO): Health, Education and Welfare/Food and Agriculture Organization
* Prepared as Package Directs

Food and Description	Measure or Quantity	Calories	Carbo- hydrates (grams)
(French's)	1.2-oz. pkg.	166	16.0
*(Kraft)	1 oz.	61	4.1
Stroganoff:			
(Durkee)	1.2-oz. pkg.	90	18.0
*(Durkee)	1 cup	820	6.5
(French's)	1¾-oz. pkg.	213	26.0
Sweet & Sour:			
(Durkee)	2-oz. pkg.	230	45.0
(French's)	2-oz. pkg.	223	55.0
Tartar (Lawry's)	.6-oz. pkg.	64	9.8
Teriyaki (French's)	1.6-oz. pkg.	136	27.0
White:			
(Durkee)	1-oz. pkg.	158	35.0
*(Durkee)	1 cup	218	41.0
*(Kraft)	1 oz.	44	2.5
SAUERKRAUT, canned:			
(USDA) solids & liq.	1 cup (8.3 oz.)	42	9.4
(USDA) drained solids	1 cup (5 oz.)	31	6.2
(Del Monte) solids & liq.	1 cup (8 oz.)	55	10.7
(Libby's) solids & liq.	⅛ of 32-oz. can	17	4.0
(Stokely-Van Camp) Bavarian style, solids & liq.	½ cup (4.2 oz.)	35	7.0
(Stokely-Van Camp) chopped or shredded	½ cup (4.2 oz.)	25	4.5
SAUERKRAUT JUICE, canned (USDA)	½ cup (4.3 oz.)	12	2.8
SAUSAGE (See also individual kinds):			
(USDA) Brown & serve, before browning	1 oz.	111	.8
(USDA) Brown & serve, after browning	1 oz.	120	.8
Cow-Boy Jo's, beef	⅝ oz.	81	.9
Cow-Boy Jo's, beef, smoked	¼ oz.	42	.3
(Hormel) Brown 'n serve	.8-oz. piece	78	.2
(Lowry's) pickled, hot	1¼ oz.	110	1.4
(Lowrey's) pickled, Polish	⅝ oz.	50	.4
(Oscar Mayer) Smokie links	1.5-oz. link	136	.6

Food and Description	Measure or Quantity	Calories	Carbo-hydrates (grams)
(Swift) *Brown 'n Serve*, after browning:			
Bacon & sausage	.7-oz. link	72	.4
Beef	.7-oz. link	86	.5
Kountry Kured	.7-oz. link	86	.3
Original	.7-oz. link	77	.5
(Wilson) *New England Brand*	1 oz.	52	.2
SAUTERNES:			
(Barton & Guestier) French white Bordeaux, 13% alcohol	3 fl. oz.	95	7.6
(Barton & Guestier) haut, French white Bordeaux, 13% alcohol	3 fl. oz.	99	8.7
(Gallo) 12% alcohol	3 fl. oz.	50	.9
(Gallo) haut, 12% alcohol	3 fl. oz.	67	2.1
(Gold Seal) dry, 12% alcohol	3 fl. oz.	82	.4
(Gold Seal) semi-soft, 12% alcohol	3 fl. oz.	87	2.6
(Great Western) Aurora, 12% alcohol	3 fl. oz.	79	4.5
(Italian Swiss Colony) 12% alcohol	3 fl. oz. (2.9 oz)	59	1.2
(Louis M. Martini) dry, 12.5% alcohol	3 fl. oz.	90	.2
(Mogen David) cream, 12% alcohol	3 fl. oz.	45	6.2
(Mogen David) dry, American, 12% alcohol	3 fl. oz.	30	1.8
(Taylor) 12.5% alcohol	3 fl. oz.	81	4.8
SCALLION (See ONION, GREEN)			
SCALLOP:			
Raw, muscle only (USDA)	4 oz.	92	3.7
Steamed (USDA)	4 oz.	127	DNA

(USDA): United States Department of Agriculture
(HEW/FAO): Health, Education and Welfare/Food and Agriculture Organization
* Prepared as Package Directs

Food and Description	Measure or Quantity	Calories	Carbohydrates (grams)
Frozen:			
(USDA) Breaded, fried, reheated	4 oz.	220	11.9
(Mrs. Paul's) batter fried	½ of 7-oz. pkg.	204	20.9
(Mrs. Paul's) breaded & fried	½ of 7-oz. pkg.	206	22.5
SCHNAPPS, PEPPERMINT:			
(DeKuyper) 60 proof	1 fl. oz.	79	7.5
(Garnier) 60 proof	1 fl. oz.	83	8.4
(Hiram Walker) 60 proof	1 fl. oz.	78	7.2
(Leroux) 60 proof	1 fl. oz.	87	9.2
***SCOTCH BROTH,** canned (Campbell)	8-oz. serving	80	8.8
SCOTCH SOUR COCKTAIL:			
(National Distillers) *Duet,* 12½% alcohol	8-fl.-oz. can	272	25.6
SCRAPPLE (USDA)	4 oz.	244	16.6
SCREWDRIVER:			
Canned:			
(National Distillers) *Duet,* 12½% alcohol	8-fl.-oz. can	288	25.6
(Party Tyme) 12½% alcohol	2 fl. oz.	69	6.4
Mix:			
(Bar-Tender's)	⅝-oz. serving	70	17.4
(Holland House)	.6-oz. pkg.	69	17.0
SCUP (See **PORGY**)			
SEA BASS, WHITE, raw, meat only (USDA)	4 oz.	109	0.
SEAFOOD PLATTER, frozen (Mrs. Paul's) combination, with potato puffs	9-oz. pkg.	514	57.0
***SECOND NATURE** (Avoset), egg substitute, refrigerated	3 T. (1½ fl. oz.)	38	1.8

Food and Description	Measure or Quantity	Calories	Carbo-hydrates (grams)
SEGO, diet food:			
Bars, all flavors	1-oz. bar	138	12.0
Canned:			
Chocolate and milk chocolate	10-fl.-oz. can	225	39.0
Very butterscotch, very banana, very strawberry, very vanilla	10-fl.-oz. can	225	35.0
Vanilla	10-fl.-oz. can	225	33.0
Very chocolate malt	10-fl.-oz. can	225	40.0
SERUTAN (J.B. Williams):			
Toasted granules	1 tsp.	6	1.3
Concentrated powder	1 tsp.	5	1.3
Fruit flavored powder	1 tsp.	6	1.5
SESAME SEEDS, dry (USDA):			
Whole	1 oz.	160	6.1
Hulled	1 oz.	165	5.0
SHAD (USDA):			
Raw, whole	1 lb. (weighed whole)	370	0.
Raw, meat only	4 oz.	193	0.
Cooked, home recipe:			
Baked with butter or margarine & bacon slices	4 oz.	229	0.
Creole	4 oz.	172	1.8
Canned, solids & liq.	4 oz.	172	0.
SHAD, GIZZARD, raw (USDA):			
Whole	1 lb. (weighed whole)	299	0.
Meat only	4 oz.	227	0.

(USDA): United States Department of Agriculture
(HEW/FAO): Health, Education and Welfare/Food and Agriculture Organization
* Prepared as Package Directs

Food and Description	Measure or Quantity	Calories	Carbohydrates (grams)
SHAKE 'N BAKE, seasoned coating mix:			
Chicken	2⅜-oz. pkg.	287	41.5
Chicken, barbecue style	3¾-oz. pkg.	377	83.2
Chicken, crispy country mild	2.4-oz. pkg.	321	50.1
Chicken, Italian flavor	2.4-oz. pkg.	294	41.4
Fish	2-oz. pkg.	234	33.9
Hamburger	2-oz. pkg.	169	33.2
Pork	2.4-oz.	255	47.1
Pork & ribs, barbecue style	2.9-oz. pkg.	314	60.1
& homestyle gravy mix:			
Beef	3.1-oz. pkg.	304	51.4
Chicken	4-oz. pkg.	424	67.4
Pork	3.7-oz. pkg.	327	67.4
SHALLOT, raw (USDA):			
With skin	1 oz.	18	4.2
With skin removed	1 oz.	20	4.8
SHERBET (See also individual kinds):			
(Dean) 1.7% fat	¼ pt. (3.3 oz.)	137	30.6
(Meadow Gold), all flavors	¼ pt.	120	13.7
(Sealtest):			
Lemon, *Light 'n Lively*	¼ pt.	130	29.0
Lime, *Light 'n Lively*	¼ pt.	130	29.0
Orange	¼ pt. (3.1 oz.)	120	26.5
Orange, *Light 'n Lively*	¼ pt.	130	30.0
Pineapple, *Light 'n Lively*	¼ pt.	130	29.0
Rainbow, *Light 'n Lively*	¼ pt.	130	29.0
Red Raspberry, *Light 'n Lively*	¼ pt.	130	28.0
Strawberry, *Light 'n Lively*	¼ pt.	130	30.0
SHERRY:			
(Gallo) 20% alcohol	3 fl. oz.	88	2.7
(Gallo) 16% alcohol	3 fl. oz.	76	3.3
(Gold Seal) 19% alcohol	3 fl. oz.	139	4.6
(Great Western) Solera, 18% alcohol	3 fl. oz.	120	8.5
Cocktail (Gold Seal) 19% alcohol	3 fl. oz.	122	1.6
Cocktail (Petri)	3 fl. oz.	102	

Food and Description	Measure or Quantity	Calories	Carbo-hydrates (grams)
Cream:			
(Gallo) 20% alcohol	3 fl. oz.	111	8.4
(Gallo) Old Decanter, Livingston, 20% alcohol	3 fl. oz.	117	12.8
(Gold Seal) 19% alcohol	3 fl. oz.	158	9.4
(Great Western) Solera, 18% alcohol	3 fl. oz.	141	12.2
(Louis M. Martini) 19.5% alcohol	3 fl. oz.	138	1.2
(Taylor) 17.5% alcohol	3 fl. oz.	138	13.2
(Williams & Humbert) Canasta, 20½% alcohol	3 fl. oz.	150	5.4
Dry:			
(Gallo) 20% alcohol	3 fl. oz.	84	1.8
(Gallo) Old Decanter, very dry, 20% alcohol	3 fl. oz.	87	2.1
(Great Western) Solera, 18% alcohol	3 fl. oz.	109	4.6
(Italian Swiss Colony-Gold Medal) 19.7% alcohol	3 fl. oz.	104	1.7
(Louis M. Martini) 19.5% alcohol	3 fl. oz.	138	1.2
(Taylor) 19.5% alcohol	3 fl. oz.	104	2.8
(Williams & Humbert) Carlito Amontillado, 20½% alcohol	3 fl. oz.	120	4.5
(Williams & Humbert) Cedro, 20½% alcohol	3 fl. oz.	120	4.5
(Williams & Humbert) Dos Cortados, 20½% alcohol	3 fl. oz.	120	4.5
(Williams & Humbert) Pando, 17% alcohol	3 fl. oz.	120	4.5
Dry Sack (Williams & Humbert) 20½% alcohol	3 fl. oz.	120	4.5

(USDA): United States Department of Agriculture
(HEW/FAO): Health, Education and Welfare/Food and Agriculture Organization
* Prepared as Package Directs

Food and Description	Measure or Quantity	Calories	Carbohydrates (grams)
Medium:			
(Great Western) cooking, 18% alcohol	3 fl. oz.	111	6.4
(Italian Swiss Colony-Gold Medal) 19.7% alcohol	3 fl. oz.	106	2.6
(Taylor) 17.5% alcohol	3 fl. oz.	123	9.0
SHERRY FLAVORING			
(French's)	1 tsp.	17	
SHORTENING (See **FAT**)			
SHREDDED WHEAT:			
(Nabisco):			
Biscuit	¾-oz. biscuit	80	17.0
Biscuit	⅞-oz. biscuit	90	19.0
Spoon Size	⅔ cup (1 oz.)	110	23.0
(Quaker)	.7-oz. biscuit	52	11.0
SHRIMP:			
Raw:			
Whole (USDA)	1 lb. (weighed in shell)	285	4.7
Meat only (USDA)	4 oz.	103	1.7
Canned:			
(USDA) Wet pack, solids & liq.	4 oz.	91	.9
(USDA) Dry pack or drained	4 oz.	132	.8
(Bumble Bee) Water pack, solids & liq.	4½-oz. can	90	.9
(Icy Point), cocktail, tiny, drained	4½-oz. can	148	.8
(Pillar Rock) cocktail, drained	4½-oz. can	148	.8
Cooked, French-fried (USDA)	4 oz.	255	11.3
Frozen:			
Raw (Gorton) breaded	¼ of 1-lb. bag	158	23.0
Cooked (Mrs. Paul's) breaded & fried	½ of 6-oz. pkg.	199	16.1

Food and Description	Measure or Quantity	Calories	Carbo-hydrates (grams)
SHRIMP CAKE (Mrs. Paul's) frozen:			
Breaded & fried	½ of 6-oz. pkg.	158	19.0
Breaded & fried, thins	½ of 10-oz. pkg.	311	30.3
SHRIMP COCKTAIL, canned:			
(Sau-Sea)	4-oz. jar	107	20.6
(Sea Snack)	4-oz. jar	110	14.8
SHRIMP PASTE, canned (USDA)	1 oz.	51	.4
SHRIMP PUFF, frozen (Durkee)	1 piece	44	3.0
SHRIMP SOUP: Canned:			
*(Campbell) cream of, condensed	10-oz. serving	210	17.0
(Crosse & Blackwell)	½ of 13-oz. can	92	6.5
(Snow) New England, condensed	⅓ of 15-oz. size	109	15.0
*Frozen (USDA):			
Prepared with equal volume water	1 cup (8.5 oz.)	158	8.4
Prepared with equal volume milk	1 cup (8.6 oz.)	243	15.2
SHRIMP STICKS, frozen (Mrs. Paul's)	½ of 8-oz. pkg.	244	27.6
SIDE CAR COCKTAIL MIX (Holland House), canned	1½ fl. oz.	66	16.5
SIP 'N SLIM COCKTAIL MIX (Holland House), canned	2 fl. oz.	19	5.1

(USDA): United States Department of Agriculture
(HEW/FAO): Health, Education and Welfare/Food and Agriculture
         Organization
* Prepared as Package Directs

Food and Description	Measure or Quantity	Calories	Carbo-hydrates (grams)
SKATE, raw, meat only (USDA)	4 oz.	111	0.
SLENDER (Carnation):			
Bars:			
Chocolate	1 bar	138	11.5
Cinnamon and vanilla	1 bar	138	12.0
Dry:			
Chocolate	1-oz. pkg.	110	20.0
Chocolate malt	1-oz. pkg.	110	20.0
Coffee	1-oz. pkg.	110	21.0
Dutch chocolate	1-oz. pkg.	110	20.0
French vanilla	1-oz. pkg.	110	21.0
Wild Strawberry	1-oz. pkg.	110	21.0
Liquid, all flavors	10-fl.-oz. can	225	34.0
SLOE GIN (See GIN, SLOE)			
SLOPPY JOE:			
Canned:			
(Libby's) beef	¼ of 15¼-oz. can	176	9.1
(Libby's) pork	¼ of 15¼-oz. can	150	8.5
(Morton House) barbecue sauce with beef	⅛ of 15-oz. can	240	19.0
Frozen:			
(Banquet) *Cooking Bag*	5-oz. bag	199	11.2
(Green Giant) with tomato sauce & beef, *Toast Topper*	5-oz. serving	160	15.0
SLOPPY JOE SEASONING MIX:			
(Ann Page)	1½-oz. pkg.	127	28.8
(Durkee)	1½-oz. pkg.	118	29.0
*(Durkee)	1¼ cups	727	30.0
(Durkee) pizza flavor	1-oz. pkg.	99	12.0
*(Durkee) pizza flavor	1¼ cups	746	26.0
(French's)	1½-oz. pkg.	128	32.0
*(Kraft)	1 oz.	47	1.8
(Lawry's)	1½-oz. pkg.	139	27.7

Food and Description	Measure or Quantity	Calories	Carbo-hydrates (grams)
SMELT, Atlantic, jack & bay (USDA):			
Raw, whole	1 lb. (weighed whole)	244	0.
Raw, meat only	4 oz.	111	0.
Canned, solids & liq.	4 oz.	227	0.
SMOKIE SAUSAGE:			
(Hormel)	.8-oz. piece	75	.4
(Vienna)	2½-oz. serving	196	.9
(Wilson)	1 oz.	84	.5
SNACK (See CRACKER, POPCORN, POTATO CHIP, etc.)			
SNAIL, raw (USDA):			
Unspecified kind	4 oz.	102	2.3
Giant African	4 oz.	83	5.0
SNAPPER (See RED SNAPPER)			
SNO BALL (Hostess)	1½-oz. cake	140	25.1
SOAVE WINE, Italian white (Antinori) 12% alcohol	3 fl. oz.	84	6.3
SOFT DRINK:			
Sweetened:			
Apple (Shasta) red	6 fl. oz.	112	28.2
Birch beer:			
(Pennsylvania Dutch)	6 fl. oz.	84	19.7
(Yukon Club)	6 fl. oz.	89	22.3
Bitter lemon:			
(Canada Dry)	6 fl. oz.	77	19.2
(Hoffman)	6 fl. oz.	85	21.3
(Schweppes)	6 fl. oz.	84	20.3

(USDA): United States Department of Agriculture
(HEW/FAO): Health, Education and Welfare/Food and Agriculture
            Organization
* Prepared as Package Directs

Food and Description	Measure or Quantity	Calories	Carbo-hydrates (grams)
Bubble Up	6 fl. oz.	73	18.4
Cherri-Berri (Hoffman)	6 fl. oz .	91	22.8
Cherry:			
(Canada Dry) wild	6 fl. oz.	96	24.0
(Cliquot Club)	6 fl. oz.	94	23.0
(Cott)	6 fl. oz.	94	23.0
(Key Food)	6 fl. oz.	81	20.1
(Mission)	6 fl. oz.	94	23.0
(Shasta) black	6 fl. oz.	84	21.2
(Yoo-Hoo) high protein	6 fl. oz.	100	18.9
Chocolate:			
(Cott) cream	6 fl. oz.	92	22.0
(Mission) cream	6 fl. oz.	92	22.0
(Yoo-Hoo) high protein	6 fl. oz.	100	18.9
Club soda (all brands)	6 fl. oz.	0	0.
Coconut (Yoo-Hoo) high protein	6 fl. oz.	100	18.9
Coffee (Hoffman)	6 fl. oz.	70	17.5
Cola:			
Coca-Cola	6 fl. oz.	73	18.5
(Cott)	6 fl. oz.	83	20.0
Jamaica (Canada Dry)	6 fl. oz.	79	19.8
(Mission)	6 fl. oz.	83	20.0
Mr. Cola	6 fl. oz.	79	20.3
(Nedick's)	6 fl. oz.	81	20.1
Pepsi-Cola	6 fl. oz.	79	19.9
RC (Royal Crown) with a twist	6 fl. oz.	74	20.5
(Royal Crown)	6 fl. oz.	78	19.5
(Shasta)	6 fl. oz.	76	19.4
(Shasta) cherry	6 fl. oz.	76	19.4
Cream:			
(Canada Dry) vanilla	6 fl. oz.	96	24.0
(Cott)	6 fl. oz.	88	22.0
(Dr. Brown's)	6 fl. oz.	84	20.9
(Key Food)	6 fl. oz.	84	20.9
(Kirsch)	6 fl. oz.	77	19.6
(Nedick's)	6 fl. oz.	84	20.9
(Shasta)	6 fl. oz.	80	20.3
(Waldbaum)	6 fl. oz.	84	20.9
Dr. Brown's Cel-Ray Tonic	6 fl. oz.	66	16.5
Dr. Pepper	6 fl. oz.	71	17.4

Food and Description	Measure or Quantity	Calories	Carbo-hydrates (grams)
Flip	6 fl. oz.	75	18.4
Fruit Mix (Hoffman)	6 fl. oz.	89	22.3
Fruit Mix (Nedick's)	6 fl. oz.	89	22.3
Ginger ale:			
(Canada Dry)	6 fl. oz.	65	15.6
(Cliquot Club)	6 fl. oz.	62	15.0
(Cott)	6 fl. oz.	62	15.0
(Dr. Brown's)	6 fl. oz.	60	15.0
(Fanta)	6 fl. oz.	63	15.8
(Hoffman) pale dry	6 fl. oz.	58	14.6
(Nedick's) pale dry	6 fl. oz.	60	15.0
(Schweppes)	6 fl. oz.	66	16.3
(Shasta)	6 fl. oz.	65	16.5
(Waldbaum)	6 fl. oz.	60	15.0
Ginger beer (Schweppes)	6 fl. oz.	72	16.8
Grape:			
(Canada Dry) concord	6 fl. oz.	96	24.0
Grapette	6 fl. oz.	91	23.4
(Hoffman)	6 fl. oz.	93	23.2
(Key Food)	6 fl. oz.	87	21.9
(Nedick's)	6 fl. oz.	93	23.2
(Schweppes)	6 fl. oz.	97	15.7
(Waldbaum)	6 fl. oz.	87	21.9
(Yoo-Hoo) high protein	6 fl. oz.	100	18.9
Grapefruit:			
(Cott)	6 fl. oz.	83	20.0
(Hoffman)	6 fl. oz.	81	20.2
(Mission)	6 fl. oz.	83	20.0
(Shasta)	6 fl. oz.	88	22.3
Half & half:			
(Key Food)	6 fl. oz.	77	19.4
(Waldbaum's)	6 fl. oz.	77	19.4
(Yukon Club)	6 fl. oz.	89	22.1
Hi Spot (Canada Dry)	6 fl. oz.	74	18.6
Lemon:			
(Cliquot Club; Cott; Mission)	6 fl. oz.	74	18.0
(Royal Crown)	6 fl. oz.	89	22.2

(USDA): United States Department of Agriculture
(HEW/FAO): Health, Education and Welfare/Food and Agriculture Organization
* Prepared as Package Directs

Food and Description	Measure or Quantity	Calories	Carbohydrates (grams)
Lemon-lime:			
(Dr. Brown's; Hoffman's; Key Food; Nedick's; Waldbaum; Yukon Club)	6 fl. oz.	74	18.4
(Shasta)	6 fl. oz.	73	18.4
Lime (Yukon Club)	6 fl. oz.	64	16.1
Mountain Dew	6 fl. oz.	89	22.1
Moxie	6 fl. oz.	89	12.0
Mr. PiBB	6 fl. oz.	70	18.8
Orange:			
(Canada Dry) Sunripe	6 fl. oz.	90	14.1
(Cliquot Club; Cott; Mission)	6 fl. oz.	103	25.0
(Hoffman)	6 fl. oz.	93	23.2
(Key Food)	6 fl. oz.	86	21.5
(Kirsch)	6 fl. oz.	88	21.9
(Nedick's)	6 fl. oz.	91	22.6
(Schweppes) Sparkling	6 fl. oz.	89	22.0
(Shasta)	6 fl. oz.	88	22.2
(Yoo-Hoo) high protein	6 fl. oz.	100	18.9
Pineapple:			
(Hoffman; Kirsch; Nedick's)	6 fl. oz.	89	22.3
(Yoo-Hoo) high protein	6 fl. oz.	100	18.9
Quinine or Tonic Water:			
(Canada Dry)	6 fl. oz.	70	16.1
(Dr. Brown's; Hoffman's; Schweppes)	6 fl. oz.	66	16.5
(Shasta)	6 fl. oz.	57	14.4
Raspberry:			
(Cliquot Club; Cott; Mission)	6 fl. oz.	98	24.0
(Dr. Brown's) black	6 fl. oz.	86	21.5
(Shasta) wild	6 fl. oz.	84	21.2
Red creme (Schweppes)	6 fl. oz.	86	21.3
Root beer:			
Barrelhead (Canada Dry)	6 fl. oz.	79	19.8
(Cliquot Club; Cott; Mission)	6 fl. oz.	85	21.0
(Dad's)	6 fl. oz.	79	19.6

Food and Description	Measure or Quantity	Calories	Carbo-hydrates (grams)
(Hires)	6 fl. oz.	75	18.8
(Nedick's)	6 fl. oz.	77	19.4
(Nehi)	6 fl. oz.	94	23.2
Rooti (Canada Dry)	6 fl. oz.	79	19.8
(Schweppes)	6 fl. oz.	79	19.3
Sarsaparilla:			
(Hoffman)	6 fl. oz.	83	22.2
(Yukon Club)	6 fl. oz.	89	22.2
Seven-Up	6 fl. oz.	73	18.0
Sour mix (Shasta)	6 fl. oz.	65	16.5
Sprite	6 fl. oz.	71	18.0
Strawberry:			
(Canada Dry) California	6 fl. oz.	89	22.3
(Cliquot Club; Cott; Mission)	6 fl. oz.	98	20.0
(Shasta)	6 fl. oz.	80	20.3
(Yoo-Hoo) high protein	6 fl. oz.	100	18.9
(Yukon Club)	6 fl. oz.	92	23.0
Teem	6 fl. oz.	71	17.7
Tee Up	6 fl. oz.	64	16.1
Tahitian Treat (Canada Dry)	6 fl. oz.	96	24.1
Tiki (Shasta)	6 fl. oz.	80	20.3
Tom Collins or Collins mix:			
(Canada Dry; Yukon Club)	6 fl. oz.	60	15.0
(Dr. Brown's; Hoffman)	6 fl. oz.	64	16.1
(Shasta)	6 fl. oz.	65	16.5
Tropical Punch (Yukon Club)	6 fl. oz.	90	22.5
Vanilla (Yoo-Hoo) high protein	6 fl. oz.	100	18.9
Vanilla Cream (Canada Dry)	6 fl. oz.	88	22.0
Vodka Mix (Shasta)	6 fl. oz.	65	16.5

(USDA): United States Department of Agriculture
(HEW/FAO): Health, Education and Welfare/Food and Agriculture Organization
* Prepared as Package Directs

Food and Description	Measure or Quantity	Calories	Carbohydrates (grams)
Whiskey Sour Mix			
(Shasta)	6 fl. oz.	65	16.5
Wink (Canada Dry)	6 fl. oz.	91	22.7
Dietetic or low calorie:			
Apple (Shasta) red	6 fl. oz.	1	.3
Bubble Up	6 fl. oz.	1	.2
Cherry:			
(Cliquot Club; Cott; Mission)	6 fl. oz.	2	.3
(Dr. Brown's; Hoffman; Key Food; Waldbaum; Yukon Club) black	6 fl. oz.	2	.4
(No-Cal; Shasta)	6 fl. oz.	0	0
(Tab)	6 fl. oz.	2	<.1
Chocolate:			
(No-Cal)	6 fl. oz.	2	<.1
(Shasta)	6 fl. oz.	0	0
Chocolate mint (No-Cal)	6 fl. oz.	2	<.1
Citrus, *Flair*	6 fl. oz.	1	.2
Coffee:			
(Hoffman)	6 fl. oz.	3	.8
(No-Cal)	6 fl. oz.	2	.3
Cola:			
(Canada Dry)	6 fl. oz.	<1	.6
(Cliquot Club; Cott; Mission)	6 fl. oz.	2	.1
Diet Rite	6 fl. oz.	<1	Tr.
(No-Cal)	6 fl. oz.	0	<.1
Pepsi, diet	6 fl. oz.	<1	<.1
Pepsi Light	6 fl. oz.	26	6.4
RC	6 fl. oz.	<1	Tr.
(Shasta) regular & cherry	6 fl. oz.	0	0.
(Yukon Club)	6 fl. oz.	1	.3
Tab	6 fl. oz.	<1	<.1
Cream:			
(Cliquot Club; Cott; Mission)	6 fl. oz.	3	.5
(Dr. Brown's; Hoffman; Key Food; Waldbaum; Yukon Club)	6 fl. oz.	1	.2

Food and Description	Measure or Quantity	Calories	Carbo-hydrates (grams)
(No-Cal)	6 fl. oz.	0	<.1
(Shasta)	6 fl. oz.	0	0.
Dr. Brown's Cel-Ray Tonic	6 fl. oz.	1	.2
Dr. Pepper	6 fl. oz.	2	.4
Fresca	6 fl. oz.	1	0.
Ginger ale:			
(Canada Dry)	6 fl. oz.	<1	0.
(Dr. Brown's; Hoffman; Key Food; Waldbaum) pale dry	6 fl. oz.	1	.2
(No-Cal)	6 fl. oz.	0	Tr.
(Shasta)	6 fl. oz.	0	0.
Tab	6 fl. oz.	2	<.1
(Yukon Club)	6 fl. oz.	1	.4
Grape:			
(Dr. Brown's; Hoffman; Key Food; Waldbaum)	6 fl. oz.	2	.4
(No-Cal; Shasta)	6 fl. oz.	0	0.
Tab	6 fl. oz.	2	0.
Grapefruit:			
(Cliquot Club; Cott; Mission)	6 fl. oz.	3	.7
(Hoffman)	6 fl. oz.	2	.4
(Shasta)	6 fl. oz.	1	.3
Half & half (Hoffman)	6 fl. oz.	3	.8
Lemon (Cliquot Club; Cott; Mission)	6 fl. oz.	3	.5
Lemon-Lime:			
Diet Rite	6 fl. oz.	2	.4
(Hoffman)	6 fl. oz.	1	.2
(Shasta)	6 fl. oz.	0	0.
Tab	6 fl. oz.	2	0.
Mr. Pipp	6 fl. oz.	<1	<.1
Orange:			
(Cliquot Club; Cott)	6 fl. oz.	2	.3

(USDA): United States Department of Agriculture
(HEW/FAO): Health, Education and Welfare/Food and Agriculture Organization
* Prepared as Package Directs

Food and Description	Measure or Quantity	Calories	Carbo-hydrates (grams)
(*Diet Rite*; Dr. Brown's; Hoffman; Key Food; Waldbaum)	6 fl. oz.	1	.2
(No-Cal; Shasta)	6 fl. oz.	0	0.
Tab	6 fl. oz.	<1	0.
Quinine or tonic (No-Cal; Shasta)	6 fl. oz.	0	0.
Raspberry:			
(Dr. Brown's; Hoffman; Key Foods; Waldbaum) black	6 fl. oz.	2	.4
(No-Cal) black	6 fl. oz.	2	<.1
(Shasta) wild	6 fl. oz.	0	0.
Red Pop (No-Cal)	6 fl. oz.	0	0.
Root beer:			
Barrelhead (Canada Dry)	6 fl. oz.	<1	.8
(Cliquot Club; Cott; Mission; Yukon Club)	6 fl. oz.	<1	.1
(Dad's; Hoffman)	6 fl. oz.	<1	.2
(No-Cal)	6 fl. oz.	0	Tr.
(Shasta) draft	6 fl. oz.	0	0.
Tab	6 fl. oz.	<1	<.1
Seven-Up	6 fl. oz.	1	.6
Shape-Up (No-Cal)	6 fl. oz.	0	0.
Sprite	6 fl. oz.	2	0.
Strawberry:			
(Cliquot Club; Cott; Mission)	6 fl. oz.	3	.5
(Hoffman)	6 fl. oz.	<1	.2
(Shasta)	6 fl. oz.	0	0.
Tab	6 fl. oz.	2	0.
Tea (No-Cal)	6 fl. oz.	0	0.
Tiki (Shasta)	6 fl. oz.	0	0.
TNT (No-Cal)	6 fl. oz.	0	0.
SOLE (USDA):			
Raw, whole	1 lb. (weighed whole)	118	0.
Meat only	4 oz.	90	0.

Food and Description	Measure or Quantity	Calories	Carbo-hydrates (grams)
Frozen:			
(Gorton) in lemon butter	⅓ of 9-oz. pkg.	147	2.0
(Mrs. Paul's) fillets, breaded & fried	½ of 8-oz. pkg.	225	21.8
(Ship Ahoy) fillet, thawed	1-lb. pkg.	309	0.
(Weight Watchers) 2-compartment meal	9½-oz. meal	208	14.0
(Weight Watchers) 3-compartment meal	16-oz. meal	245	14.1
SORGHUM (USDA):			
Grain	1 oz.	94	20.7
Syrup	1 T. (.7 oz.)	54	12.2
SORREL (See **DOCK**)			
SOUP (See individual listings by kind)			
SOUP GREENS (Durkee)	2½-oz. jar	216	43.0
SOURSOP, raw (USDA):			
Whole	1 lb. (weighed with skin & seeds)	200	50.3
Flesh only	4 oz.	74	18.5
SOUSE (USDA)	1 oz.	51	.3
SOUTHERN COMFORT:			
80 proof	1 fl. oz.	79	3.4
90 proof	1 fl. oz.	87	3.5
100 proof	1 fl. oz.	96	3.5
SOYBEAN:			
(USDA):			
Young seeds:			
Raw	1 lb. (weighed in pod)	322	31.7

(USDA): United States Department of Agriculture
(HEW/FAO): Health, Education and Welfare/Food and Agriculture
Organization
* Prepared as Package Directs

Food and Description	Measure or Quantity	Calories	Carbo-hydrates (grams)
Boiled, drained	4 oz.	134	11.5
Canned, solids & liq.	4 oz.	85	7.1
Canned, drained solids	4 oz.	117	8.4
Mature seeds, dry:			
Raw	1 lb.	1828	152.0
Raw	1 cup (7.4 oz.)	846	70.4
Cooked	4 oz.	147	12.2
Dry roasted:			
(Soy Ahoy)	1 oz.	139	6.0
(Soytown)	1 oz.	139	6.0
Oil roasted:			
(Soy Ahoy)	1 oz.	152	4.8
(Soy Ahoy) barbecue or garlic	1 oz.	152	4.8
(Soytown)	1 oz.	152	4.8
SOYBEAN CURD or TOFU (USDA):			
Regular	4 oz.	82	2.7
Cake	4.2-oz. cake	86	2.9
SOYBEAN FLOUR (See FLOUR)			
SOYBEAN GRITS, high fat (USDA)	1 cup (4.9 oz.)	524	46.0
SOYBEAN MILK (USDA):			
Fluid	4 oz.	37	1.5
Powder	1 oz.	122	7.9
SOYBEAN PROTEIN (USDA)	1 oz.	91	4.3
SOYBEAN PROTEINATE (USDA)	1 oz.	88	2.2
SOYBEAN SPROUT (See BEAN SPROUT)			
SOY SAUCE (See SAUCE)			

Food and Description	Measure or Quantity	Calories	Carbohydrates (grams)
SPAGHETTI. Plain spaghetti products are essentially the same in caloric value and carbohydrate content on the same weight basis. The longer the cooking, the more water is absorbed and this affects the nutritive value (USDA):			
Dry	1 oz.	105	21.3
Dry, broken	1 cup (2.5 oz.)	262	53.4
Cooked:			
8-10 minutes, "al dente"	1 cup (5.1 oz.)	216	43.9
8-10 minutes, "al dente"	4 oz.	168	34.1
14-20 minutes, tender	1 cup (4.9 oz.)	155	32.2
14-20 minutes, tender	4 oz.	126	26.1
SPAGHETTI MEAL:			
Canned (Franco-American) with meat sauce	7¾-oz. serving	220	26.0
Canned (Franco-American) with tomato sauce & cheese	½ of 14¾-oz. can	170	33.0
Frozen:			
(Banquet)	11½-oz. dinner	450	62.9
(Morton) & meatball	11-oz. dinner	344	59.4
(Swanson) & meatball	12½-oz. dinner	410	57.0
(Swanson) *Hungry Man*, & meatballs	18½-oz. dinner	660	83.0
Mix:			
*(Ann Page) Italian style	¼ of 8-oz. pkg.	205	37.4
*(Kraft) deluxe, with meat sauce	4 oz.	151	23.1
SPAGHETTI & FRANKFURTERS, canned (Franco-American) in tomato sauce, *Spaghetti-Os*	½ of 14¾-oz. can	210	26.0

(USDA): United States Department of Agriculture
(HEW/FAO): Health, Education and Welfare/Food and Agriculture
    Organization
* Prepared as Package Directs

Food and Description	Measure or Quantity	Calories	Carbohydrates (grams)
SPAGHETTI & MEATBALLS in TOMATO SAUCE:			
Home recipe (USDA)	1 cup (8.7 oz.)	332	38.7
Canned, regular pack:			
(USDA)	1 cup (8.8 oz.)	258	28.5
(Franco-American)	7¼-oz. can	210	23.0
(Franco-American) Spaghetti-Os	½ of 14¾-oz. can	210	24.0
(Hormel)	15-oz. can	348	20.0
(Libby's)	½ of 15-oz. can	178	27.5
Canned, dietetic or low calorie (Dia-Mel)	8-oz. can	200	24.0
Frozen (Green Giant)	9-oz. entree	280	30.0
SPAGHETTI with MEAT SAUCE, frozen:			
(Banquet)	8-oz. entree	311	31.3
(Kraft)	12½-oz. pkg.	343	48.9
SPAGHETTI SAUCE (See also SPAGHETTI SAUCE MIX):			
Clam:			
(Buitoni) red	4 oz.	106	1.4
(Buitoni) white	4 oz.	140	2.2
(Ragu) chopped	5 oz.	110	14.0
Marinara (Ann Page)	¼ of 15½-oz. jar	70	12.3
Marinara (Prince)	4 oz. serving	80	12.4
Meat-flavored (Ann Page)	¼ of 15½-oz. jar	81	12.3
Meat:			
(Buitoni)	4 oz. serving	111	5.0
(Prince)	½ cup (4.9 oz.)	101	11.0
(Ragu)	5-oz. serving	115	14.0
(Ragu) extra thick & zesty	5-oz. serving	130	14.0
(Ronzoni)	4-oz. serving	87	11.0
Meatless or plain:			
(Ann Page) with mushroom	¼ of 15½-oz. jar	75	12.5
(Ann Page) plain	¼ of 15½-oz. jar	76	12.9
(Prince)	½ cup (4.6 oz.)	90	11.4
(Ragu)	5-oz. serving	105	14.0
(Ragu) extra thick & zesty	5-oz. serving	120	13.0
(Ronzoni)	4-oz. serving	78	13.0

Food and Description	Measure or Quantity	Calories	Carbo-hydrates (grams)
Mushroom:			
(Prince)	4-oz. serving	77	11.3
(Ragu)	5-oz. serving	105	13.0
(Ragu) extra thick & zesty	5-oz. serving	110	14.0
Pepperoni (Ragu)	5-oz. serving	120	14.0
Dietetic (Featherweight) low sodium	4½-oz. serving	60	8.0
SPAGHETTI SAUCE MIX:			
(Ann Page) with mushrooms	1½-oz. pkg.	125	26.7
(Ann Page) without mushrooms	1½-oz. pkg.	128	27.0
(Durkee)	1½-oz. pkg.	85	20.0
*(Durkee)	2½ cups	224	52.0
(Durkee) mushroom	1.2-oz. pkg.	69	16.0
*(Durkee) mushroom	2⅔ cups	208	48.0
(French's) Italian style	1½-oz. pkg.	121	26.8
(French's) with mushroom	1⅜-oz. pkg.	125	19.0
(Lawry's) with mushrooms	1½-oz. pkg.	147	22.6
*(Spatini)	2-oz. serving	80	4.0
*(Wyler)	½ cup	21	3.9
SPAM (Hormel):			
Regular	3 oz.	260	3.2
& cheese	3 oz.	260	2.1
Spread	1 oz.	80	0.
SPANISH MACKEREL, raw (USDA):			
Whole	1 lb. (weighed whole)	490	0.
Meat only	4 oz.	201	0.
SPECIAL K, cereal (Kellogg's)	1¼ cups (1 oz.)	110	21.0

(USDA): United States Department of Agriculture
(HEW/FAO): Health, Education and Welfare/Food and Agriculture
              Organization
* Prepared as Package Directs

Food and Description	Measure or Quantity	Calories	Carbo hydrate (grams)
SPINACH:			
Raw (USDA):			
Untrimmed	1 lb. (weighed with large stems & roots)	85	14.0
Trimmed or packaged	1 lb.	118	19.5
Trimmed, whole leaves	1 cup (1.2 oz.)	9	1.4
Trimmed, chopped	1 cup (1.8 oz.)	14	2.2
Boiled, whole leaves, drained (USDA)	1 cup (5.5 oz.)	36	5.6
Canned, regular pack:			
(USDA) solids & liq.	½ cup (4.1 oz.)	22	3.5
(USDA) drained solids	½ cup	27	4.0
(Del Monte) solids & liq.	½ cup (4.1 oz.)	28	3.4
(Libby's) solids & liq.	½ cup (4.2 oz.)	23	3.6
Canned, dietetic or low calorie:			
(USDA) low sodium, solids & liq.	4 oz.	24	3.9
(USDA) low sodium, drained solids	4 oz.	29	4.5
(Blue Boy) solids & liq.	4-oz. serving	22	2.4
(Featherweight) low sodium, solids & liq.	½ cup	30	4.0
Frozen:			
(USDA) chopped, boiled, drained	4 oz.	26	4.2
(Birds Eye) creamed	⅓ of 9-oz. pkg.	60	6.0
(Birds Eye) chopped	⅓ pkg.	20	3.0
(Birds Eye) leaf	⅓ pkg.	20	3.0
(Green Giant) creamed	½ cup	95	10.5
(Green Giant) in butter sauce	½ cup	45	3.0
(Green Giant) souffle, *Bake 'n Serve*	1 cup	300	27.0
(Green Giant) in cheese sauce	1 cup	140	14.0
SPINY LOBSTER (See **CRAYFISH**)			
SPLEEN, raw (USDA):			
Beef & calf	4 oz.	118	0.

Food and Description	Measure or Quantity	Calories	Carbohydrates (grams)
Hog	4 oz.	121	0.
Lamb	4 oz.	130	0.

SPONGE CAKE (See CAKE, Sponge)

SQUAB, pigeon, raw (USDA):
Dressed	1 lb. (weighed with feet, inedible viscera & bones)	569	0.
Meat & skin	4 oz.	333	0.
Meat only	4 oz.	161	0.
Light meat only, without skin	4 oz.	141	0.
Giblets	1 oz.	44	.3

SQUASH SEEDS, dry (USDA):
In hull	4 oz.	464	12.6
Hulled	1 oz.	157	4.3

SQUASH, SUMMER:
Fresh (USDA):
Crookneck & straightneck, yellow:
Whole	1 lb. (weighed untrimmed)	89	19.1
Boiled, drained, diced	½ cup (3.6 oz.)	15	3.2
Boiled, drained, slices	½ cup (3.1 oz.)	13	2.7

Scallop, white & pale green:
Whole	1 lb. (weighed untrimmed)	93	22.7
Boiled, drained, mashed	½ cup (4.2 oz.)	19	4.5

Zucchini & cocazelle, green:
Whole	1 lb. (weighed untrimmed)	73	15.5

(USDA): United States Department of Agriculture
(HEW/FAO): Health, Education and Welfare/Food and Agriculture Organization
* Prepared as Package Directs

Food and Description	Measure or Quantity	Calories	Carbo-hydrates (grams)
Boiled, drained slices	½ cup (2.7 oz.)	9	1.9
Canned (Del Monte) zucchini, in tomato sauce	½ cup (4.1 oz.)	37	7.9
Frozen:			
(USDA) unthawed	4 oz.	24	5.3
(USDA) boiled, drained	4 oz.	24	5.3
(Birds Eye) sliced	⅓ pkg.	18	3.0
(Birds Eye) zucchini	⅓ pkg.	16	3.0
(Green Giant) in cheese sauce	½ cup	60	8.0
(Mrs. Paul's) zucchini parmesan	½ of 12-oz. pkg.	493	93.2
(Mrs. Paul's) zucchini sticks, batter fried	½ of 9-oz. pkg.	186	23.2
SQUASH, WINTER:			
Fresh (USDA):			
Acorn:			
Whole	1 lb. (weighed with skin & seeds)	152	38.6
Baked, flesh only, mashed	½ cup (3.6 oz.)	56	14.3
Boiled, mashed	½ cup (4.1 oz.)	39	9.7
Butternut:			
Whole	1 lb. (weighed with skin & seeds)	171	44.4
Baked, flesh only	4 oz.	77	19.8
Boiled, flesh only	4 oz.	46	11.8
Hubbard:			
Whole	1 lb. (weighed with skin & seeds)	117	28.1
Baked, flesh only	4 oz.	57	13.3
Baked, mashed, flesh only	½ cup (3.6 oz.)	51	11.7
Boiled, flesh only, diced	½ cup (4.2 oz.)	35	8.1
Boiled, flesh only, mashed	½ cup (4.3 oz.)	37	8.4
Frozen:			
(USDA) heated	½ cup (4.2 oz.)	46	11.0
(Birds Eye)	⅓ pkg.	50	11.0
SQUID, raw, meat only (USDA)	4 oz.	95	1.7

Food and Description	Measure or Quantity	Calories	Carbo-hydrates (grams)
STARCH (See **CORNSTARCH**)			
***SQUOZE** (Pillsbury) all flavors	8 fl. oz.	40	10.0
***START**, instant breakfast drink	½ cup	60	14.0
***STOCKPOT SOUP** (Campbell) condensed, vegetable & beef	10-oz. serving	120	13.0
STOMACH, PORK, scalded (USDA)	4 oz.	172	0.
STRAINED FOOD (See **BABY FOOD**)			
STRAWBERRY:			
(USDA):			
Fresh, whole	1 lb. (weighed with caps & stems)	161	36.6
Fresh, whole, capped	1 cup (5.1 oz.)	53	12.1
Canned, unsweetened or low calorie, water pack, solids & liq.	4 oz.	25	6.4
Frozen (Birds Eye):			
Halves	½ cup (5.3 oz.)	170	48.0
Quick thaw	5 oz.	110	30.0
Sliced	5 oz.	180	48.0
Whole	4 oz.	70	20.0
STRAWBERRY DRINK MIX (Wyler's)	3-oz. pouch	338	84.6
STRAWBERRY FRUIT DRINK, canned (Hi-D)	6 fl. oz.	89	22.0

(USDA): United States Department of Agriculture
(HEW/FAO): Health, Education and Welfare/Food and Agriculture Organization
* Prepared as Package Directs

Food and Description	*Measure or Quantity*	*Calories*	*Carbohydrates (grams)*
STRAWBERRY ICE CREAM:			
(Breyer's)	¼ pt.	130	17.0
(Breyer's) twin	¼ pt.	140	20.0
(Dean) 10.5% fat	1 cup (5.6 oz.)	336	40.0
(Meadow Gold) 10% fat	½ pt.	252	32.0
(Sealtest)	¼ pt.	130	18.0
(Swift's) sweet cream	½ cup (2¼ oz.)	124	15.3
STRAWBERRY JELLY:			
Sweetened (Smucker's)	1 T.	53	13.5
Dietetic or low calorie (Featherweight)	1 T.	14	4.0
STRAWBERRY PIE:			
Home recipe (USDA)	⅙ of 9″ pie (5.6 oz.)	313	48.8
(Tastykake) creme	4-oz. pie	356	50.7
Frozen:			
(Banquet) cream	⅙ of 14-oz. pie	169	22.5
(Morton) cream	⅙ of 16-oz. pie	182	22.0
STRAWBERRY PIE FILLING:			
(Comstock)	½ cup	154	36.7
(Wilderness)	21-oz. can	738	180.9
STRAWBERRY PRESERVES or JAM:			
Sweetened:			
(Bama)	1 T. (.7 oz.)	54	13.5
(Smucker's)	1 T. (.7 oz.)	52	13.5
Dietetic or low calorie:			
(Dia-Mel)	1 tsp. (6 grams)	2	0.
(Diet Delight)	1 T. (.6 oz.)	13	3.3
(Featherweight)	1 T.	14	3.0
(Kraft)	1 oz.	36	8.9
(Louis Sherry) wild	1 tsp.	2	0.
(Tillie Lewis)	1 tsp (5 grams)	4	1.0
STRAWBERRY-RHUBARB PIE FILLING (Lucky Leaf)	8 oz.	258	62.8

Food and Description	Measure or Quantity	Calories	Carbo-hydrates (grams)
STRAWBERRY SYRUP:			
Sweetened (Smucker's)	1 T. (.6 oz.)	45	11.6
Dietetic or low calorie (Featherweight)	1 T.	14	3.0
STUFFING MIX:			
Chicken:			
*Stove Top	½ cup	180	20.0
*(Uncle Ben's) Stuff'n Such, without butter	½ cup	123	24.8
*(Uncle Ben's) Stuff'n Such, with butter	½ cup	198	24.8
Cornbread:			
(Pepperidge Farm)	8-oz. pkg.	880	168.0
*Stove Top	½ cup	170	20.0
*(Uncle Ben's) Stuff'n Such, without butter	½ cup	129	26.9
*(Uncle Ben's) Stuff'n Such, with butter	½ cup	205	26.9
Herb seasoned (Pepperidge Farm)	8-oz. pkg.	880	168.0
*Pork, Stove Top	½ cup	170	20.0
*With rice, Stove Top	½ cup	180	23.0
*Sage (Uncle Ben's):			
Without butter	½ cup	124	24.9
With butter	½ cup	198	24.9
White bread, Mrs. Cubbison's	1 oz.	101	20.5
STURGEON (USDA):			
Raw, section	1 lb. (weighed with skin & bones)	362	0.
Raw, meat only	4 oz.	107	0.
Smoked	4 oz.	169	0.
Steamed	4 oz.	181	0.
SUCCOTASH:			
Canned:			
(Libby's) whole kernel	¼ of 16-oz. can	70	16.0

(USDA): United States Department of Agriculture
(HEW/FAO): Health, Education and Welfare/Food and Agriculture Organization
* Prepared as Package Directs

Food and Description	Measure or Quantity	Calories	Carbo-hydrates (grams)
(Libby's) cream style	½ cup (4.6 oz.)	97	23.0
(Stokely-Van Camp) solids & liq.	½ cup (4.5 oz.)	85	17.5
Frozen:			
(USDA) boiled, drained	½ cup (3.4 oz.)	89	19.7
(Birds Eye)	⅓ pkg.	80	17.0
SUCKER, CARP, raw (USDA):			
Whole	1 lb. (weighed whole)	196	0.
Meat only	4 oz.	126	0.
SUCKER, including **WHITE MULLET,** raw (USDA):			
Whole	1 lb. (weighed whole)	203	0.
Meat only	4 oz.	118	0.
SUET, raw (USDA)	1 oz.	242	0.
SUGAR, beet or cane (there are no differences in calories and carbohydrates among brands) (USDA):			
Brown:			
Regular	1 lb.	1692	437.3
Brownulated	1 cup (5.4 oz.)	567	146.5
Firm-packed	1 cup (7.5 oz.)		
Firm-packed	1 T. (.5 oz.)	48	12.5
Confectioners':			
Unsifted	1 cup (4.3 oz.)	474	122.4
Unsifted	1 T. (8 grams)	30	7.7
Sifted	1 cup (3.4 oz.)	366	94.5
Sifted	1 T. (6 grams)	23	5.9
Stirred	1 cup (4.2 oz.)	462	119.4
Stirred	1 T. (8 grams)	29	7.5
Granulated	1 lb.	1746	451.3
Granulated	1 cup (6.9 oz.)	751	194.0
Granulated	1 T. (.4 oz.)	46	11.9
Granulated	1 lump (1⅛″ x ¾″ x ⅜″, 6 grams)	23	6.0

Food and Description	Measure or Quantity	Calories	Carbo-hydrates (grams)
Maple	1 lb.	1579	408.0
Maple	1¾″ x 1¼″ x ½″ piece (1.2 oz.)	104	27.0
SUGAR APPLE, raw (USDA):			
Whole	1 lb. (weighed with skin & seeds)	192	48.4
Flesh only	4 oz.	107	26.9
SUGAR CRISP, cereal (Post)	⅞ cup (1 oz.)	110	25.0
SUGAR FROSTED FLAKES, cereal (Kellogg's)	⅔ cup (1 oz.)	110	26.0
SUGAR POPS, cereal (Kellogg's)	1 cup (1 oz.)	110	16.0
SUGAR SMACKS, cereal (Kellogg's)	¾ cup (1 oz.)	110	25.0
SUGAR SUBSTITUTE:			
Sprinkle Sweet (Pillsbury)	1 tsp.	2	.5
Sugar-Like (Dia-Mel)	1-gram packet	3	1.0
Sug'r Like (Featherweight)	1 tsp.	2	1.0
Superose (Whitlock)	1-gram packet	4	.9
Sweet'ner (Weight Watchers)	1-gram packet	3	1.0
Sweetness & Light	1 tsp. (1 gram)	4	.9
Sweet'n-it (Dia-Mal) liquid	5 drops	0	0.
*Sweet*10* (Pillsbury)	⅛ tsp.	0	0.
SUNFLOWER SEED:			
(USDA) in hulls	4 oz. (weighed in hull)	343	12.2
(USDA) hulled	1 oz.	159	5.6
(Flavor House) dry roasted	1 oz.	179	4.0
(Frito-Lay's)	1 oz.	181	4.7

(USDA): United States Department of Agriculture
(HEW/FAO): Health, Education and Welfare/Food and Agriculture
        Organization
* Prepared as Package Directs

Food and Description	Measure or Quantity	Calories	Carbo- hydrates (grams)
(Planters) dry roasted	1 oz.	159	5.9
(Planters) hulled	1 oz.	164	5.4
SUNFLOWER SEED FLOUR (See **FLOUR**)			
SUNNY DOODLES (Drake's)	1.1-oz. cake	102	17.1
SUZY Q (Hostess):			
Banana	2¼-oz. cake	244	38.4
Chocolate	2½-oz. cake	240	36.5
SWAMP CABBAGE (USDA):			
Raw, whole	1 lb. (weighed untrimmed	107	9.8
Boiled, trimmed, drained	4 oz.	24	4.4
SWEETBREADS (USDA):			
Beef, raw	1 lb.	939	0.
Beef, braised	4 oz.	363	0.
Calf, raw	1 lb.	426	0.
Calf, braised	4 oz.	191	0.
Hog (See **PANCREAS**)			
Lamb, raw	1 lb.	426	0.
Lamb, braised	4 oz.	198	0.
SWEET POTATO:			
Raw (USDA):			
All kinds, unpared	1 lb. (weighed whole)	419	96.6
All kinds, pared	4 oz.	129	29.8
Firm-fleshed, Jersey types, pared	4 oz.	116	25.5
Soft-fleshed, Puerto Rico variety, pared	4 oz.	133	31.0
Baked (USDA) peeled after baking	3.9-oz. sweet potato (5″ x 2″)	155	35.8
Baked (USDA) peeled after boiling	5-oz. sweet potato (5″ x 2″)	168	38.7

Food and Description	Measure or Quantity	Calories	Carbo- hydrates (grams)
Candied (USDA) home recipe	6.2-oz. sweet potato (3½" x 2¼")	294	59.8
Canned, regular pack:			
(USDA) in syrup, solids & liq.	4 oz.	129	31.2
(USDA) vacuum or solid pack	½ cup (3.8 oz.)	118	27.1
(King Pharr)	½ cup	118	22.5
(King Pharr) yam	½ cup	114	27.0
Canned, dietetic pack, without added sugar & salt	4 oz.	52	12.2
Dehydrated flakes (USDA) dry	½ cup (2 oz.)	220	52.2
*Dehydrated flakes (USDA) prepared with water	½ cup (4.4 oz.)	120	28.5
Frozen:			
(Green Giant) glazed	½ cup	170	32.5
(Mrs. Paul's) candied with apple	⅛ of 12-oz. pkg.	165	37.2
(Mrs. Paul's) candied, yellow	⅛ of 12-oz. pkg.	184	44.3
SWEET POTATO PIE:			
Home recipe (USDA)	⅛ of 9" pie (5.4 oz.)	324	36.0
(Tastykake)	4-oz. pie	359	50.0
SWEETSOP (See SUGAR APPLE)			
SWISS ROLE (Drake's)	3-oz. roll	376	52.9
SWISS STEAK, frozen (Swanson)	10-oz. dinner	350	19.0
SWORDFISH (USDA):			
Raw, meat only	1 lb.	535	0.

(USDA): United States Department of Agriculture
(HEW/FAO): Health, Education and Welfare/Food and Agriculture Organization
* Prepared as Package Directs

Food and Description	Measure or Quantity	Calories	Carbo-hydrates (grams)
Broiled, with butter or margarine	3" x 3" x ½" steak (4.4 oz.)	218	0.
Canned, solids & liq.	4 oz.	116	0.
SYLVANDER WINE (Louis M. Martini) 12½% alcohol	3 fl. oz.	90	.2
SYRUP (See individual listings by kind, such as **PANCAKE & WAFFLE SYRUP**, or by brand name, such as **LOG CABIN**)			

T

TABASCO SAUCE (McIlhenny)	¼ tsp. (1 gram)	<1	<.1
TACO:			
(Ortega)	1 taco	220	13.0
(Patio)	¼-oz. taco	179	15.1
(Patio) cocktail	½-oz. taco	39	4.8
Filling, canned (Gebhardt)	1 oz.	63	3.0
Seasoning mix:			
(Durkee)	1.1-oz. pkg.	67	15.0
*(Durkee)	1 cup	641	7.5
(French's)	1¾-oz. pkg.	50	30.0
(Lawry's)	1¼-oz. pkg.	120	21.8
Shell (Ortega)	1 shell	54	3.8
TAMALE, canned:			
(Armour Star)	15½-oz. can	620	63.2
(Derby) beef, with sauce	1 tamale (2.2 oz.)	120	6.5
(Gebhardt)	2 oz.	110	20.0
(Hormel) beef	1 tamale (2.1 oz.)	80	4.9
(Wilson)	15½-oz. can	601	63.3
TAMARIND, fresh (USDA):			
Whole	1 lb. (weighed with pods & seeds)	520	136.1
Flesh only	4 oz.	271	70.9

Food and Description	Measure or Quantity	Calories	Carbohydrates (grams)
TANDY CAKE (Tastykake):			
Chocolate	⅔-oz. cake	147	21.0
Choc-O-Mint	.6-oz. cake	102	13.0
Dandy Kake	.6-oz. cake	102	13.0
Karamel	⅔-oz. cake	100	12.2
*TANG, instant breakfast drink:			
Grape	½ cup (4 oz.)	60	15.0
Grapefruit	½ cup (4 fl. oz.)	50	13.0
Orange	½ cup (4 fl. oz.)	60	14.0
TANGELO, fresh (USDA):			
Juice from whole fruit	1 lb. (weighed with peel, membrane & seeds)	104	24.6
Juice	½ cup (4.4 oz.)	51	12.0
TANGERINE or MANDARIN ORANGE: Fresh:			
Whole (USDA)	1 lb. (weighed with peel, membrane & seeds)	154	38.9
Whole (USDA)	4.1-oz. tangerine (2⅜″ dia.)	39	10.0
Peeled (Sunkist)	1 large tangerine (4.1 oz.)	39	10.0
Sections, without membranes (USDA)	1 cup (6.8 oz.)	89	22.4
Canned, regular pack (Del Monte) solids & liq.	¼ of 22-oz. can	106	25.3
Canned, dietetic or low calorie:			
(Diet Delight) solids & liq.	½ cup (4.3 oz.)	51	11.7

(USDA): United States Department of Agriculture
(HEW/FAO): Health, Education and Welfare/Food and Agriculture Organization
* Prepared as Package Directs

Food and Description	Measure or Quantity	Calories	Carbohydrates (grams)
(Featherweight) water pack, solids & liq.	½ cup	30	6.0
(Tillie Lewis)	½ cup (4.3 oz.)	44	11.0
TANGERINE JUICE:			
Fresh (USDA)	½ cup (4.4 oz.)	53	12.5
Canned, unsweetened (USDA)	½ cup (4.4 oz.)	53	12.6
Canned, sweetened (USDA)	½ cup (4.4 oz.)	62	14.9
Frozen:			
*(USDA)	½ cup (4.4 oz.)	57	13.4
*(Minute Maid) sweetened	6 fl. oz.	85	20.8
TAPIOCA, dry, quick cooking, granulated:			
(USDA)	1 cup (5.4 oz.)	535	131.3
(USDA)	1 T. (10 grams)	35	8.6
TAPIOCA PUDDING:			
Home recipe (USDA) apple	½ cup (4.4 oz.)	146	36.8
Home recipe (USDA) cream	½ cup (2.9 oz.)	110	14.0
Canned:			
(Betty Crocker)	½ cup (4.3 oz.)	150	22.0
(Del Monte)	5-oz. container	174	30.1
(Hunt's) *Snack Pack*	5-oz. can	130	23.0
Mix:			
(Ann Page) chocolate	¼ of 3½-oz. pkg.	97	22.6
(Ann Page) vanilla	¼ of 3¼-oz. pkg.	89	22.3
*(My-T-Fine) vanilla	½ cup (5 oz.)	130	28.0
TARO, raw (USDA):			
Tubers, whole	1 lb. (weighed with skin)	373	90.3
Tubers, skin removed	4 oz.	111	26.9
Leaves & stems	1 lb.	181	33.6
TARRAGON (French's)	1 tsp.	5	.7
TAUTUG or BLACKFISH, raw (USDA):			
Whole	1 lb. (weighed whole)	149	0.
Meat only	4 oz.	101	0.

Food and Description	Measure or Quantity	Calories	Carbo-hydrates (grams)
TEA (See also **TEA MIX, ICED**):			
Bag (Lipton)	1 bag	0	0.
Bag (Tender Leaf)	1 bag	1	
Bottle (Lipton)	10 fl. oz.	140	35.0
Canned (Lipton) lemon-flavored	12 fl. oz.	130	32.0
Canned (Lipton) lemon-flavored, sugar free	12 fl. oz.	2	0.
Instant:			
(USDA) dry powder, slightly sweetened	1 tsp.	1	.4
*(USDA) beverage, slightly sweetened	1 cup (8.4 oz.)	5	.9
*(Lipton) lemon-flavored	1 cup (8 fl. oz.)	4	1.0
*(Lipton) 100% tea	8 fl. oz.	0	0.
Nestea	1 tsp. (.6 grams)	0	0.
(Tender Leaf)	1 tsp.	1	
TEAM, cereal	1 cup (1 oz.)	110	24.0
TEA MIX, ICED:			
Regular:			
(A&P) *Our Own*, lemon-flavored	1 tsp. (1.5 grams)	6	1.4
*(A&P) *Our Own*, lemon-flavored with sugar	8 fl. oz.	85	21.2
*(Lipton) lemon-flavored	8 fl. oz.	60	16.0
Nestea, lemon-flavored	8 fl. oz.	20	.2
Nestea, lemon-flavored with sugar	6 fl. oz.	70	17.0
*(Salada) all flavors	1 cup	57	13.6
*(Wyler's)	1 cup	56	14.0
Dietetic or low calorie:			
(Ann Page)	1 tsp. (1.5 grams)	6	1.4
*(Lipton) lemon-flavored	8 fl. oz.	2	0.

(USDA): United States Department of Agriculture
(HEW/FAO): Health, Education and Welfare/Food and Agriculture
           Organization
* Prepared as Package Directs

Food and Description	Measure or Quantity	Calories	Carbo-hydrates (grams)
TEMPTYS (Tastykake):			
Butter creme	⅔-oz. cake	94	12.9
Chocolate	⅔-oz. cake	95	17.1
Lemon	⅔-oz. cake	95	17.3
TENDERGREEN (See **MUSTARD SPINACH**)			
TEQUILA (See **DISTILLED LIQUOR**)			
TEXTURED VEGETABLE PROTEIN:			
Breakfast links, *Morningstar Farms*	.8-oz. link	54	2.3
Breakfast patties, *Morningstar Farms*	1.3-oz. pattie	98	4.9
Breakfast slices, *Morningstar Farms*	1-oz. slice	50	1.0
Chili seasoning (Williams)	4-oz. pkg.	428	47.4
Hamburger seasoning (Williams)	4-oz. pkg.	385	53.6
Meatloaf seasoning (Williams)	4-oz. pkg.	393	54.2
Pathmark Plus:			
Dry	⅓ oz.	28	3.0
*Prepared	4 oz.	178	2.9
Sloppy Joe seasoning (Williams)	4-oz. pkg.	382	55.8
*Sloppy Joe seasoning (Williams)	4 oz.	186	9.2
Spaghetti sauce (Williams)	4-oz. pkg.	366	56.5
*Spaghetti sauce (Williams)	4-oz. serving	118	7.6
Taco seasoning (Williams)	4-oz. pkg.	378	48.7
THUNDERBIRD WINE (Gallo):			
14% alcohol	3 fl. oz.	86	8.1
20% alcohol	3 fl. oz.	106	7.5
THURINGER, sausage:			
(USDA)	1 oz.	87	.5
(Hormel)	1 oz.	100	<1.0

Food and Description	Measure or Quantity	Calories	Carbohydrates (grams)
(Oscar Mayer) summer sausage	.8-oz. slice	79	.2
(Oscar Mayer) summer sausage, beef	.8-oz. slice	73	.5
THYME, dried (French's)	1 tsp.	5	1.0
TIA MARIA, liqueur (Hiram Walker) 63 proof	1 fl. oz.	92	10.0
TIGER TAILS (Hostess)	4.4-oz. piece	444	76.2
TILEFISH (USDA):			
Raw, whole	1 lb. (weighed whole)	183	0.
Baked, meat only	4 oz.	156	0.
TOASTER CAKE:			
(Nabisco) all varieties	1.7-oz. piece	190	35.0
(Thomas') fresh or frozen, *Toast-r-Cake:*			
Blueberry	1.3-oz. cake	110	17.5
Bran	1 piece	112	19.6
Corn	1.3-oz. cake	116	18.3
TOASTY O's, cereal	1 oz.	113	19.9
TODDLER FOOD (See **BABY FOOD**)			
TOFFEE KRUNCH BAR (Sealtest)	3 fl. oz.	150	12.0
TOFU (See **SOYBEAN CURD**)			

(USDA): United States Department of Agriculture
(HEW/FAO): Health, Education and Welfare/Food and Agriculture Organization
* Prepared as Package Directs

Food and Description	Measure or Quantity	Calories	Carbo-hydrates (grams)
TOMATO:			
Fresh (USDA):			
Green whole, untrimmed	1 lb. (weighed with core & stem end)	99	21.1
Green, trimmed, unpeeled	4 oz.	27	5.8
Ripe:			
Whole, eaten with skin	1 lb.	100	21.3
Whole, peeled	1 lb. (weighed with skin, stem ends & hard core)	88	18.8
Whole, peeled	1 med. (2″ x 2½″, 5.3 oz.)	33	7.0
Whole, peeled	1 small (1¾″ x 2½″, 3.9 oz.)	24	5.2
Sliced, peeled	½ cup (3.2 oz.)	20	4.2
Boiled (USDA)	½ cup (4.3 oz.)	31	6.7
Canned, regular pack:			
(USDA) whole, solids & liq.	½ cup (4.2 oz.)	25	5.1
(Contadina):			
Diced in puree	4 oz.	40	9.0
Sliced, baby	4 oz.	40	8.5
Stewed	1 cup	70	18.0
Whole, round & pear	1 cup	50	11.0
(Del Monte) stewed, solids & liq.	½ cup (4.2 oz.)	39	8.2
(Del Monte) wedges, solids & liq.	½ cup (4.1 oz.)	35	7.2
(Del Monte) whole, peeled, solids & liq.	½ cup (4.2 oz.)	27	5.3
(Hunt's) stewed	4 oz.	30	7.0
(Hunt's) whole, peeled	4 oz.	20	5.0
(Libby's) stewed	½ of 16-oz. can	60	35.5
(Libby's) whole, peeled, solids & liq.	½ of 16-oz. can	43	9.8
(Stokely-Van Camp) stewed, solids & liq.	½ cup (4.2 oz.)	35	7.5
(Stokely-Van Camp) whole, solids & liq.	½ cup (4.3 oz.)	25	5.0
Canned, dietetic or low calorie:			
(USDA) low sodium	4 oz.	23	4.8

Food and Description	Measure or Quantity	Calories	Carbohydrates (grams)
(Blue Boy)	4 oz.	25	4.8
(Diet Delight) whole, peeled	½ cup (4.3 oz.)	25	5.0
(Featherweight) low sodium	½ cup	20	4.0
(Featherweight) low sodium, stewed	½ cup	35	9.0
(Tillie Lewis)	½ cup (4.3 oz.)	24	6.1
TOMATO JUICE:			
Canned, regular pack:			
(USDA)	½ cup (4.3 oz.)	23	5.2
(Campbell)	6-fl.-oz. can	35	8.0
(Del Monte)	6 fl. oz.	36	7.4
(Libby's)	6 fl. oz.	33	7.5
(Sacramento)	5½ fl. oz.	33	7.7
(Stokely-Van Camp)	½ cup (4.2 oz.)	23	4.5
Canned, dietetic or low calorie:			
(USDA)	4 oz. (by wt.)	22	4.9
(Blue Boy)	4 oz. (by wt.)	24	4.5
(Diet Delight)	6 fl. oz. (6.4 oz.)	36	7.5
(Featherweight)	½ of 12-oz. can	35	8.0
(Tillie Lewis)	6 fl. oz. (6.4 oz.)	36	7.3
Concentrate (USDA) canned	4 oz. (by wt.)	86	19.4
*Concentrate (USDA) canned, diluted with 3 parts water by volume	4 oz. (by wt.)	23	5.1
Dehydrated (USDA)	1 oz.	86	19.3
*Dehydrated (USDA)	½ cup (4.3 oz.)	24	5.4
TOMATO JUICE COCKTAIL:			
(USDA)	4 oz. (by wt.)	14	5.7
(USDA)	6-oz. can	139	31.6
(Sacramento) Peppy	½ cup (4.3 oz.)	28	6.6
(Sacramento) *Tomato Plus*	5½-fl.-oz. can	49	9.9
Snap-E-Tom	6 fl. oz.	38	6.8

(USDA): United States Department of Agriculture
(HEW/FAO): Health, Education and Welfare/Food and Agriculture Organization
* Prepared as Package Directs

Food and Description	Measure or Quantity	Calories	Carbo- hydrates (grams)
TOMATO PASTE, canned:			
(USDA)	6-oz. can	139	31.6
(USDA)	½ cup (4.6 oz.)	106	24.0
(USDA)	1 T. (.6 oz.)	13	3.0
(Contadina)	6-oz. can	150	35.0
(Del Monte)	6-oz. can	164	33.8
(Hunt's)	6 oz.	140	28.0
Dietetic (Cellu) low sodium	⅛ cup	75	17.5
TOMATO PRESERVE			
(Smucker's)	1 T. (.7 oz.)	53	13.5
TOMATO PUREE:			
Canned, regular pack:			
(USDA)	1 cup (8.8 oz.)	98	22.2
(Contadina) heavy	1 cup	120	27.0
Canned, dietetic or low calorie:			
(USDA)	8 oz.	88	20.0
(Cellu) low sodium	1 cup	80	20.0
TOMATO SAUCE:			
Canned, regular pack:			
(Contadina)	1 cup	90	19.0
(Del Monte)	1 cup (8 oz.)	85	17.0
(Del Monte) with mushrooms	1 cup	103	21.4
(Del Monte) with onions	1 cup	109	23.0
(Del Monte) with tomato tidbits	1 cup	130	5.7
(Hunt's) with bits	8 oz.	60	14.0
(Hunt's) with cheese	8 oz.	100	18.0
(Hunt's) with herbs	8 oz.	180	26.0
(Hunt's) with mushrooms	8 oz.	80	18.0
(Hunt's) with onions	8 oz.	45	10.0
(Hunt's) plain	8 oz.	30	14.0
(Hunt's) *Prima Salsa:*			
Regular	8 oz.	220	40.0
With meat	8 oz.	240	40.0
With mushroom	8 oz.	220	40.0
(Hunt's) special	8 oz.	80	18.0
(Libby's)	8-oz. can	82	19.6
(Stokely-Van Camp)	1 cup (9 oz.)	70	13.0

Food and Description	Measure or Quantity	Calories	Carbo-hydrates (grams)
TOMATO SOUP:			
Canned, regular pack:			
(USDA) condensed	8 oz. (by wt.)	163	28.8
*(USDA) prepared with equal volume water	1 cup (8.6 oz.)	88	15.7
*(USDA) prepared with equal volume milk	1 cup (8.8 oz.)	172	22.5
*(Ann Page)	1 cup	73	14.1
*(Ann Page) & rice	1 cup	115	20.1
*(Campbell) condensed, made with equal volume milk	10-oz. serving	210	27.0
*(Campbell) & beef, *Noodle-Os,* condensed	10-oz. serving	160	24.0
*(Campbell) bisque, condensed	10-oz. serving	140	27.0
*(Campbell) & rice, old fashioned, condensed	10-oz. serving	130	26.0
(Campbell) Royale, *Soup For One*	7¾-oz. can	180	33.0
(Progresso)	1 cup (8 oz.)	110	23.0
Canned, dietetic or low calorie:			
(Campbell) low sodium	7¼-oz. can	130	22.0
(Dia-Mel)	8-oz. serving	50	11.0
(Featherweight) low sodium	8-oz. can	120	18.0
Mix:			
(USDA) vegetable, with noodles	1 oz.	98	17.9
*(Lipton) *Cup-a-Soup*	6 fl. oz.	70	13.0
*(Nestlé's) *Souptime*	6 fl. oz.	70	13.0
(Wyler's) cream of	1-oz. pkg.	96	19.0
TOMCOD, ATLANTIC, raw (USDA):			
whole	1 lb. (weighed whole)	136	0.
Meat only	4 oz.	87	0.

(USDA): United States Department of Agriculture
(HEW/FAO): Health, Education and Welfare/Food and Agriculture Organization
* Prepared as Package Directs

Food and Description	Measure or Quantity	Calories	Carbo-hydrates (grams)
TOM COLLINS:			
Canned (Party Tyme) 10% alcohol	2 fl. oz.	58	5.9
Mix (Party Tyme)	½-oz. pkg.	50	13.3
TONGUE (USDA):			
Beef, medium fat, raw, untrimmed	1 lb.	714	1.4
Beef, medium fat, braised	4 oz.	277	.5
Calf, raw, untrimmed	1 lb.	454	3.1
Calf, braised	4 oz.	181	1.1
Hog, raw, untrimmed	1 lb.	741	1.7
Hog, braised	4 oz.	287	.6
Lamb, raw, untrimmed	1 lb.	659	1.7
Lamb, braised	4 oz.	288	.6
Sheep, raw, untrimmed	1 lb.	877	7.9
Sheep, braised	4 oz.	366	2.7
TONGUE, CANNED:			
Pickled (USDA)	1 oz.	76	<.1
Potted or deviled (USDA)	1 oz.	82	.2
(Hormel)	1 oz. (12-oz. can)	67	<.1
TOPPING:			
Sweetened:			
Butterscotch (Kraft)	1 T.	57	12.4
Butterscotch (Smucker's)	1 T. (.7 oz.)	64	16.3
Caramel (Kraft)	1 T.	54	12.7
Caramel (Smucker's)	1 T.	64	16.1
Cherry (Smucker's)	1 T.	59	15.0
Chocolate:			
(Kraft)	1 oz.	73	18.0
Fudge (Hershey's)	1 T. (.5 oz.)	49	7.3
Fudge (Kraft)	1 T.	68	10.9
Fudge (Smucker's)	1 T.	62	14.8
Milk (Smucker's)	1 T. (.7 oz.)	66	14.8
Mint, fudge (Smucker's)	1 T. (.7 oz.)	62	14.8
Marshmallow (Kraft)	1 T.	38	9.4
Mint (Marzetti)	1 T.	38	9.4
Pecan (Kraft)	1 oz.	122	13.6
Pineapple (Kraft)	1 oz.	80	19.7
Strawberry (Kraft)	1 oz.	80	19.7
Walnut (Kraft)	1 oz.	113	14.3

Food and Description	Measure or Quantity	Calories	Carbo- hydrates (grams)
Dietetic or low calorie:			
Chocolate (Diet Delight)	1 T. (.6 oz.)	10	2.1
Chocolate (Tillie Lewis)	1 T. (.5 oz.)	8	2.0
TOPPING, WHIPPED:			
(USDA) pressurized	1 cup (2.5 oz.)	190	9.0
(USDA) pressurized	1 T. (4 grams)	10	Tr.
(Birds Eye) *Cool Whip,* non-dairy	1 T.	14	1.0
(Kraft)	1 oz.	79	4.3
(Lucky Whip)	1 T.	12	.5
Richwhip, frozen, liquid	1 T. (¼ oz.)	20	1.2
(Rich's) *Spoon 'n Serve*	1 T. (4 grams)	14	1.1
(Rich's) *Whip Topping*	¼ oz.	20	1.2
(Sealtest) *Big Top*	1.5 fl. oz.	15	.7
(Sealtest) *Zip Whip,* real cream	1 T. (.4 oz.)	8	1.0
TOPPING, WHIPPED, MIX:			
Regular:			
*(Dream Whip)	1 T.	10	1.0
Dry (Lucky Whip)	1 oz.	159	16.0
*(Lucky Whip)	1 T.	10	1.0
Dietetic or low calorie:			
*(D-Zerta)	1 T.	8	0.
*(Featherweight)	1 T.	6	1.0
TORTILLA:			
(USDA)	.7-oz. tortilla	42	9.7
(Amigos)	1-oz. tortilla	111	19.7
TOTAL, cereal (General Mills)	1 cup (1 oz.)	110	23.0
TOWEL GOURD, raw (USDA):			
Unpared	1 lb. (weighed with skin)	69	15.8
Pared	4 oz.	20	4.6

(USDA): United States Department of Agriculture
(HEW/FAO): Health, Education and Welfare/Food and Agriculture
    Organization
* Prepared as Package Directs

Food and Description	Measure or Quantity	Calories	Carbo-hydrates (grams)
TREET (Armour)	1 oz.	84	.3
TRIPE:			
Beef, commercial (USDA)	4 oz.	113	0.
Beef, pickled (USDA)	4 oz.	70	0.
Canned (Libby's)	¼ of 24-oz. can	296	1.2
TRIPLE JACK WINE (Gallo)			
20% alcohol	3 fl. oz.	102	6.5
TRIPLE SEC LIQUEUR:			
(Bols) 78 proof	1 fl. oz.	101	8.8
(Garnier) 60 proof	1 fl. oz.	83	8.5
(Hiram Walker) 80 proof	1 fl. oz.	105	9.8
(Leroux) 80 proof	1 fl. oz.	102	8.9
TRIX, cereal (General Mills)	1 cup (1 oz.)	110	25.0
TROPICAL PUNCH DRINK,			
bottled (Wagner's)	6 fl. oz.	101	25.2
TROUT:			
Brook, fresh, whole (USDA)	1 lb. (weighed whole)	224	0.
Brook, fresh, meat only (USDA)	4 oz.	115	0.
Lake (See **LAKE TROUT**)			
Rainbow (USDA):			
Fresh, meat with skin	4 oz.	221	0.
Canned	4 oz.	237	0.
Frozen (1000 Springs):			
Boned	5-oz. trout	135	2.7
Dressed	5-oz. trout	164	3.2
Boned & breaded	5-oz. trout	245	
TUNA:			
Raw (USDA) bluefin, meat only	4 oz.	164	0.
Raw (USDA) yellowfin, meat only	4 oz.	151	0.
Canned in oil:			
(USDA) solids & liq.	6½-oz. can	530	0.

Food and Description	Measure or Quantity	Calories	Carbohydrates (grams)
(USDA) drained solids	6½-oz. can	309	0.
(Breast O'Chicken) solids & liq.	6½-oz. can	427	0.
(Bumble Bee) drained solids	½ cup (3 oz.)	167	0.
(Carnation) solids & liq.	6½-oz. can	427	0.
(Chicken of the Sea):			
Solids & liq., chunk light	6½-oz. can	405	<1.8
Drained solids, chunk light	6½-oz. can	294	0.
(Icy Point):			
Drained solids, chunk, light	6½-oz. can	280	0.
Drained solids, solid, white	7-oz. can	286	0.
(Pillar Rock):			
Drained solids, solid, white	7-oz. can	286	0.
Drained solids, chunk, light	6½-oz. can	280	0.
(Star Kist):			
Solids & liq., chunk, light	6½-oz. can	450	0.
Solids & liq., flakes or grated	6¼-oz. can	440	0.
Solids & liq., solid, white	7-oz. can	520	0.
Solids & liq., chunk, white	6½-oz. can	480	0.
Canned in water:			
(USDA) solids & liq.	6½-oz. can	234	0.
(Breast O' Chicken)	6½-oz. can	211	0.
(Carnation) solids & liq.	6½-oz. can	211	0.
(Star Kist):			
Solids & liq., chunk, white	6½-oz. can	240	0.
Solids & liq., solid, light	7-oz. can	220	0.

(USDA): United States Department of Agriculture
(HEW/FAO): Health, Education and Welfare/Food and Agriculture
         Organization
* Prepared as Package Directs

Food and Description	Measure or Quantity	Calories	Carbo-hydrates (grams)
Solids & liq., solid, light	7-oz. can	240	0.
Solids & liq., chunk, light	6½-oz. can	200	0.
*TUNA HELPER (General Mills):			
Country Dumplings noodles	⅕ pkg.	230	31.0
Creamy noodles	⅕ pkg.	280	30.0
Creamy rice	⅕ pkg.	250	33.0
Newberg-style macaroni	⅕ pkg.	240	29.0
Noodles & cheese sauce	⅕ pkg.	230	28.0
TUNA & PEAS, frozen (Green Giant) creamed, Toast Topper-	5-oz. serving	140	11.0
TUNA PIE, frozen:			
(Banquet)	8-oz. pie	479	42.7
(Morton)	8-oz. pie	373	36.4
TUNA SALAD:			
Home recipe (USDA) made with tuna, celery, mayonnaise, pickle, onion & egg	4 oz.	194	4.0
Canned (Carnation) Spreadable	1½-oz. serving	81	3.2
TURBOT, GREENLAND, raw (USDA):			
Whole	1 lb. (weighed whole)	344	0.
Meat only	4 oz.	166	0.
TURBOT MEAL, frozen (Weight Watchers):			
2-compartment meal	8-oz. meal	316	12.0
Stuffed, 3-compartment	16-oz. meal	420	25.9
TURKEY:			
Raw (USDA) ready-to-cook	1 lb. (weighed with bones)	722	0.
Raw (USDA) light meat	4 oz.	132	0.

Food and Description	Measure or Quantity	Calories	Carbo- hydrates (grams)
Raw (USDA) dark meat	4 oz.	145	0.
Raw (USDA) skin only	4 oz.	459	0.
Roasted (USDA):			
Flesh, skin & giblets	From 13½-lb. raw ready-to-cook turkey	9678	0.
Flesh & skin	From 13½-lb. raw ready-to-cook turkey	7872	0.
Flesh & skin	4 oz.	253	0.
Meat only:			
Chopped	1 cup (5 oz.)	268	0.
Diced	4 oz.	200	0.
Light	4 oz.	200	0.
Light	1 slice (4″ x 2″ x ¼″, 3 oz.)	75	0.
Dark	4 oz.	230	0.
Dark	1 slice (2½″ x 1⅝″ x ¼″, .7 oz.)	43	0.
Skin only	1 oz.	128	0.
Giblets, simmered (USDA)	2 oz.	132	.9
Canned, boned:			
(USDA)	4 oz.	229	0.
(Lynden Farms) solids & liq.	5-oz. jar	230	0.
(Lynden Farms) & noodle	15-oz. can	463	34.0
(Swanson) with broth	5-oz. can	220	0.
(Wilson) roast, *Tender Made*	4 oz.	117	0.
TURKEY DINNER, frozen:			
(USDA) sliced turkey, mashed potato, peas	12-oz. dinner	381	43.2
(Banquet)	11-oz. dinner	293	27.8
(Banquet) *Man Pleaser*	19-oz. dinner	629	73.8
(Morton)	11-oz. dinner	338	39.4

(USDA): United States Department of Agriculture
(HEW/FAO): Health, Education and Welfare/Food and Agriculture
    Organization
* Prepared as Package Directs

Food and Description	Measure or Quantity	Calories	Carbo-hydrates (grams)
(Morton) sliced, *Country Table*	15-oz. dinner	514	89.5
(Swanson)	11½-oz. dinner	360	45.0
(Swanson) *Hungry Man*	19-oz. dinner	740	80.0
(Swanson) 3-course	16-oz. dinner	520	60.0
(Weight Watchers) sliced breast, 3-compartment	16-oz. dinner	350	26.8
TURKEY ENTREE, frozen:			
(Morton) sliced, *Country Table*	12½-oz. entree	390	34.9
(Swanson) with gravy, dressing & whipped potatoes	8¾-oz. entree	260	27.0
(Swanson) *Hungry Man*	13¼-oz. entree	380	35.0
TURKEY FRICASSEE, canned (Lynden Farms)	14½-oz. can	366	28.8
TURKEY GIZZARD (USDA):			
Raw	4 oz.	178	1.2
Simmered	4 oz.	222	1.2
TURKEY PIE:			
Home recipe (USDA) baked	⅓ of 9″ pie	550	42.2
Frozen:			
(USDA) unheated	8 oz.	447	45.6
(Banquet)	8-oz. pie	415	40.6
(Morton)	8-oz. pie	375	31.8
(Swanson)	8-oz. pie	450	40.0
(Swanson) *Hungry Man*	16-oz. pie	790	60.0
TURKEY, POTTED (USDA)	1 oz.	70	0.
TURKEY SALAD, canned (Carnation)	1½-oz. serving	86	3.0
TURKEY SOUP, canned:			
(USDA) condensed, & noodle	8 oz. (by wt.)	147	15.9
*(USDA) condensed, prepared with equal volume water	1 cup (8.8 oz.)	82	8.8

Food and Description	Measure or Quantity	Calories	Carbo-hydrates (grams)
*(Ann Page) & noodle	1 cup	129	17.8
*(Ann Page) & vegetable	1 cup	63	8.9
(Campbell) *Chunky*	18½-oz. can	320	34.0
*(Campbell) & noodle, condensed	10-oz. serving	80	10.0
(Lynden Farms) broth	1 cup (8 oz.)	14	0.
Dietetic (Campbell) low sodium	7½-oz. can	170	14.0
TURKEY TETRAZZINI, frozen (Weight Watchers)	13-oz. meal	401	51.0
TURMERIC (French's)	1 tsp.	7	1.3
TURNIP (USDA):			
Fresh, without tops	1 lb. (weighed with skins)	117	25.7
Fresh, pared, diced	½ cup (2.4 oz.)	20	4.4
Fresh, pared, slices	½ cup (2.3 oz.)	19	4.2
Boiled, drained, diced	½ cup (2.8 oz.)	18	3.8
Boiled, drained, mashed	½ cup (4 oz.)	26	5.6
TURNIP GREENS, leaves & stems:			
Fresh (USDA)	1 lb. (weighed untrimmed)	107	19.0
Boiled (USDA) in small amount water, short time, drained	½ cup (2.5 oz.)	14	2.6
Boiled (USDA) in large amount water, long time, drained	½ cup (2.5 oz.)	14	2.4
Canned (USDA) solids & liq.	½ cup (4.1 oz.)	21	3.7
Canned (Stokely-Van Camp) chopped	½ cup (4.1 oz.)	23	3.5
Frozen:			
(USDA) boiled, drained	½ cup (2.9 oz.)	19	3.2
(Birds Eye) chopped	⅓ pkg.	20	2.0

(USDA): United States Department of Agriculture
(HEW/FAO): Health, Education and Welfare/Food and Agriculture Organization
* Prepared as Package Directs

Food and Description	Measure or Quantity	Calories	Carbohydrates (grams)
(Birds Eye) chopped, with sliced turnip	⅓ pkg.	20	3.0
TURNOVER (See individual kinds)			
TURTLE, GREEN (USDA):			
Raw, in shell	1 lb. (weighed in shell)	97	0.
Raw, meat only	4 oz.	101	0.
Canned	4 oz.	120	0.
20/20 WINE (Mogen David) 20% alcohol	3 fl. oz.	105	9.8
TWINKIE (Hostess):			
Regular	1½-oz. cake	147	26.1
Devil's food	1½-oz. cake	150	24.7
TWISTER, wine (Gallo) 20% alcohol	3 fl. oz.	109	8.2
VALPOLICELLA WINE, Italian red (Antinori)	3 fl. oz.	84	6.3
VANDERMINT, Dutch liqueur (Park Avenue Imports) 60 proof	1 fl. oz.	90	10.2
VANILLA EXTRACT (Virginia Dare) 34% alcohol	1 tsp.	10	Tr.
VANILLA ICE CREAM (See also individual brand names):			
(Borden):			
10.5% fat	¼ pt. (2.3 oz.)	132	15.8
Lady Borden, 14% fat	¼ pt. (2.5 oz.)	162	17.0
(Breyer's):			
Plain	¼ pt.	150	16.0
& strawberry	¼ pt.	150	20.0

Food and Description	Measure or Quantity	Calories	Carbohydrates (grams)
(Dean):			
10.1% fat	1 cup (5.3 oz.)	296	33.8
12% fat	1 cup (5.6 oz.)	341	34.9
(Meadow Gold) 10% fat	¼ pt.	126	15.0
(Prestige) French	¼ pt. (2.6 oz.)	183	15.8
(Sealtest):			
Cherry	¼ pt.	130	17.0
Fudge royale	¼ pt. (2.3 oz.)	150	20.0
Party Slice	¼ pt. (2.3 oz.)	140	16.0
& red raspberry & orange sherbet	¼ pt.	130	21.0
10.2% fat	¼ pt. (2.3 oz.)	150	16.0
(Swift's) sweet cream	½ cup (2.3 oz.)	127	15.7
VANILLA ICE MILK,			
(Borden) *Lite Line*	¼ pt.	108	17.2
***VANILLA PIE,** mix			
(Pillsbury) marble, no bake	⅙ of pie	390	49.0
VANILLA PUDDING:			
Home recipe (USDA) blancmange, with starch base	½ cup (4.5 oz.)	142	20.4
Canned, regular pack:			
(Betty Crocker)	½ cup (5 oz.)	190	29.0
(Del Monte)	5-oz. container	189	32.1
(Hunt's) *Snack Pack*	5-oz. can	190	26.0
(Royal) *Creamerino*	5-oz. container	217	31.0
(Thank You)	½ cup (4.5 oz.)	169	29.2
Canned, dietetic or low calorie, *Sego*	½ of 8-oz. can	125	19.5
Chilled:			
(Breakstone)	5-oz. container	252	32.5
(Sanna)	4¼-oz. container	172	25.7
(Sealtest)	4-oz. serving	125	20.9
Frozen (Rich's)	4½-oz. container	199	27.5

(USDA): United States Department of Agriculture
(HEW/FAO): Health, Education and Welfare/Food and Agriculture Organization
* Prepared as Package Directs

Food and Description	Measure or Quantity	Calories	Carbohydrates (grams)
VANILLA PUDDING or PIE FILLING MIX:			
Sweetened:			
(Ann Page) regular	¼ of 3⅛-oz. pkg.	84	21.0
(Ann Page) cherry	¼ of 3¼-oz. pkg.	86	21.4
*(Jell-O) regular, French	½ cup	180	30.0
*(Jell-O) regular, plain	½ cup	170	27.0
*(Jell-O) instant	½ cup	180	31.0
*(Jell-O) instant, French	½ cup	180	30.0
*(My-T-Fine) regular	½ cup	133	28.0
*(Royal) regular	½ cup (5.1 oz.)	163	26.4
*(Royal) instant	½ cup (5.1 oz.)	176	28.8
Dietetic or low calorie:			
*(D-Zerta)	½ cup	70	13.0
*(Estee)	½ cup	85	16.0
VANILLA RENNET MIX			
(Junket):			
Powder, dry	1 oz.	116	28.0
*Powder	4 oz.	108	14.7
Tablet, dry	1 tablet	1	.2
*Tablet, & sugar	4 oz.	101	13.5
VEAL, medium fat (USDA):			
Chuck, raw	1 lb. (weighed with bone)	628	0.
Chuck, braised, lean & fat	4 oz.	266	0.
Flank, raw	1 lb. (weighed with bone)	1410	0.
Flank, stewed, lean & fat	4 oz.	442	0.
Foreshank, raw	1 lb. (weighed with bone)	368	0.
Foreshank, stewed, lean & fat	4 oz.	245	0.
Loin, raw	1 lb. (weighed with bone	681	0.
Loin, broiled, medium done, chop, lean & fat	4 oz.	265	0.
Plate, raw	1 lb. (weighed with bone)	828	0.
Plate, stewed, lean & fat	4 oz.	344	0.
Rib, raw, lean & fat	1 lb. (weighed with bone)	723	0.

Food and Description	Measure or Quantity	Calories	Carbo- hydrates (grams)
Rib, roasted, medium done, lean & fat	4 oz.	305	0.
Round & rump, raw	1 lb. (weighed with bone)	573	0.
Round & rump, broiled, steak or cutlet, lean & fat	4 oz. (weighed without bone)	245	0.
VEAL DINNER or ENTREE, frozen:			
(Banquet) buffet, parmigian with tomato sauce	2-lb. pkg.	1563	119.1
(Banquet) *Cooking Bag,* parmigian	5-oz. bag	287	19.5
(Banquet) dinner, parmigian	11-oz. dinner	421	42.1
(Green Giant) parmigiana, breaded	7-oz. entree	310	19.0
(Morton) parmigiana	10¼-oz. dinner	335	46.6
(Swanson) parmigiana	12¼-oz. dinner	460	41.1
(Swanson) parmigiana, *Hungry Man*	20½-oz. dinner	910	70.0
VEGETABLE BOUILLON:			
(Herb-Ox)	1 cube	6	.5
MBT	6-gram packet	12	2.0
(Steero)	1 cube	4	<.1
(Wyler's)	1 cube	7	.3
VEGETABLE FAT (See FAT)			
VEGETABLE JUICE COCKTAIL, canned:			
(USDA)	4 oz. (by wt.)	19	4.1
V-8 (Campbell) regular and spicy hot	6 fl. oz.	35	8.0
V-8 (Campbell) low sodium	6 fl. oz.	35	8.0

(USDA): United States Department of Agriculture
(HEW/FAO): Health, Education and Welfare/Food and Agriculture
    Organization
* Prepared as Package Directs

Food and Description	Measure or Quantity	Calories	Carbo-hydrates (grams)
VEGETABLES, MIXED:			
Canned, regular pack:			
(Chun King) Chinese, drained	1 cup	20	3.1
(Del Monte) solids & liq.	½ cup (4 oz.)	38	6.9
(Del Monte) drained solids	½ cup (3.2 oz.)	41	7.4
(Hung's) chop suey	4 oz.	20	3.0
(Libby's) solids & liq.	½ cup (4.2 oz.)	41	9.8
(Stokely-Van Camp) solids & liq.	½ cup (4.3 oz.)	40	8.5
(Veg-All)	½ cup (4 oz.)	39	7.8
Canned, dietetic or low calorie:			
(Cellu) low sodium	½ cup	35	8.0
(Featherweight) low sodium	½ cup	35	8.0
Frozen:			
(USDA) boiled, drained	½ cup (3.2 oz.)	58	12.2
(Birds Eye):			
Jubilee	⅓ pkg.	120	17.0
5-minute style	⅓ pkg.	60	11.0
Americana Recipe:			
New England style	⅓ of 10-oz. pkg.	60	11.0
New Orleans creole style	⅓ of 10-oz. pkg.	70	13.0
Pennsylvania Dutch style	⅓ of 10-oz. pkg.	40	7.0
San Francisco style	⅓ of 10-oz. pkg.	45	6.0
Wisconsin Country style	⅓ of 10-oz. pkg.	40	6.0
International style with seasoned sauces:			
Bavarian style beans & spaetzle	⅓ pkg.	50	10.0
Chinese style	⅓ pkg.	20	5.0
Danish	⅓ pkg.	30	9.0
Hawaiian with pineapple	⅓ pkg.	40	12.0
Italian style	⅓ pkg.	45	8.0
Japanese style	⅓ pkg.	40	9.0
Parisian style	⅓ pkg.	30	7.0
Stir Fry:			
Cantonese style	⅓ pkg.	50	10.0

Food and Description	Measure or Quantity	Calories	Carbo-hydrates (grams)
Chinese style	⅓ pkg.	35	7.0
Hawaiian style	⅓ pkg.	45	10.0
Japanese style	⅓ pkg.	30	6.0
Mandarin style	⅓ pkg.	30	6.0
(Green Giant):			
Regular	½ cup	45	8.0
In butter sauce	½ cup	65	8.5
Chinese style	½ cup	65	10.0
Japanese style	½ cup	15	11.0
Hawaiian style	½ cup	100	16.5
(Kounty Kist):			
Regular	½ cup	45	8.0
California blend	½ cup	15	2.5
(Le Sueur):			
Pea, pea pod & water chestnuts in sauce	1 cup	180	20.0
Pea, onion & carrots in butter sauce	1 cup	160	20.0

VEGETABLE OYSTER (See SALSIFY)

VEGETABLE SOUP:

Canned, regular pack:			
*(USDA) beef, prepared with equal volume water	1 cup (8.6 oz.)	78	9.6
*(USDA) with beef broth, prepared with equal volume water	1 cup (8.8 oz.)	80	13.8
*(USDA) vegetarian, prepared with equal volume water	1 cup (8.6 oz.)	78	13.2
*(Ann Page) with beef stock	1 cup	130	20.0
*(Ann Page) vegetarian	1 cup	70	12.3
*(Campbell)	10-oz. serving	100	17.0
*(Campbell) beef	10-oz. serving	90	10.0
(Campbell) *Chunky*	19-oz. can	280	44.0

(USDA): United States Department of Agriculture
(HEW/FAO): Health, Education and Welfare/Food and Agriculture Organization
* Prepared as Package Directs

Food and Description	Measure or Quantity	Calories	Carbo-hydrates (grams)
*(Campbell) *Noodle-Os*	10-oz. serving	90	13.0
*(Campbell) old fashioned	10-oz. serving	90	11.0
(Campbell) Old World, *Soup For One*	7¾-oz. can	125	18.0
*(Campbell) vegetarian	10-oz. serving	90	16.0
*(Manischewitz)	8 fl. oz.	63	10.2
Canned, dietetic or low calorie:			
(Campbell) low sodium	7¼-oz. can	90	15.0
(Campbell) beef, low sodium	7¼-oz. can	80	8.0
*(Claybourne)	8-oz. serving	104	4.0
*(Dia-Mel)	8-oz. serving	60	12.0
(Featherweight) & beef	8-oz. can	180	28.0
*Frozen (USDA) with beef, prepared with equal volume water	8-oz. (by wt.)	79	7.7
Mix:			
*(Lipton):			
Alphabet vegetable, *Cup-a-Soup*	6 fl. oz.	40	6.0
*Vegetable beef	8 fl. oz.	60	9.0
Vegetable beef, *Cup-a-Soup*	6 fl. oz.	60	9.0
*Vegetable beef with shells	8 fl. oz.	100	18.0
*Vegetable, country	8 fl. oz.	70	13.0
*Vegetable, Italian	8 fl. oz.	100	19.0
Vegetable, Spring *Cup-a-Soup*	6 fl. oz.	45	7.0
*(Wyler's):			
Regular	6 fl. oz.	42	7.2
Chicken	6 fl. oz.	28	4.3
VEGETABLE STEW, canned (Hormel) *Dinty Moore*	8-oz. serving	170	19.5
"VEGETARIAN FOODS":			
Canned or dry:			
Big franks, drained (Loma Linda)	1.9-oz. frank	112	4.9

Food and Description	Measure or Quantity	Calories	Carbo-hydrates (grams)
Chili, canned (Worthington)	½ cup (4.9 oz.)	190	20.0
Chili beans (Loma Linda)	½ cup (4.7 oz.)	146	21.1
Choplet, canned (Worthington)	1.6-oz. slice	50	3.0
Cutlet, canned (Worthington)	2.2-oz. slice	63	2.6
Dinner cuts, drained (Loma Linda)	1.6-oz. cut	51	2.7
Dinner cuts, no salt added (Loma Linda)	1.6-oz. cut	45	2.6
FriChik (Worthington)	1.6-oz. piece	95	1.0
Granburger (Worthington)	6 T. (1.2 oz.)	129	12.0
Gravy Quik (Loma Linda):			
Brown	.7-oz. packet	69	11.0
Country	.7-oz. packet	70	11.5
Mushroom	.7-oz. packet	69	11.5
Onion	.7-oz. packet	72	12.7
Smoky bits	.8-oz. packet	67	10.8
Linketts, drained (Loma Linda)	1.3-oz. link	71	3.6
Little links (Loma Linda)	.8-oz. link	42	1.4
Non-meat balls (Worthington)	.6-oz. meatball	40	2.3
Numete, canned (Worthington)	½″ slice (2.4 oz.)	160	9.0
Nutena (Loma Linda)	½″ slice (2.5 oz.)	198	7.9
Peanuts & soya, canned (USDA)	4 oz.	269	15.2
Proteena (Loma Linda)	½″ slice (2.6 oz.)	158	5.6
Protose, canned (Worthington)	½″ slice (2.7 oz.)	190	7.0
Redi-burger (Loma Linda)	½″ slice (2.5 oz.)	150	9.0
Sandwich spread (Loma Linda)	1 T. (.6 oz.)	27	2.0
Saucettes (Worthington)	1.2-oz. link	65	1.5

(USDA): United States Department of Agriculture
(HEW/FAO): Health, Education and Welfare/Food and Agriculture Organization
* Prepared as Package Directs

Food and Description	Measure or Quantity	Calories	Carbohydrates (grams)
Savorex (Loma Linda)	1 oz.	51	4.5
Skallops (Worthington) drained	½ cup (3 oz.)	70	3.0
Soyagen, all purpose powder (Loma Linda)	1 T. (10 grams)	48	4.7
Soyalac, concentrate, liquid (Loma Linda)	1 cup (9 oz.)	327	33.8
Soyalac, powder (Loma Linda)	1 oz.	136	12.4
Soyalac, ready-to-use (Loma Linda)	1 cup	640	63.1
Soyalac, ready-to-use (Loma Linda)	1 cup (8.5 oz.)	156	16.1
Soyameat (Worthington):			
Beef-like slices	1-oz. slice	55	1.5
Chicken-like, diced	¼ cup (2 oz.)	120	2.0
Chicken-like, sliced	1.1-oz. slice	65	1.0
Salisbury steak-like slices	2.3-oz. slice	160	2.0
Soyamel (Worthington)	1 oz.	145	15.2
Soyamel, low fat (Worthington)	1 oz.	110	14.0
Spaghetti sauce (Loma Linda)	½ cup (4 oz.)	325	63.1
Stew pac, drained (Loma Linda)	2 oz.	69	5.7
Super-Links (Worthington)	1.9-oz. link	120	4.0
Tender bits (Loma Linda)	.6-oz. piece	20	2.2
Tender rounds, drained (Loma Linda)	1-oz. round	47	2.6
Vegeburger (Loma Linda)	½ cup (3.9 oz.)	124	7.7
Vegeburger, no salt added (Loma Linda)	½ cup (3.9 oz.)	132	7.0
Vegelona (Loma Linda)	½" slice (3.3 oz.)	157	12.5
Vegetable steak, canned (Worthington)	1.3-oz. piece	40	2.8
Vegetarian burger, canned (Worthington)	⅛ cup (3.3 oz.)	121	6.0
Vega-Links, canned (Worthington)	1.1-oz. link	70	1.5
Vita-Burger (Loma Linda)	1 pattie	76	6.9

Food and Description	Measure or Quantity	Calories	Carbo-hydrates (grams)
Wheat protein, nuts or peanuts, canned (USDA)	4 oz.	240	20.1
Wheat protein, vegetable oil, canned (USDA)	4 oz.	214	5.9
Wheat & soy protein, soy or other vegetable oil, canned (USDA)	4 oz.	170	10.8
Wheat & soy protein, canned (USDA)	4 oz.	118	8.6
Wheat protein, canned (USDA)	4 oz.	124	10.0
Worthington 209, turkey-like flavor	1.1-oz. slice	75	1.5
Frozen:			
Beef-Like Roll (Worthington)	2½-oz. slice	140	4.0
Beef-Like Slices (Worthington)	1-oz. slice	60	2.0
Beef pie (Worthington)	8-oz. pie	470	51.0
Bologna (Loma Linda)	½" slice (3 oz.)	197	6.2
Breakfast links (Loma Linda)	.7-oz. link	44	1.4
Breakfast sausage (Loma Linda)	1½" piece (3 oz.)	208	4.8
Burger patties (Loma Linda)	3-oz. pattie	221	11.4
Chicken (Loma Linda)	½" slice (3 oz.)	179	5.5
Chicken pie (Worthington)	8-oz. pie	450	42.0
Chicken-Like Roll (Worthington)	2½-oz. piece	170	2.0
Chicken-Like Slices (Worthington)	1-oz. slice	70	1.0
Chic-Ketts (Worthington)	½ cup (3 oz.)	180	6.0
Corned Beef-Like Roll (Worthington)	2½-oz. piece	190	6.0

(USDA): United States Department of Agriculture
(HEW/FAO): Health, Education and Welfare/Food and Agriculture Organization
* Prepared as Package Directs

Food and Description	Measure or Quantity	Calories	Carbo-hydrates (grams)
Corned Beef-Like, sliced (Worthington)	.5-oz. slice	40	2.3
Croquettes (Worthington)	1 croquette (1 oz.)	75	5.0
Fillets (Worthington)	1.7-oz. piece	108	5.0
FriPats (Worthington)	2.5-oz. piece	180	3.0
Meatballs (Loma Linda)	.8-oz. meatball	46	2.2
Prosage Links (Worthington)	.8-oz. link	60	1.7
Prosage Patties (Worthington)	1.3-oz. pattie	100	3.5
Prosage, sliced (Worthington)	⅜" slice (1.2 oz.)	85	3.5
Roast Beef (Loma Linda)	½" slice (3 oz.)	194	3.8
Sizzle Burger (Loma Linda)	2.5-oz. burger	180	10.0
Smoked Beef-Like Roll (Worthington)	2½-oz. piece	170	7.0
Smoked Beef-Like Luncheon Slice (Worthington)	.3-oz. slice	2	1.0
Smoked Turkey-Like Roll (Worthington)	2½-oz. piece	180	3.0
Smoked Turkey-Like Slices (Worthington)	.7-oz. slice	50	.8
Stakelets (Worthington)	3-oz. piece	180	8.0
Stripples (Worthington)	.3-oz. strip	25	.8
Tuno (Worthington)	2-oz. serving	90	3.0
Turkey (Loma Linda)	½" slice	181	4.8
Wham, roll (Worthington)	2½-oz. piece	140	4.0
Wham, sliced (Worthington)	.8-oz. slice	47	1.3
VENISON, raw, lean meat only (USDA)	4 oz.	143	0.
VERMOUTH:			
Dry:			
(C&P) 19% alcohol	3 fl. oz.	90	3.0
(Gallo) 18% alcohol	3 fl. oz.	75	1.7
(Great Western) 16% alcohol	3 fl. oz.	87	1.6
(Lejon) 18.5% alcohol	3 fl. oz.	99	2.2

Food and Description	Measure or Quantity	Calories	Carbohydrates (grams)
(Noilly Pratt) 19% alcohol	3 fl. oz.	101	1.6
(Taylor) 17% alcohol	3 fl. oz.	99	3.0
Rosso (Gancia) 21% alcohol	3 fl. oz.	153	6.9
Sweet:			
(C&P) 16% alcohol	3 fl. oz.	120	14.4
(Gallo) 18% alcohol	3 fl. oz.	118	12.3
(Great Western) 16% alcohol	3 fl. oz.	132	12.4
(Lejon) 18.5% alcohol	3 fl. oz.	134	11.4
(Noilly Pratt) 16% alcohol	3 fl. oz.	128	12.1
(Taylor) 17% alcohol	3 fl. oz.	132	12.3
White (Gancia) 16.8% alcohol	3 fl. oz.	132	7.8
White (Lejon) 18.5% alcohol	3 fl. oz.	101	2.6
VICHYSSOISE SOUP (Crosse & Blackwell)	½ can (6½ oz.)	94	9.4
VIENNA SAUSAGE, canned:			
(USDA)	1 oz.	68	<.1
(Hormel)	.6-oz. sausage	42	.5
(Libby's) in barbeque sauce	.7-oz. sausage	50	.5
(Libby's) in beef broth	.7-oz. sausage	45	.2
(Wilson)	1 oz.	85	<.1
VILLA ANTINORI, Italian white wine, 12½% alcohol	3 fl. oz.	87	6.3
VINEGAR:			
Cider:			
(USDA)	½ cup (4.2 oz.)	17	7.1
(USDA)	1 T. (.5 oz.)	2	.9
Distilled:			
(USDA)	½ cup (4.2 oz.)	14	6.0
(USDA)	1 T. (.5 oz.)	2	.8
Red or white wine (Regina):			
Champagne	½ cup	1	.3
Red, plain or with garlic	¼ cup	1	.3

(USDA): United States Department of Agriculture
(HEW/FAO): Health, Education and Welfare/Food and Agriculture
           Organization
* Prepared as Package Directs

Food and Description	Measure or Quantity	Calories	Carbo-hydrates (grams)
VINESPINACH or BASELLA, raw (USDA)	4 oz.	22	3.9
VIN KAFE (Lejon) 19.7% alcohol	3 fl. oz.	183	22.8
VIN ROSE (See **ROSE WINE**)			
VIRGIN SOUR MIX (Party Tyme)	½-oz. pkg.	50	13.3
VODKA, unflavored (See **DISTILLED LIQUOR**)			
VODKA & TONIC, canned (Party Tyme) 10% alcohol	2 fl. oz.	55	5.1
VOIGNY WINE (Chanson) 13% alcohol	3 fl. oz.	96	7.5

W

Food and Description	Measure or Quantity	Calories	Carbo-hydrates (grams)
WAFER (See **COOKIE** or **CRACKER**)			
WAFFLE:			
Home recipe (USDA)	7" waffle (2.6 oz.)	209	28.1
Frozen:			
(USDA)	1.6-oz. waffle (8 in 13-oz. pkg.)	116	19.3
(USDA)	.8-oz. waffle (6 in 5-oz. pkg.)	61	10.1
(Aunt Jemima) jumbo	1¼-oz. waffle	86	13.6
(Downyflake):			
Blueberry or jumbo	1 waffle	85	16.0
Regular	1 waffle	55	10.5
(Eggo):			
Blueberry	1.4 oz. waffle	130	18.0
Bran	2-oz. waffle	170	20.0
Plain	1.4-oz. waffle	120	17.0
Strawberry	1.4-oz. waffle	130	18.0

Food and Description	Measure or Quantity	Calories	Carbo-hydrates (grams)
WAFFLE MIX (USDA) (See also **PANCAKE & WAFFLE MIX**):			
Dry, complete mix	1 oz.	130	18.5
*Prepared with water	2.6-oz. waffle (½″ x 4½″ x 5½″, 7″ dia.)	229	30.2
Dry, incomplete mix	1 oz.	101	21.5
*Prepared with egg & milk	2.6-oz. waffle (7″ dia.)	206	27.2
*Prepared with egg & milk	7.1-oz. waffle (9″ x 9″ x ⅝″, 1⅛ cup batter)	550	72.4
WAFFLE SYRUP (See **SYRUP** and also individual names such as **LOG CABIN**)			
WALNUT:			
(USDA):			
Black, in shell, whole	1 lb. (weighed in shell)	627	14.8
Black, shelled, whole	4 oz. (weighed whole)	712	16.8
Black, chopped	½ cup (2.1 oz.)	377	8.9
English or Persian, in shell, whole	1 lb. (weighed in shell)	1329	32.2
English or Persian, shelled, whole	4 oz.	738	17.9
English or Persian, chopped	½ cup (2.1 oz.)	391	9.5
English or Persian, halves	½ cup (1.8 oz.)	326	7.9
(Diamond) halves & pieces	1 cup (3.5 oz.)	679	12.8
(Hammon's) kernels	4 oz.	746	11.6

(USDA): United States Department of Agriculture
(HEW/FAO): Health, Education and Welfare/Food and Agriculture Organization
* Prepared as Package Directs

Food and Description	Measure or Quantity	Calories	Carbo-hydrates (grams)
WATER CHESTNUT, CHINESE, raw (USDA):			
Whole	1 lb. (weighed unpeeled)	272	66.4
Peeled	4 oz.	90	21.5
WATERCRESS, raw (USDA):			
Untrimmed	½ lb. (weighed untrimmed)	40	6.2
Trimmed	½ cup (.6 oz.)	3	.5
WATERMELON, fresh (USDA):			
Whole	1 lb. (weighed with rind)	54	13.4
Wedge	2-lb. wedge (4″ x 8″ measured with rind)	111	27.3
Slice	½ slice (12.2 oz., ¾″ x 10″)	41	10.2
Diced	1 cup (5.6 oz.)	42	10.2
WATERMELON RIND (Crosse & Blackwell)	1 T. (.6 oz.)	38	9.3
WAX GOURD, raw (USDA):			
Whole	1 lb. (weighed with skin & cavity contents)	41	9.4
Flesh only	4 oz.	15	3.4
WEAKFISH (USDA):			
Raw, whole	1 lb. (weighed whole)	263	0.
Broiled, meat only	4 oz.	236	0.
WELSH RAREBIT:			
Home recipe (USDA)	1 cup (8.2 oz.)	415	14.6
Canned (Snow)	½ cup (4 oz.)	171	7.8
Frozen (Green Giant) with cheddar & swiss cheese, *Toast Topper*	5-oz. serving	220	12.0

Food and Description	Measure or Quantity	Calories	Carbo-hydrates (grams)
WESTERN DINNER, frozen:			
(Banquet)	11-oz. dinner	417	32.4
(Morton) *Round-Up*	11¾-oz. dinner	424	33.4
(Swanson)	11¾-oz. dinner	460	41.0
(Swanson) *Hungry Man*	17¾-oz. dinner	890	77.0
WEST INDIAN CHERRY (See **ACEROLA**)			
WHALE MEAT, raw (USDA)	4 oz.	177	0.
WHEAT **CHEX,** cereal (Ralston Purina)	⅔ cup (1 oz.)	110	23.0
WHEATENA, dry	¼ cup (1.1 oz.)	112	22.5
WHEAT FLAKES ,cereal, crushed (USDA)	1 cup (2.5 oz.)	248	56.4
WHEAT GERM, crude, commercial, milled (USDA)	1 oz.	103	13.2
WHEAT GERM CEREAL:			
(USDA)	¼ cup (1 oz.)	110	14.0
(Kretschmer):			
Regular	¼ cup (1 oz.)	110	13.0
With sugar & honey	¼ cup (1 oz.)	110	17.0
WHEATIES, cereal (General Mills)	1 cup (1 oz.)	110	23.0
WHEAT, ROLLED (USDA):			
Uncooked	1 cup (3.1 oz.)	296	66.3
Cooked	1 cup (7.7 oz.)	163	36.7
WHEAT, SHREDDED, cereal (See **SHREDDED WHEAT**)			

(USDA): United States Department of Agriculture
(HEW/FAO): Health, Education and Welfare/Food and Agriculture Organization
* Prepared as Package Directs

Food and Description	Measure or Quantity	Calories	Carbohydrates (grams)
WHEAT, WHOLE-GRAIN (USDA), hard red spring	1 oz.	94	19.6
WHEAT, WHOLE-MEAL, cereal (USDA):			
Dry	1 oz.	96	20.5
Cooked	4 oz.	51	10.7
WHEY (USDA):			
Dry	1 oz.	99	20.8
Fluid	1 cup (8.6 oz.)	63	12.4
WHISKEY or WHISKY (See DISTILLED LIQUOR)			
WHISKEY SOUR:			
(Hiram Walker)	3 fl. oz.	177	12.0
(National Distillers) *Duet,* 12½% alcohol	8-fl.-oz. can	256	17.6
Mix:			
(Bar-Tender's)	1 serving (⅝ oz.)	70	17.2
(Holland House) dry	.6-oz. pkg.	69	17.0
(Holland House) liquid	1½ fl. oz.	82	19.5
(Party Tyme)	½-oz. pkg.	50	13.5
WHITEFISH, LAKE (USDA):			
Raw, whole	1 lb. (weighed whole)	330	0.
Raw, meat only	4 oz.	176	0.
Baked, stuffed, made with bacon, butter, onion, celery & bread crumbs, home recipe	4 oz.	244	6.6
Smoked	4 oz.	176	0.
WHITEFISH & PIKE (See GEFILTE FISH)			
WIENER (See FRANKFURTER)			
WILD BERRY, fruit drink (Hi-C)	6 fl. oz.	88	22.0

Food and Description	Measure or Quantity	Calories	Carbo-hydrates (grams)
WILDBERRY DRINK, canned (Ann Page)	1 cup (8.7 oz.)	124	30.9
WILD RICE, raw (USDA)	½ cup (2.9 oz.)	289	61.7
WINE (most wines are listed by kind, brand, vineyard, region or grape name):			
Cooking, Sauterne (Regina)	¼ cup	2	.5
Cooking, Sherry (Regina)	¼ cup	19	4.7
Dessert (USDA) 18.8% alcohol	3 fl. oz.	122	6.9
Dessert (Petri)	3 fl. oz.	124	
Flavored (Petri)	3 fl. oz.	124	
Red (Mogen David) 12% alcohol	3 fl. oz.	24	1.8
Table:			
(USDA) 12.2% alcohol	3 fl. oz.	75	3.7
(Petri) Vino Bianco, 12% alcohol	3 fl. oz.	66	2.1
(Petri) Vino Rosso, 13% alcohol	3 fl. oz.	64	1.5
(United Vintners) *Vino Primo Wine,* 12% alcohol	3 fl. oz.	66	1.6
WON TON SOUP, canned (Mow Sang)	10-oz. can	134	21.0
WORCESTERSHIRE SAUCE (See **SAUCE,** Worcestershire)			
WRECKFISH, raw, meat only (USDA)	4 oz.	129	0.

(USDA): United States Department of Agriculture
(HEW/FAO): Health, Education and Welfare/Food and Agriculture Organization
* Prepared as Package Directs

Food and Description	Measure or Quantity	Calories	Carbo-hydrates (grams)

Y

YAM (USDA):
Raw, whole	1 lb. (weighed with skin)	394	90.5
Raw, flesh only	4 oz.	115	26.3
Canned & frozen (See **SWEET POTATO**)			

YAM BEAN, raw (USDA):
Unpared tuber	1 lb. (weighed unpared)	225	52.2
Pared tuber	4 oz.	62	14.5

YANKEE DOODLES (Drake's)
	1.1-oz. piece	109	15.6

YEAST:
Baker's:
Compressed (USDA)	1 oz.	24	3.1
Compressed (Fleischmann's)	⅗-oz. cake	19	1.9
Dry (USDA)	1 oz.	80	11.0
Dry (USDA)	1 pkg. (7 grams)	20	2.7
Dry (Fleischmann's)	¼ oz. (pkg. or jar)	24	2.9
Brewer's dry, debittered (USDA)	1 oz.	80	10.9
Brewer's dry, debittered (USDA)	1 T. (8 grams)	23	3.1

YELLOWTAIL, raw, meat only (USDA)
	4 oz.	156	0.

YODEL (Drake's)
	.9-oz. roll	116	14.6

YOGURT:
Made from whole milk (USDA)	½ cup (4.3 oz.)	76	6.0
Made from partially skimmed milk, plain or			

Food and Description	Measure or Quantity	Calories	Carbo-hydrates (grams)
vanilla:			
(USDA)	½ cup (4.3 oz.)	61	6.3
(USDA)	8-oz. container	113	11.8
Plain:			
(Alta-Dena) *Maya*	1 container	210	18.0
(Alta-Dena) *Naja*	1 container	180	20.0
(Borden) Swiss style	5-oz. container	82	9.9
(Borden) Swiss style	8-oz. container	131	15.9
(Breakstone)	8-oz. container	141	12.7
(Breakstone)	1 T. (.5 oz.)	9	.8
(Breyer's)	1 cup	180	17.0
(Dannon)	8-oz. container	140	14.0
(Dean)	8-oz. container	143	18.4
(Sealtest) *Light 'n Lively*	1 cup	150	18.0
Apple cinnamon			
(Breakstone)	8-oz. container	229	39.9
Apple crisp (New Country)	8-oz. container	240	41.4
Apricot:			
(Breyer's)	1 cup	270	47.0
(Dannon)	8-oz. container	245	43.4
(Sealtest) *Light 'n Lively*	1 cup	250	48.0
Apricot crunch (New Country)	8-oz. container	251	42.5
Banana:			
(Breyer's)	1 cup	270	47.0
(Dannon)	8-oz. container	245	43.4
(Dannon) *Danny-in-a-Cup*	1 cup	210	42.0
Blueberry:			
(Breakstone)	8-oz. container	252	46.3
(Breyer's)	1 cup	270	47.0
(Dannon)	8-oz. container	245	43.4
(Dannon) *Danny Parfait*	½ cup	160	35.0
(Dean)	8-oz. container	259	50.6
(Meadow Gold) Swiss style	8-oz. container	245	49.0
(Sealtest) *Light 'n Lively*	1 cup	250	49.0
(Sanna) *Swiss Miss*	4-oz. container	125	19.0

(USDA): United States Department of Agriculture
(HEW/FAO): Health, Education and Welfare/Food and Agriculture
        Organization
* Prepared as Package Directs

Food and Description	Measure or Quantity	Calories	Carbohydrates (grams)
Blueberry ripple (New Country)	8-oz. container	238	42.0
Boysenberry:			
(Dannon)	8-oz. container	245	43.4
(Dannon) *Danny Bar,* carob coated	2½-fl.-oz. bar	130	15.0
(Dannon) *Danny Yo*	3½-oz. serving	115	21.0
(Meadow Gold)	8-oz. container	249	54.0
Cherry:			
(Breyer's) black	1 cup	270	47.0
(Dannon)	8-oz. container	245	43.4
(Dannon) *Danny-in-a-Cup*	1 cup	210	42.0
(Dannon) *Danny Parfait*	½ cup	160	35.0
(Dean)	8-oz. container	245	47.9
(Sealtest) *Light 'n Lively,* black	1 cup	240	45.0
Cherry supreme (New Country)	8-oz. container	240	43.0
Chocolate (Dannon) *Danny Yo*	3½-oz. serving	115	21.0
Coffee (Dannon)	8-oz. container	200	33.1
Date walnut (New Country)	8-oz container	257	42.6
Dutch apple (Dannon)	8-oz. container	245	43.4
Flavored (Alta-Dena) *Maya*	1 container	280	39.0
Flavored (Alta-Dena) *Naja*	1 container	250	40.0
French vanilla ripple (New Country)	8-oz. container	239	41.2
Fruit crunch (New Country)	8-oz. container	241	41.1
Hawaiian salad (New Country)	8-oz. container	252	42.1
Honey (Dannon)	8-oz. container	245	43.4
Lemon:			
(Dannon)	8-oz. container	200	33.1
(Dannon) *Danny Yo*	3½-oz. serving	115	21.0
(Sealtest) *Light 'n Lively*	8-oz. container	250	47.0
Lemon ripple (New Country)	8-oz. container	238	42.0
Mandarin orange (Borden) Swiss style	8-oz. container	227	45.9
Mandarin orange (Sealtest) *Light 'n Lively*	1 cup	240	46.0

Food and Description	Measure or Quantity	Calories	Carbo-hydrates (grams)
Orange (Dean)	8-oz. container	311	62.9
Orange-pineapple (Breyer's)	1 cup	270	47.0
Peach:			
(Borden) Swiss style	5-oz. container	138	27.8
(Borden) Swiss style	8-oz. container	221	44.5
(Breyer's)	1 cup	270	47.0
(Dannon)	8-oz. container	245	43.4
(Dannon) *Danny Parfait*	½ cup	160	35.0
(Dean)	8-oz. container	259	49.1
(Meadow Gold)	8-oz. container	249	54.0
(Sealtest) *Light 'n Lively*	8-oz. container	250	48.0
Peach melba (Sealtest) *Light 'n Lively*	1 cup	250	48.0
Peaches 'n Cream (New Country)	8-oz. container	241	42.5
Pineapple:			
(Breakstone)	8-oz. container	220	37.9
(Breyer's)	1 cup	270	47.0
(Dean)	8-oz. container	265	48.7
(Meadow Gold)	8-oz. container	249	54.0
(Sealtest) *Light 'n Lively*	1 cup	250	50.0
Pineapple-cherry (Axelrod)	8-oz. container	229	42.4
Pineapple-orange (Dannon):			
Regular	8-oz. container	245	43.4
Danny-in-a-Cup	1 cup	210	42.0
Danny Parfait	½ cup	160	35.0
Prune whip:			
(Breakstone)	8-oz. container	231	41.1
(Dannon)	8-oz. container	245	43.4
Raspberry:			
(Borden) Swiss style	5-oz. container	147	29.5
(Borden) Swiss style	8-oz. container	236	47.2
(Breakstone)	8-oz. container	249	45.8
(Breyer's)	1 cup	270	47.0
(Dannon) red	8-oz. container	245	43.4
(Dannon) red, *Danny Bar*, chocolate coated	2½ fl. oz.	130	15.0

(USDA): United States Department of Agriculture
(HEW/FAO): Health, Education and Welfare/Food and Agriculture Organization
* Prepared as Package Directs

Food and Description	Measure or Quantity	Calories	Carbo-hydrates (grams)
(Dannon) red, *Danny-in-a-Cup*	1 cup	210	42.0
(Dannon) red, *Danny Parfait*	½ cup	160	35.0
(Dannon) red, *Danny Yo*	3½-oz. serving	115	21.0
(Dean) red	8-oz. container	272	53.6
(Meadow Gold) Swiss style	8-oz. container	245	49.0
(Sealtest) red, *Light 'n Lively*	1 cup	230	43.0
Raspberry ripple (New Country)	8-oz. container	238	42.0
Strawberry:			
(Borden) Swiss style	5-oz. container	142	27.8
(Borden) Swiss style	8-oz. container	227	44.5
(Breakstone)	8-oz. container	225	43.5
(Breyer's)	1 cup	270	47.0
(Dannon)	8-oz. container	245	43.4
(Dannon) *Danny Bar*	2½ fl. oz.	70	13.0
(Dannon) *Danny Bar*, chocolate coated	2½ fl. oz.	130	15.0
(Dannon) *Danny Flip*, with strawberry topping	5 fl. oz.	180	39.0
(Dannon) *Danny Parfait*	½ cup	160	35.0
(Dannon) *Danny-Yo*	3½-oz. serving	115	21.0
(Dean)	8-oz. container	256	46.8
(Meadow Gold)	8-oz. container	249	54.0
(Meadow Gold) Swiss style	8-oz. container	245	49.0
(Sanna) *Swiss Miss*	4-oz. container	125	19.0
(Sealtest) *Light 'n Lively*	1 cup	250	47.0
Strawberry supreme (New Country)	8-oz. container	238	42.0
Vanilla:			
(Borden) Swiss style	5-oz. container	148	28.4
(Borden) Swiss style	8-oz. container	235	45.4
(Breakstone)	8-oz. container	195	29.5
(Breyer's)	1 cup	230	32.0
(Dannon)	8-oz. container	200	33.1
(Dannon) *Danny Bar*	2½-fl.-oz. bar	60	10.0
(Dannon) *Danny Bar*, carob coated	2½-fl.-oz. bar	120	12.0

Food and Description	Measure or Quantity	Calories	Carbo-hydrates (grams)
(Dannon)			
Danny-in-a-Cup	1 cup	180	33.0
(Dannon) *Danny Flip* with red raspberry topping	5 fl. oz.	170	35.0
(Dannon) *Danny Sampler*	2 fl. oz.	70	14.0
(Dannon) *Danny-Yo*	3½-oz. serving	115	21.0

YOGURT CHIFFON PIE, frozen, (Sara Lee) *Light & Luscious*:

Blueberry	⅛ of pie	120	20.4
Cherry	⅛ of pie	121	21.1
Strawberry	⅛ of pie	118	19.4

Z

ZINFANDEL WINE:

(Inglenook) Estate, 12% alcohol	3 fl. oz.	58	.3
(Inglenook) vintage, 12% alcohol	3 fl. oz.	59	.3
(Italian Swiss Colony) 13% alcohol	3 fl. oz.	61	.9
(Louis M. Martini) 12½% alcohol	3 fl. oz.	90	.2

ZITI, frozen:

(Buitoni) baked, with sauce	4 oz.	128	21.4
(Ronzoni) baked	4½-oz. serving	130	19.0

ZUCCHINI (See **SQUASH, SUMMER**)

ZWIEBACK:

(USDA)	1 oz.	120	21.1
(Gerber)	.2-oz. piece	30	5.3
(Nabisco)	.3-oz. piece	30	5.0

(USDA): United States Department of Agriculture
(HEW/FAO): Health, Education and Welfare/Food and Agriculture Organization
* Prepared as Package Directs

Bibliography

Dawson, Elsie H., Gilpin, Gladys L., and Fulton, Lois H. *Average weight of a measured cup of various foods.* U.S.D.A. ARS 61–6, February 1969. 19 pp.

Leung, W. T. W., Busson, F., and Jardin, C. *Food composition table for use in Africa.* U.S. Department of Health, Education and Welfare and Food and Agriculture Organization of the United Nations. 1968. 306 pp.

Leung, W. T. W., Butrum, R. V., and Chang, F. H. *Food composition table or use in East Asia.* U.S. Department of Health, Education and Welfare and Food and Agriculture Organization of the United Nations. December 1972. 334 pp.

Merrill, A. L. and Watt, B. K., *Energy value of foods—basis and derivation.* U.S.D.A. Handb. 74, 105 pp. 1955.

Pecot, Rebecca K., Jaeger, Carol M., and Watt, Bernice K., *Proximate composition of beef from carcass to cooked meat: Method of derivation and tables of values.* U.S.D.A. Home Economics Research Report 31, 32 pp. 1965.

Pecot, Rebecca K. and Watt, Bernice K., *Food yields: Summarized by different stages of preparation.* U.S.D.A. Handb. 102, 93 pp. 1956.

U.S.D.A. Nutritive value of foods. Home and Garden Bul. 72, 36 pp. 1964 and revised edition, 1970. 41 pp.

U.S.D.A. Unpubl. Data 1969.

Watt, Bernice K., Merrill, Annabel L., et. al., *Composition of foods: Raw, processed, prepared.* U.S.D.A. Agriculture Handb. 8, 190 pp. 1963.

About the Author

BARBARA KRAUS received a Master's in Anthropology from New York University with a concentration in the study of food habits. She was also the author of *The Cookbook of the United Nations* and *The Cookbook to Serve 2, 6 or 24.* Also available in Signet editions are *The Barbara Kraus Calorie Guide to Brand Names & Basic Foods, The Barbara Kraus Carbohydrate Guide to Brand Names & Basic Foods, The Barbara Kraus Dictionary of Protein,* and *The Barbara Kraus Guide to Fiber in Foods.*

SIGNET Books for Your Reference Shelf

☐ **MEDICAL REPORTS FROM** *Weight Watchers® Magazine*, **Foreword by Jean Nidetch,** founder, Weight Watchers International, Inc. Here is a book that explodes a multitude of common myths as it shows that overweight is not just a problem affecting your social life and appearance, but a major medical threat. (#W6465—$1.50)

☐ **CONSUMER GUIDE®—RATING THE DIETS by Theodore Berland and the editors of Consumer Guide®.** For anyone who wants to lose weight and keep it off, and for everyone confused by the countless diet fads, here, at last, is a book that presents the total picture of the dieting scene, complete with up-to-date advice from nutritionists and medical experts. (#E8940—$2.25)*

☐ **LET'S EAT RIGHT TO KEEP FIT by Adelle Davis.** Sensible, practical advice from America's foremost nutrition authority as to what vitamins, minerals and food balances you require, and the warning signs of diet deficiencies.
(#E8979—$2.75)

☐ **LET'S COOK IT RIGHT by Adelle Davis.** Completely revised and updated, this is the celebrated cookbook dedicated to good health, good sense and good eating. Contains 400 easy-to-follow, basic recipes, a table of equivalents and an index.
(#E7711—$2.50)

☐ **EATING IS OKAY! A Radical Approach to Weight Loss: The Behavioral Control Diet by Henry A. Jordon, M.D., Leonard S. Levitz, Ph.D., and Gordon M. Kimbrell, Ph.D.** You can get thin and stay thin by changing your life style—say the doctors of the phenomenally successful Behavioral Weight Control Clinic. (#W7926—$1.50)

* Price slightly higher in Canada

Buy them at your local bookstore or use this convenient coupon for ordering.

THE NEW AMERICAN LIBRARY, INC.,
P.O. Box 999, Bergenfield, New Jersey 07621

Please send me the SIGNET BOOKS I have checked above. I am enclosing
$_____ (please add 50¢ to this order to cover postage and handling).
Send check or money order—no cash or C.O.D.'s. Prices and numbers are
subject to change without notice.

Name _____

Address _____

City_____ State_____ Zip Code_____
Allow 4-6 weeks for delivery.
This offer is subject to withdrawal without notice.